FINANCIAL AND MANAGERIAL CONTROL

A Health Care Perspective

Edward J. Lusk
The Wharton School
University of Pennsylvania
and
Janice Gannon Lusk
The Wharton School
University of Pennsylvania

Aspen Systems Corporation
Germantown, Maryland
1979

Library of Congress Cataloging in Publication Data

Lusk, Edward J.
Financial and managerial control:
a health care perspective

Includes bibliographical references and index.
1. Health facilities—Finance. 2. Health
facilities—Accounting. I. Lusk, Janice G., joint
author. II. Title.
RA971.3.L87 338.4'7'3621 78-10606
ISBN 0-89443-036-X

Library of Congress Catalog Card Number: 78-10606
ISBN: 0-89443-036-X

Printed in the United States of America

1 2 3 4 5

Dedicated to
the Memory of

Robert D. Eilers

He that soweth little shall reap little;
and he that soweth plenteously shall reap
plenteously.
Let every man do according as he is
disposen in his heart,
not grudgingly —

2 Cor ix.6,7 part.

Table of Contents

Preface

The focus of this text is on the generation of control information. Various financial and managerial control problems of health care institutions have been considered. In writing the various chapters, we have been careful to select original material which would be useful in developing control insights for both academic presentations and practitioner reference.

Since the accounting system is one important source of control information, various aspects of the accounting model (discussed in Appendix A) are examined. Chapters 2, 3, 4, and 6 discuss the accounting for cash, accounts receivable, inventory, and working capital and examine the control and management information which may be generated through the accounting system. The remaining chapters of the text do not rely upon the formal accounting system as a means of generating control information. Chapters 7–10, 12, 13, and 14 are organized to provide insights into the techniques and models which may be used to generate control information.

In order to provide a fully developed text in the area of control, we felt it important to discuss the institution's long-range planning or budgeting process. Chapter 5 discusses the accounting for and selection of long-term debt alternatives to finance major investment activities of the institution. Chapter 11 discusses a model which may be useful in selecting various capital investments.

The text therefore provides material which focuses only on control (Chapters 1, 2, 3, 4, 6, 7, 8, the first half of 9, 10, 12, 13, and 14) and material which focuses on control and examines the planning function (Chapters 1, 2, 3, 4, 5, 6, 7, 8, 9, 10, 11, 12, and 14). We believe that either alternative will provide a satisfactory examination of the material on either the semester or quarter system.

The questions and problems following each chapter have been selected to examine in greater detail particular points discussed in the chapters. A full understanding of the message of this text cannot be obtained without attempting to answer these questions and problems. They should be viewed as an important opportunity to further develop the chapter's theme. Where we felt it was important, solutions and partial solutions have been included. We encourage the readers to contribute exercises and problems which might be useful in subsequent editions. Of course, proper credit will be given in the text should one of these contributions be used. Any comments on the text also would be greatly appreciated. We believe that learning only occurs through critical analysis, and consequently, your feedback is important in developing subsequent editions.

Edward J. Lusk & Janice Gannon Lusk
December, 1978

Acknowledgments

The material presented in this text has been accumulated over a considerable period of time. During this time many students and other individuals have made various contributions which, in one form or another, found their way into the text. Our sincere and profound gratitude is due these individuals. Notable among them are Steven Berkowitz, William Hamilton, Ron Howe, Margaret Kauffman, Tony Kovner, Mark Lebo, Sam Mitchell, Warren Reid, and Joe Streleckis. A special thanks goes to R. Neal Gilbert of the Blyth, Eastman and Dillon Health Care Funding, Inc., who contributed valuable information used to prepare the debt management section of Chapter 5.

We wish to thank Linda Pisa for her patience in typing many drafts of this text. The final copy of the manuscript was edited and prepared by Mary McCutcheon, whose patience and talents are boundless.

A special note of thanks to our mothers, Rita Gannon and Florence Lusk, for being the way they are; some of it rubbed off.

Chapter 1

Control: An Analytical Perspective

If you don't know where you're going, any map will do.

A. Rappaport

Ideally, a comprehensive examination of the various techniques, models, and systems of control relevant in the health care environment should consider all of the institution's internal and external interactions. Unfortunately, this task is well beyond current measurement capabilities. Therefore, this text examines the analytic aspects of control, focusing on control information which can be generated by particular techniques, models, and control systems. It will not be possible to examine these techniques, models, and control systems as integrated subsystems, or to specify how this control information affects the behavior of the institution's decision makers.

THE BEHAVIORAL DIMENSION OF CONTROL

Although the effect of individual interactions on institutional control processes should be integrated with the analytic examination of control, the current state of the behavioral sciences precludes this integration. However, a simple model of an institution's behavioral system can provide a background for the control analysis undertaken in this text. This model, developed below, should be helpful in ascertaining the possible behavioral implications of the various techniques, models, and systems of control examined in subsequent chapters.

Behavioral Model: An Unbalanced Optimization

Two assumptions underlie the behavioral model. The first is that two groups, one medical and the other administrative, are involved in the institutional resource conversion process. The second is that each group has a well specified, although not necessarily measurable, objective function.

The Medical Group

The medical group affects resource conversion through its three general activities: health care delivery, research, and teaching. By engaging in these activities, the medical group attempts to maximize its utility. Hence, the medical group's objective function can be noted as:

$$\max \phi^M(\alpha_1, \alpha_2, \alpha_3)$$

where: ϕ^M is a utility function for the medical group and
$\alpha_{1,2,3}$ represents health care delivery, research, and teaching, respectively.

The notation max ϕ^M means that the medical group takes actions to affect health care delivery, research, and teaching such that the aggregate utility of the group is maximized.

However, the medical group's actions are restricted or constrained by the particular state of the institution concerning such factors as current patient volume and mix, revenue and research funds available, and size of the institution. These constraints may be represented as:

$$\begin{aligned} f_1(\alpha_1, \alpha_2, \alpha_3) &\leq \hat{\beta}_1 \\ \vdots \quad & \quad \vdots \\ f_n(\alpha_1, \alpha_2, \alpha_3) &\leq \hat{\beta}_n \end{aligned}$$

where: f_i, $i=1,2,\cdots n$ represents the way that health care delivery (α_1), research (α_2), and teaching (α_3) utilize resource β_i and
$\hat{\beta}_i$, $i=1,2\ldots n$ represents an actual amount of resource β_i.

The model assumes that one of the constraints, f_k, concerns cost, and that $\hat{\beta}_k$ is the maximum cost which can be incurred over the short-range planning period.

The Administrative Group

The administrative group affects the resource conversion process with cost controls that are used to monitor resource utilization. By controlling costs, the administrative group maximizes its utility. Hence, the administrative group's objective function can be noted as:

$$\max \phi^A(g(\hat{\beta}_k))$$

where: ϕ^A is a utility function for the administrative group and
$g(\hat{\beta}_k)$ is a function of the expected cost, $\hat{\beta}_k$, for the control period (see Problem 1-2).

However, the administrative group's ability to maximize its utility is also subject to a number of constraints, including the three represented as follows:

$$h_1(g(\hat{\beta}_k)) \geq C_1(\alpha_1)$$
$$h_2(g(\hat{\beta}_k)) \geq C_2(\alpha_2)$$
$$h_3(g(\hat{\beta}_k)) \geq C_3(\alpha_3)$$

where: h_i, $i=1,2,3$ are composite functions of the expected cost for health care delivery, research, and teaching, respecitvely, and
$C_i(\alpha_i)$, $i=1,2,3$ represent the minimum acceptable level of health care delivery (α_1), research (α_2), and teaching (α_3) given $\hat{\beta}_k$.

Hence, the administrative group cannot alter costs through $g(\hat{\beta}_k)$ in such a way as to inhibit the attainment of the minimum acceptable level of health care delivery, research, and teaching.

Model Interactions

The model interrelationships may be specified as follows:

Medical

$$\max \phi^M(\alpha_1, \alpha_2, \alpha_3)$$
subject to:
$$f_1(\alpha_1, \alpha_2, \alpha_3) \leq \hat{\beta}_1$$
$$\vdots$$
$$f_k(\alpha_1, \alpha_2, \alpha_3) \leq \hat{\beta}_k \leftarrow$$
$$\vdots$$
$$f_n(\alpha_1, \alpha_2, \alpha_3) \leq \hat{\beta}_n$$

Administrative

$$\max \phi^A(g(\hat{\beta}_k))$$
subject to:
$$h_1(g(\hat{\beta}_k)) \geq C_1(\alpha_1) \leftarrow$$
$$h_2(g(\hat{\beta}_k)) \geq C_2(\alpha_2) \leftarrow$$
$$h_3(g(\hat{\beta}_k)) \geq C_3(\alpha_3); \leftarrow$$
Other constraints.

As indicated, the specific arguments of the medical objective function appear in the constraint set of the administrative model ($C_1(\alpha_1)$, $C_2(\alpha_2)$, $C_3(\alpha_3)$), and the specific argument of the administrative objective function appears in the constraint set of the medical model ($\hat{\beta}_k$). This property, called periodic interdependency, is useful in understanding the problems of control in health care institutions.

In a decision system where periodic interdependency exists, if one group or coalition dominates the organization's decision network, that group will eventually control the system. For example, assume that the medical and administrative groups have an equal degree of organizational power. Given this balance, each group can effectively take actions to maximize its utility. However, if the medical group attains a power advantage and uses it to expand the institution's base of technology (and the required support staff), then the costs required to support the new minimum acceptable level of α_1, α_2 and α_3 will increase. This increased level of medical activity shifts the constraints of the administrative model so that the administrative group must now attempt to control $g(\hat{\beta}_k)$ given a general increase in the level of institutional costs. As the medical group continues to expand costs in pursuit of its objectives, the administrative group's chance of effectively pursuing its cost control objectives declines, causing the medical group's concern for the cost constraint to dissipate further (see Problem 1-1).

This caricature is not suggested as an analytical model. It does, however, point out the behavioral frame of reference of the managers of health care institutions. This tendency toward imbalance and its control implications should be kept in mind as the various aspects of control are discussed in subsequent chapters.

External Factors Currently Affecting the Resource Conversion Process

The optimization model interactions discussed typify the interrelationships that existed in health care insitutions through the late 1960s. Although the same tendencies exist today, other factors such as the following may become important in temporarily suppressing them.

- Third party reimbursement policymakers have become increasingly aware of the obvious cost implications of retrospective reimbursement.
- Subsequent to this awareness and, in some respect, in a coordinative effort with third party payers, various regional, state, and federal agencies (e.g., health systems agencies (HSAs) and state advisory boards (SABs)) have made attempts to control costs.
- Third party payers have redefined reimbursable costs incurred to deliver a particular service.

- Disreputable physicians who have scandalously abused the reimbursement system have been prosecuted and jailed in various jurisdictions.
- Health care professionals have begun to realize that the physician's salary is eventually, although indirectly, related to effective cost management.
- Alternatives to the traditional health care delivery system, such as health maintenance organizations (HMOs), have been developed.

These factors have established new constraints that have caused physicians and administrators to rethink their previous group interrelationships and have created an environment which has stimulated interest in the role of the physician in the economic management of the institution.

THE PURPOSE OF THE TEXT

The time is now right to move forward, to study, and to begin the development of techniques, models, and control systems necessary to achieve resource control in the health care delivery field. However, a note of realism is appropriate. Resource control is complex, even in organizations not beset with the numerous complications often characterizing resource control in health care institutions. This text is just the beginning. The considerations herein will be restricted to things that seem reasonable in today's environment. However, the material discussed is not developed within a specific legislative framework. Most of the concepts, techniques, and models (excepting certain material in the Appendices to Chapters 5 and 9) were developed from management principles and could be used to guide an institution's resource control process in any legislative context. In summary, the text will focus on the provision of decision-relevant information, rather than on the specification of a prescription for behavior.

Problems

Problem 1-1. The other side to the optimization model caricature on page 3 may be stated as follows:

> True, costs have increased, but not because of a system's imbalance. Cost increases are to be expected given the rate of inflation, the rate of price increases due to technological innovation and the dependence of the medical profession on expensive technology.

Also, if the administrative group maximizes its utility by controlling costs, it can maximize its utility just as well at an increased level of cost. In fact, the more costs there are to control, the better the chance to control effectively.

Finally, the real problem is not the propensity for imbalance, but rather the effects of malpractice suits on spending. An institution cannot afford to be without a full complement of the most sophisticated technology.

Required

a. Discuss this viewpoint.
b. Formulate a simple model to characterize the system's interactions embodied by this viewpoint.
c. Contrast this model with the model in the chapter and discuss the cost control implications for each point where the models differ.

Problem 1-2. One possible form of $g(\hat{\beta}_k)$ is: minimize $(\hat{\beta}_k - \bar{\beta}_k)^2$.

where: $\hat{\beta}_k$ represents the maximum expected cost for the control period, and
$\bar{\beta}_k$ represents the actual cost incurred during the control period.

Discuss the control and behavioral implications of this form of utility argument. Formulate three other functional arguments and discuss their control and behavioral implications.

Problem 1-3. Discuss the following statement: Members of the administrative group should not concern themselves with cost control because cost is a professional area of control. Their primary function is to design and maintain an accounting system that will yield the maximum reimbursement within the rules of the third party payers.

Chapter 2

Cash

Distrust and caution are the parents of security.

B. Franklin

The control and management of cash assets are fundamental to the efficient operation of any organization. Controlling and managing cash are particularly important in health care institutions, where it is often believed that effective financial management and humanitarianism are incompatible goals. The first section of this chapter examines the controls most often used to safeguard cash; the second outlines the basic elements of effective cash management in health care institutions.[1]

CASH CONTROL

Cash controls are needed to avoid the loss, misappropriation, or theft of cash maintained by the institution. Two aspects of cash control important in developing an effective cash management system are a voucher system and reconciliations of internal cash records, with cash accounts kept externally. The voucher system is an ex ante control over cash disbursements. However, to expedite the disbursement of small amounts of cash, a petty cash fund is often used. The reconciliation of internal cash records with cash accounts kept externally is a means of controlling cash receipts and cash disbursements ex post which may take two forms—a bank reconciliation or a proof of cash.

Voucher System

To control the accumulation of assets, most institutions (1) specify individuals in the organization who have the authority to acquire assets, and

(2) set dollar limits beyond which particular individuals have no authority to contract for the acquisition of assets. These limits are often related to the degree of responsibility an individual has in the organization. Usually, individual limits are fairly low. As the costs of assets become relatively large, joint or multiple authorizations are required to secure assets.

For example, the financial manager of the cardiology department may be able to authorize purchases of $300 or less. For amounts between $300 and $500, a second authorizing signature may be required from one of the staff physicians whose primary appointment is cardiology. For amounts over $500, but not exceeding $1,000, the chief of cardiology's authorization also may be required. Finally, for amounts in excess of $1,000, the approval of the hospital planning committee may be required. These limits may vary among the hospital departments, with more autonomous departments traditionally having higher limits.

The voucher system is merely the formal documentation of this authorization process. A voucher is a form which has one section for the purchase order or cash disbursement information (vendor and description of the asset to be acquired) and another section for the authorizing signatures. Usually a purchase order or cash disbursement cannot be initiated unless a valid voucher is presented to the purchasing department, or to the cash disbursements clerk.

The voucher system is often integrated into the organization's resource control system, which ordinarily encompasses purchasing (voucher system), cash disbursements (voucher system and check register), and resource control (internal control and asset safeguarding systems). A typical arrangement for purchase and cash disbursement control is represented in Figure 2-1.

An effective voucher system is one which performs the following functions:

1. documents (with prenumbered forms) the organizational purchase authority system,
2. is integrated into the organizational information networks,
3. is uniformly administered to all departments, and
4. is considered by organizational members to be an integral part of the organizational control system.

As previously indicated, when a voucher system is used, all cash disbursements require a voucher. Because a voucher system requires substantial documentation, costs and benefits regarding its use should be considered. For instance, the costs of preparing a voucher for the outlay of small amounts of cash may exceed the benefits of protecting that small amount of cash. Hence, the outlay of small amounts of cash may not require a

Figure 2-1 A Purchase Control System

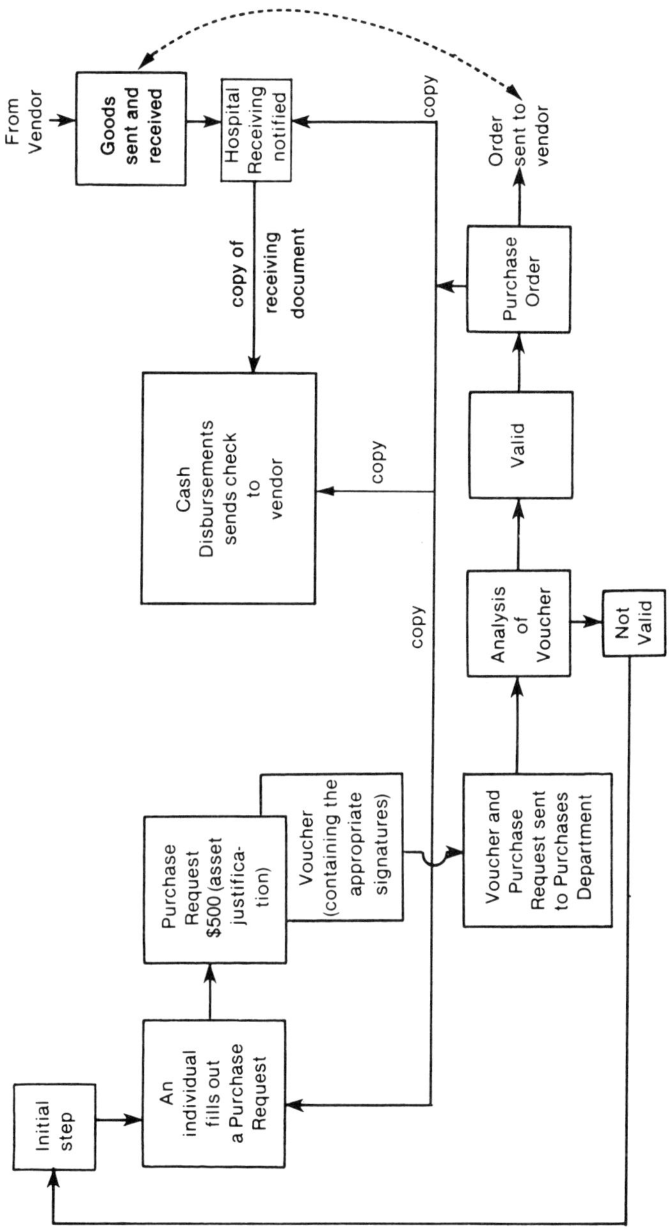

formal voucher. (In fact voucher control is rarely required for immaterial expenditures.) However, to monitor small cash disbursements the less formal petty cash fund can be used.

Petty Cash Fund

The petty cash fund usually is maintained by one individual in a department. When small amounts of cash are needed a simple, prenumbered petty cash voucher is filled out and exchanged for the required cash. When the cash in the fund is nearly exhausted, the person maintaining the fund fills out a formal voucher to obtain money to replenish the fund.

The accounting entry to establish a petty cash fund of $100 is:

Petty Cash	$100.00	
Voucher Payable		$100.00

The entry to replenish the fund for $87.00 of miscellaneous expenses paid out of the petty cash fund is:

Miscellaneous Expense	$87.00	
Voucher Payable[2]		$87.00

The sum of the petty cash vouchers and the cash remaining in the fund must always equal the original balance of the fund.

Because the petty cash fund is relatively small, safeguarding the fund generally is of little concern. The rationalization for this attitude is that even if the entire fund were stolen, the organization would only lose a minor amount of money. Most managers believe that identifying a dishonest person in the organization would be worth the amount of cash in the petty cash fund. However, theft of the entire fund is not the only way that misappropriations can occur. If fraudulent petty cash vouchers are used to deplete the fund on a daily basis and the fund is replenished weekly, the organization can lose a substantial amount of cash over the year. In general, the organization's control system must be more sensitive to the "take a little, leave a little" individual than the person who absconds with an entire asset.

The voucher system and the petty cash fund are important in safeguarding cash assets and coordinating the accumulation of other assets. However, they do not provide comprehensive cash control. To complement the voucher system, two reconciliation techniques, the bank reconciliation and the proof of cash, may be used.

Reconciling Internal and External Cash Records

A reconciliation is needed between two sets of records when some activity, which will eventually be common to both sets of records, is only recorded on one set of records at the reconciliation date. The lag between the time the institution collects cash receipts or makes cash disbursements and the time these transactions are recorded at the bank gives rise to a situation that requires a reconciliation. To verify the cash transactions recorded by the institution with those processed by the bank, a bank reconciliation or a proof of cash should be prepared.

Bank Reconciliation

The bank reconciliation verifies the cash balance reported on the organization's ledgers with the organization's cash balance at the bank. For example, assume that cash is recorded on two sets of records, cash at the bank, noted as CB, and cash on the institution's books, noted as IC. Further assume that the set of cash transactions for the period is $\{A_1, A_2, A_3, A_4, A_5\}$ and that at the beginning of the period $\mathrm{CB}(t_{n-1}) = \mathrm{IC}(t_{n-1})$, where: t_{n-1} denotes the beginning of the period. During the period the following occurs:

$$\mathrm{CB}(t_{n-1}) + (A_1, A_2, A_3) = \mathrm{CB}(t_n)$$

$$\mathrm{IC}(t_{n-1}) + (A_1, A_3, A_4, A_5) = \mathrm{IC}(t_n)$$

where: t_n denotes the end of the period.

A reconciliation could take one of the following forms:

Reconciliation I:

CB to IC $\qquad \mathrm{CB}(t_n) + (A_4, A_5) - (A_2) = \mathrm{IC}(t_n)$

Reconciliation II:

IC to CB $\qquad \mathrm{IC}(t_n) + (A_2) - (A_4, A_5) = \mathrm{CB}(t_n)$

Reconciliation III:

Reconciliation to a Correct Adjusted Balance (CAB)

$$\mathrm{CB}(t_n) + (A_4, A_5) = \mathrm{CAB}(t_n)$$
$$\mathrm{IC}(t_n) + (A_2) = \mathrm{CAB}(t_n)$$

Each of the above reconciliations would verify the corresponding cash activity between the two sets of records. However, the third reconciliation method yields the most useful information by computing the correct cash balance, which may not be recorded on either set of records. Further, this CAB reconciliation is useful because the items that reconcile $\mathrm{IC}(t_n)$ to

$CAB(t_n)$ form a list of the adjusting entries required to correct the cash balance recorded on the institution's books.

Some questions useful in providing information needed to reconcile the recorded cash activity to the correct adjusted balance are:

1. Where is the item *currently* recorded?
2. Where *would it be* recorded if there were no time difference involved in processing the transaction?
3. When the transaction is eventually recorded. will it be an addition or deduction?

Transaction information derived in response to these questions can be used to adjust the respective ending balances. Some common adjustments are outlined below:

Bank Reconciliation

(t_n)

$CB(t_n)$	$IC(t_n)$
−OC	−SC
+DT	−NSF
	+NC
$CAB(t_n)$	$CAB(t_n)$

where: OC represents outstanding checks;
DT represents deposits in transit;
SC represents bank service charges;
NSF represents not-sufficient-funds checks; and
NC represents notes collected by the bank.

The adjusting journal entries are taken from the items listed under $IC(t_n)$: (SC, NSF, NC). When these adjusting journal entries have been posted, the cash ledger balance will equal $CAB(t_n)$.

Proof of Cash

The proof of cash is an invaluable technique for ascertaining the accuracy of the recorded cash flows. In addition to verifying the cash balance reported on the institution's ledger, the proof of cash verifies the institution's receipts and disbursements with the receipts and disbursements recorded in the institution's account at the bank. Although it replaces the bank reconciliation, it is considerably more difficult to prepare (see Problem 2-9). Therefore, a bank reconciliation is usually prepared monthly, while the proof of cash is prepared only once or twice each year.

The elements required for a proof of cash are (1) a bank reconciliation for the beginning of the period, (2) a bank reconciliation for the end of the period, (3) the cash disbursements as recorded on the books and at the bank during the period, and (4) the cash receipts as recorded on the books and at the bank during the period. The reconciling items from the beginning and end of the period are used in the reconciliation of receipts and disbursements between the institution's book and bank records.

The form of the proof of cash is:

Proof of Cash Format

The Period t_{n-1} to t_n will be noted as *.

$CB(t_{n-1})$	$+R_B^*$	$-D_B^*$	$=$	$CB(t_n)$
$A_1(t_{n-1})$		$\rightarrow\Delta_1\leftarrow$		$A_1(t_n)$
$A_2(t_{n-1})$	$\rightarrow\Delta_2\leftarrow$			$A_2(t_n)$
$A_3(t_{n-1})$		$\rightarrow\Delta_3$		. . .
$A_4(t_{n-1})$		$\rightarrow\Delta_4\leftarrow$		$A_4(t_n)$
. . .	$\Delta_5\leftarrow$			$A_5(t_n)$
$IC(t_{n-1})$	$+R_I^*$	$-D_I^*$	$=$	$IC(t_n)$

Where: $R_{B,I}^*$ represents the institution's cash receipts as recorded at the bank and the institution, respectively, for the period t_{n-1} to t_n;

$D_{B,I}^*$ represents the institution's cash disbursements as recorded at the bank and the institution, respectively, for the period t_{n-1} to t_n;

$A_i(t_{n-1})$, $A_i(t_n)$ represents the ith reconciling item at period t_{n-1}, t_n, respectively; and

Δ_i represents the difference between $A_i(t_n)$ and $A_i(t_{n-1})$, computed as $A_i(t_n) - A_i(t_{n-1})$. The column in which the Δ_i is placed (receipts or disbursements) depends upon whether the reconciliation adjustment pertains to cash receipts or cash disbursements.

Cash receipts and disbursements differ between the two sets of records because transactions affecting both sets of records are not recorded simultaneously by the bank and by the institution. Consequently, some transactions are recorded on one set of records that are not recorded on the other set of records.

For a simple example of the proof of cash, assume that only two reconciling items appear in the bank reconciliation in each time period, $OC(t_{n-1}) = \$400$, $OC(t_n) = \$500$, and $DT(t_{n-1}) = \$100$, $DT(t_n) = \$150$. Given the additional information that $CB(t_{n-1}) = \$1,000$, $R_B^* = \$3,000$ and $D_B^* = \$2,500$, the proof of cash may be prepared as follows:

Proof of Cash

	Balance (t_{n-1})	R_B^* Receipts	D_B^* Disbursements[3]	Balance (t_n)
Per bank	\$1,000	\$3,000	(\$2,500)	\$1,500
DT	+ 100 ⟶	⟶ + 50 ⟵		⟵ + 150
OC	(400) ⟶		⟶ (100) ⟵	⟵ (500)
Per books	\$ 700	\$3,050	(\$2,600)	\$1,150
		R_I^*	D_I^*	

Four steps are required to prepare this proof of cash: (1) verify the cash balances recorded in the institution's ledger at time t_{n-1} and time t_n, (2) reconcile the difference between cash receipts recorded at the bank and at the institution during the period t_{n-1} to t_n, (3) reconcile the difference between cash disbursements recorded at the bank and at the institution during the period t_{n-1} to t_n, and (4) sum the receipts and disbursements columns to verify the totals with the cash receipts and disbursements recorded in the institution's ledger during the period.

The first step in completing the proof of cash is to verify the cash balances recorded on the institution's ledger at t_{n-1} and at t_n. This information is obtained directly from the bank reconciliations of the respective periods. However, the clerical accuracy of these reconciliations should be checked.

The next step in preparing the proof of cash involves reconciling the difference between the receipts recorded at the bank, R_B^*, with the receipts recorded by the institution, R_I^*. For example, since deposits in transit are receipts recorded by the institution but not yet received by the bank, the DT row of the proof of cash may yield items that reconcile, partially or totally, the difference between R_B^* and R_I^*. In the example, deposits in transit at t_n are \$150 (in other words, \$150 of cash receipts have been recorded by institution but have not been received by the bank at t_n). Therefore, $DT(t_n)$ must be added to R_B^* to reconcile R_B^* with R_I^*. However, deposits in transit at t_{n-1} were \$100. Since this \$100 was recorded as an institutional cash receipt during the period t_{n-2} to t_{n-1}, it is not included in the institution's cash receipts for the period t_{n-1} to t_n and therefore must be subtracted from R_B^* to reconcile R_B^* with R_I^*. Hence,

$$\Delta_1 = \$150 - \$100 = \$50,$$

or, summing across the row from t_{n-1} to t_n, \$100 + \$50 = \$150. This type of analysis should be completed for each item that affects cash receipts recorded at the bank or at the institution.

A similar process is followed to reconcile the difference between the cash disbursements recorded at the bank, D_B* and the cash disbursements recorded by the institution, D_I*. For example, since outstanding checks are disbursements recorded by the institution but not yet paid by the bank, the OC row of the proof of cash may yield items that partially or totally reconcile the difference between D_B* and D_I*. In this case, outstanding checks at t_n are \$500 (\$500 of checks drawn by the institution have not yet been deducted from the institution's account at the bank). Therefore, OC(t_n) must be added to D_B* to reconcile with D_I*. However, since the \$400 of outstanding checks at t_{n-1} were drawn by the institution in periods prior to the period t_{n-1} to t_n, these disbursements are not included in D_I* and must therefore be subtracted from D_B* to reconcile the two sets of records. Hence,

$$\Delta_2 = (\$500) - (\$400) = (\$100)$$

or summing across the row, (\$400) + (\$100) = (\$500). Again, this procedure should be followed for each reconciling item that affects cash disbursements.

The final step in the proof of cash involves summing the columns to assure that the totals R_I* and D_I* agree with the amounts in the institution's cash receipts and cash disbursements records for the period. In this case:

$$R_I^* = \$3{,}000 + \$50 = \$3{,}050, \text{ and}$$

$$D_I^* = (\$2{,}500) + (\$100) = (\$2{,}600).$$

If these amounts appear in the cash receipts and cash disbursements books, then the cash receipts and disbursements reconcile between the institution and the bank. If the amounts in the cash receipts and cash disbursements books are materially different from these totals, then the institution's cash control procedures should be reviewed.

In summary, the control of cash is basic to the internal control of the organization. The proof of cash and the bank reconciliation, when used with the voucher system, provide a strong, comprehensive set of controls over cash.

Bank Reconciliation and Proof of Cash: An Example

Assume the following information has been gathered for the Memorial Hospital as of June 30, 19X1:

Bank Statement
Memorial Hospital
June 30, 19X1

Beginning Balance: $1,106	Debits: $634		Credits: $1,842	Ending Balance: $2,314
	Debits			*Credits*
Check No.	*Date Paid*	*Amount*	*Date*	*Amount*
99	6/1	$ 98	6/1	$ 150
100	6/2	52	6/15	32
101	6/2	100	6/22	600
102	6/22	65	6/30	1060 CM*
103	6/21	54		
105	6/15	26		
106	6/29	70		
109	6/29	129		
110	6/29	11		
	6/23	22 NSF		
	6/30	7 SC		

*Proceeds of collection on a 180 day $1,000, 12% note receivable, due 6/30.

LEDGER INFORMATION

	Cash Disbursements		*Cash Receipts*	
Check No.	*Date Issued*	*Amount*	*Date*	*Amount*
A.J.E. 83*	5/31	$ 7		
101	6/1	100	6/15	$ 32
102	6/4	65	6/22	600
103	6/7	45	6/30	25
104	6/10	93		
105	6/13	26	Total Book Receipts $657	
106	6/18	70		
107	6/21	52		
108	6/24	68		
109	6/27	129		
110	6/27	11		
Total Book Disbursements $659				

*Adjusting journal entry to record the bank service charge for the month of May.

In addition, the following information is abstracted from the ledgers of the Memorial Hospital and derived from the bank:

1. Cash balance per the hospital general ledger was $1,063 before the adjusting journal entry on 5/31 and $1,054 on 6/30.
2. Outstanding checks as of 5/31 amounted to $200 (#52 for $50, #99 for $98, #100 for $52).
3. A cut-off bank statement for the period 7/1 to 7/10 showed a deposit of $25 on 7/1. No cash receipts were recorded on the books for that period.

Given this information, the following bank reconciliation may be prepared:

Memorial Hospital
Bank Reconciliation
Month of June, 19X1

Per Books		Per Bank	
Balance 6/30/19X1	$1,054	Balance 6/30/19X1	$2,314
Additions:		Additions:	
Proceeds of Collection		Deposits in Transit	25
on 180 day, 12% Note	1,060		$2,339
	$2,114		
Deductions:		Deductions:	
NSF Check	$ 22	O/S Checks (#52, #104,	
Service Charge	7	#107, #108)	$ 263
Transposition Error			
(Check #103)	9		
Total Deductions	$ 38	Total Deductions	$ 263
Corrected Balance	$2,076	Corrected Balance	$2,076

In analyzing the information from the books column, the following adjusting entry may be determined:

Cash	$1,022	
Miscellaneous Expense	7	
Accounts Payable	9	
Accounts Receivable	22	
Notes Receivable		$1,000
Interest Income		60

To correct the balance recorded in the cash account on June 30, 19X1. After this adjusting entry is posted the balance in cash ledger will be $2,076 (i.e., $1,054 + $1,022).

The following proof of cash also may be prepared, given the information on page 16:

Memorial Hospital
Proof of Cash
Month of June, 19X1

	Balance 5/31	Receipts	Disbursements	Balance 6/30
Per Bank	$1,106	$1,842	($634)	$2,314
Additions:				
Deposits in Transit	150	(125)		25
Deductions:				
Outstanding Checks Prior to June	(200)		150	(50)
June			(213)	(213)
Proceeds of Collection on Note		(1,060)		(1,060)
NSF Check			22	22
Service Charge			7	7
Transposition Error			9	9
Per Books	$1,056	$ 657	($659)	$1,054

Note that the cash receipts and disbursements, as reconciled, agree with the ledger totals for the month of June.

CASH MANAGEMENT

Although important, controlling or safeguarding cash will not insure (1) that the institution is making the best use of its cash, or (2) that cash will be available when cash demands arise. Organized case management is necessary to insure that the institution is maintaining cash balances of the proper size.

Effective cash management is the product of two elements: the accurate recording of cash transactions and management's ability to abstract relevant information from the accounting system. These elements are fundamental to the efficient execution of four policies required to maintain an effective cash management system: (1) cash owed for services redered should be collected in a timely manner;[4] (2) the payment of current liabilities should be carefully monitored; (3) the information required to prepare the cash budget should be developed from accurate forecasting models; and (4) cooperative banking relationships should be established and maintained.

This section first examines the recording of current liabilities and discusses management's ability to monitor the payment of current liabilities through information generated by the accounting system. Then, the four policy aspects of an effective cash management system are discussed. The section concludes with a case study that further examines the relationship between each policy and an institution's cash management system.

Payment of Current Liabilities: Net and Gross Price Methods

Careful monitoring of the payment of current liabilities is an important aspect of an effective cash management system because considerable cash savings in the form of purchase discounts often are available if sufficient cash can be generated to pay current liabilities within the discount period. Therefore, care should be taken to insure that current liabilities are accurately recorded in the institution's accounting system. In addition, information regarding purchase discounts should be recorded so that management can easily abstract the appropriate information to determine if the cash savings provided by purchase discounts are being realized.

Trade and Time Discounts

Two types of purchase discounts, (1) trade or quantity discounts and (2) time discounts may be made available to purchasers by vendors. A trade discount is a legal discount which usually varies with the quantity of goods purchased. The greater the quantity, the greater the discount per unit. Substantial savings usually can be derived through trade discounts. However, management must recognize that as purchase quantities increase, inventory carrying costs also increase (see Chapter 4). Therefore, the costs, as well as the benefits, of a trade discount must be considered before the discount is taken.

A typical statement describing a trade discount is:

> For a given unit purchase price before trade discounts, the buyer qualifies for a series of discounts, $d_1, d_2, \ldots, d_n$ depending upon the quantity, $q_1, q_2, \ldots, q_n$ to be purchased.

For example, assume that the price of a syringe is \$7.80 per unit. A vendor of syringes may offer a discount of two percent if more than 100 syringes are purchased, and an additional discount of 1.5 percent if more than 300 syringes are purchased. Assuming that a nursing agency purchases 400 syringes, the purchase price per unit would be \$7.80 × .965 = \$7.53.[5] This purchase price includes a discount of \$.27 (\$7.80 − \$7.53) per unit, or a total saving of \$108 (400 units × \$.27). These quantity discounts can be substantial, and ignoring them is often costly. However, the savings generated from taking trade discounts must always be judged against the possible increase in inventory carrying costs.

Time discounts, on the other hand, are discounts given for early payment of current liabilities. Time discount contracts are often written as

$$d/t_1;\ n/t_2,$$

where: d represents the discount which may be taken if the liability is paid before t_1 elapses:

t_1 represents some time period of short duration (perhaps 10 days) and is referred to as the discount period;

n indicates the total amount of the liability that is due before t_2 elapses; and

t_2 represents some time period of greater duration (perhaps 30 days). After t_2 has passed, the payable is considered delinquent.

Taking time discounts generally is desirable because the effective interest rate (EIR) of a given time discount, stated as

$$\text{EIR} = d\left[\frac{365}{t_1}\right],$$

almost always will be greater than the rate of interest the institution would be required to pay to borrow the funds to pay the liability within the discount period. In fact, monitoring time discounts to insure that payments are made to vendors within the discount period usually is so important that specific accounting entries are made to reflect either discount opportunities taken or discount opportunities lost.

Management must decide what information should be generated by the accounting system. If discount opportunities taken are to be identified by the accounting system, the gross price method of recording purchases and payments should be used. Conversely, if discount opportunities lost are to be identified by the accounting system, the net price method of accounting for purchases and payments should be used. Both of these methods are found in practice. However, the impact of the gross price method on effective managerial action is significantly less than the impact of the net price method.

Gross Price Method

Under the gross price method of accounting for current liabilities, if payment is made during the discount period, the discount is recorded at the time the payment is made. If the payment is made after the discount period has expired, the journal entry is made as if no discount had been offered.

For example, assume the nursing agency in the previous example purchases the 400 syringes for $7.53 each. The total account payable for this purchase is $3,012. Now, assume that two time discounts are available as follows:

5,2/15,30; net/45.

This means that if payment is made within 15 days, a discount of five percent may be taken; if payment is made within 30 days, a two percent discount may be taken. Payment, in any case, is expected within 45 days. If the agency experiences the following economic events regarding this purchase:

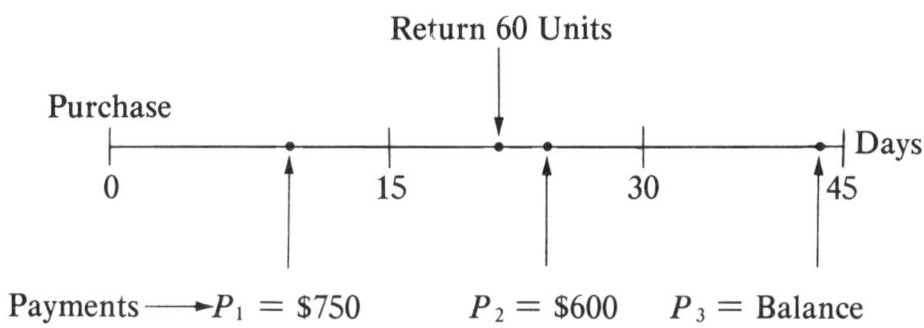

the journal entries required to record these transactions under the gross price method would be:

Inventory	$3,012.00	
Accounts Payable (·)[6]		$3,012.00
To record the purchase of 400 syringes at $7.53 each.		
Accounts Payable (·)	789.47	
Purchase Discounts Taken		39.47
Cash		750.00

To record the cash payment P_1 within the five percent discount period.		
Accounts Payable (·)	$451.80	
Inventory		$451.80
To record the return of 60 syringes.		
Accounts Payable (·)	612.24	
Purchase Discounts Taken		12.24
Cash		600.00
To record the cash payment P_2 within the two percent discount period.		
Accounts Payable (·)	1,158.49	
Cash		1,158.49
To record the payment of the balance in accounts payable after both discount periods have passed.		

Note that cash payments made within the discount period satisfy a greater amount of the account payable than the actual amount of cash tendered. For example, if the entire liability were paid within the first discount period, the amount of cash to be paid would be:

$$\$3{,}012 \times (1 - .05) = \$2{,}861.40.$$

Therefore, a cash payment of $2,861.40 satisfies a payable of $3,012. The same pattern pertains to partial payments. Hence, the amount of liability satisfied with a cash payment C at a discount rate d is:

$$\text{Accounts Payable Debit} = C/(1 - d).$$

Net Price Method

Under the net price method of accounting for accounts payable, the goods purchased are recorded net of the discount at the time of the purchase. Hence, if payment is made within the discount period, the transaction is recorded as if no discount had been offered, while if payment is made after the discount period has expired, the amount of the discount foregone is recorded. Using the facts from the previous example, the following entries would be made under the net price method:

Inventory	$2,861.40	
Accounts Payable (·)		$2,861.40
To record the purchase of 400 syringes net of the five percent purchase discount.		
Accounts Payable (·)	750.00	
Cash		750.00
To record payment P_1		
Purchase Discounts Lost	66.68	
Accounts Payable (·)		66.68
To convert the amount in the accounts payable account to a discount rate of two percent after the five percent discount period has expired.		
Accounts Payable (·)	442.76	
Inventory		442.76
To record the return of 60 syringes.		
Accounts Payable (·)	600.00	
Cash		600.00
To record payment P_2		
Accounts Payable	1,135.32	
Purchase Discounts Lost	23.17	
Cash		1,158.49
To record the final cash payment.		

In any case, where the amount of discount taken under the gross price method is added to the amount of discount lost under the net price method, the total must equal the total discount available. In the above example:

Purchase discount taken:	$ 51.71
Purchase discount lost:	$ 89.85
Purchase discount available:	$141.56.

The total purchase discount available in this example is $150.60 − $9.04 = $141.56, where $150.60 is the discount available from the purchase of 400 syringes ($3,012 × .05) and $9.04 is the discount not available owing to the return of 60 syringes during the two percent discount period ($451.80 × .02).

Summary

At the time of the purchase, the gross price method records the liability at the amount which must be paid to satisfy the entire account payable disregarding any time discounts. Therefore, under this method, the only time a difference exists between the amount of the cash payment and the associated liability is when a payment is made within the discount period. At that time, a "Purchase Discounts Taken" account is created. This account represents only the discounts actually taken. Discount opportunities foregone are not recorded under the gross price method.

Under the net price method, the liability is recorded at the minimum amount which must be paid if the entire cash payment is made within the discount period. Therefore, whenever payments are made after the discount period expires, cash greater than the amount recorded in the accounts payable account must be tendered and a "Purchase Discounts Lost" account created. This account records the amount of the discount actually foregone. Discount opportunities taken are not recorded under the net price method.

Taking advantage of discounts is economically desirable, and institutional policy should dictate that all cash payments be made within the discount period. The gross price method generates accounting information that shows when that policy has been followed, while the net price method highlights when that policy has not been followed. From a control perspective, knowing where savings are being lost is usually more useful than knowing where savings are being generated. Therefore, the preferable accounting method is the net price method.

The Policy Aspects of Effective Cash Management

Effective cash management begins with policy statements. The organization must formulate policies regarding the recording and collection of cash for services rendered, recording and payment of current liabilities, preparation of the cash budget, and nature of the institution's banking relationships. If these management policies are well formulated and well executed, the periodic sources and uses of cash should be fairly predictable and, hence, manageable.

Collection of Cash for Services Rendered

Management's policy regarding the collection of cash for services rendered should attempt to minimize the time between the rendering of service and the collection of the cash from the patient or third party payer. (Accounts receivable management is considered extensively in Chapter 3.) The most desirable collection policy, from the institution's point of view, is for the patient account to be settled at the time of discharge. However, if the institution is unable or unwilling to institute and enforce a policy requiring the collection of cash for services rendered at the time of discharge, accounts receivable must be created.

Once accounts receivable have been created, three periods of time become relevant in managing these accounts: the "in-house billing float," the time the account is outstanding, and the "mail float." The in-house billing float is the period of time between rendering the service and issuing a billing invoice. This time period can be minimized by maintaining an effective information system which is coordinated with an adequate system of internal control. The time the account is outstanding or the time between mailing the billing invoice and the cash remittance by the debtor can be minimized by an aggressive collection policy. Finally, the mail float, the period of time between the debtor's remittance and the receipt of the check by the payee's bank, can often be reduced by using lock boxes (discussed in the case study in the following section). If each of these time periods can be minimized, the goal of the accounts receivable collection policy will be realized.

Payment of Current Liabilities

Management's policy regarding the payment of current liabilities should require that two time periods be maximized. The first is the time between the date an invoice is received from a vendor and the date a check is issued which qualifies for the purchase discount. The second is the time between the issuance of a check to the vendor and the date that check clears the institution's bank account. The first time period can be maximized if information regarding the date that discount will be lost is routinely generated from the accounting system. By coordinating the issuance of checks to vendors with this information, the first time period can be maximized (see Question 2-8). The second time period can be maximized by attempting to maximize the float. A common practice used to extend float is to use out-of-state checking accounts.

Preparation of the Cash Budget

An effective cash management system also requires a cash budget that records the forecasted cash inflows from various sources and also records the forecasted demands for cash. Accurate forecasting of these cash flows can alert management to the possible need for financing cash deficits or the possible opportunities to invest cash excesses. Therefore, management policy should require that these forecasts be generated with models that are capable of providing the best estimates of cash flows. The cash budget should be prepared periodically and updated intermittently as current information is generated (see Figure 2-5).

Banking Relationships

Finally, the institution should have a policy regarding the nature of the relationship to be maintained with the banking community. Cooperative interaction with local banks may allow the institution to take advantage of numerous special banking services that may enable the institution to better manage its cash and may also aid in the preparation of the cash budget. The institution should maintain cash balances in several banks if these banks offer different services that may be useful to the institution.

CASE STUDY

This case examines the cash management system of a large urban teaching hospital. The four elements of an effective cash management system, (1) the conversion of accounts receivable, (2) the satisfaction of accounts payable, (3) the forecasting and development of the cash budget, and (4) the banking relationships, are explored in detail (see Question 2-9). The case concludes with a number of recommendations for improved cash management.

Analysis of the Conversion of Accounts Receivable

The hospital currently has $15 million of accounts receivable arising from two sources—patient accounts and nonpatient accounts. Patient accounts, which are divided into inpatient and outpatient accounts, for administrative, billing, and collection purposes, comprise 95 percent of total accounts receivable. The remaining accounts receivable arise from such nonpatient accounts as cafeteria charges, television rentals, office space charges, and miscellaneous departmental billings.

More timely conversion of the patient and nonpatient accounts receivable could significantly improve the hospital's cash position. Unfortunately, in this case, the hospital management does not exert sufficient control over nonpatient accounts receivable to effect immediate changes in the cash conversion of these inflows because many of the nonpatient accounts receivable occur under long-term contracts. In addition, the number of these debtors is large, the amount owed by each is relatively small, and the total amount of nonpatient accounts receivable is relatively minor with respect to total accounts receivable. Hence, an analysis of these accounts will not be undertaken.

However, management intervention could be beneficial in improving the cash conversion of inpatient and outpatient accounts receivable. Most of these accounts are due from third party payers, primarily Blue Cross, Medicare, and Medicaid. In addition, since 95 percent of total accounts receivable are from patient accounts, any improvement in the cash conversion of these accounts would have a substantial impact on the cash position of the hospital.

Inpatient Accounts Receivable

An examination of the inpatient revenue accounts shows that most of the hospital's revenue is derived through the creation of accounts receivable. In fact, more than 75 percent of the inpatient revenue in fiscal 19X1–X2 was derived from Blue Cross, Medicare, and Medicaid as follows:

Revenue Source	Percentage	Approximate Dollars
Blue Cross	29.68	$20,968,714
Medicare	34.66	24,487,049
Medicaid	12.73	8,993,656
All Other	22.93	16,199,886
Total	100.00	$70,649,305

Furthermore, the major third parties' contribution to total inpatient revenue is expected to increase from 77.1 percent to over 80 percent in fiscal 19X3–X4. Consequently, any action that would speed the collection of these accounts would improve the hospital's cash position.

Blue Cross, Medicare, and Medicaid reimburse the hospital for actual patient days at a standard rate which may be adjusted at any time, but is usually adjusted quarterly. Any difference between the reimbursed costs and the actual Blue Cross, Medicare, and Medicaid costs are settled at the end of the fiscal year. Hence, in addition to the opportunity loss resulting from delays in receiving reimbursements, an additional economic opportunity loss is incurred as a result of the delayed payment of differences between reimbursed costs and actual costs (see Figure 2–2).

To assist the hospital in managing its cash, Blue Cross and Medicare have recently agreed to make periodic interim payments (PIP) or automatic reimbursement payments to the hospital every two weeks, rather than as bills are received by Blue Cross and Medicare (see Question 2–10). The automatic reimbursement payments are estimated from prior period payments. These payments are adjusted and the estimates revised at the end of each quarter.

This new reimbursement procedure results in two major benefits. First, since Blue Cross and Medicare reimbursements account for 64 percent of inpatient revenue, the short-term credit requirement of the hospital can be estimated more accurately. Second, the reduction in the average

age of the Blue Cross and Medicare receivables will result in a one-time cash flow increase. If Medicaid were to participate in the PIP program, these benefits would be enhanced because cash inflows from nearly 80 percent of the hospital's revenue could be estimated more accurately and an additional one-time cash benefit of approximately $1 to $3 million would be realized (see Figure 2–3).

The collection of accounts receivable from payers other than the major insurers can be problematic. Although these accounts give rise to only 22.93 percent of inpatient revenue, they must be collected from more than 150 private insurance companies, from patients whose insurance policies provide for copayments, and from the two percent of all inpatients who have no health care insurance. Moreover, the differences in the policies offered by the various private insurance companies are bewildering. Each carrier specifies covered and noncovered procedures, different patient/insurance company copayment agreements, different limits of coverage and special documentation requirements. As a result, insurance coverage must be handled on a patient-by-patient basis. Furthermore, these private insurance companies tend to delay payment so that their resources can be maintained in income-producing investments as long as possible. These problems combine to make the timely collection of these accounts quite difficult.

Since legal action is financially infeasible in speeding the collection of accounts receivable from private insurance companies that usually pay, albeit in their own slow time, the hospital must use more subtle means of collecting these accounts. Hence, a new billing policy has recently been implemented by the hospital. Under this policy, private patients are billed for the entire cost of their hospital stay. The patients must then contact the appropriate insurance company so that their accounts can be paid. This policy is expected to improve the cash flow from patients covered by private insurance companies because these insurance companies could lose clients by withholding payments for substantial time periods. Hence, by converting the patient from a secondary payment source into an active collection agent for the hospital, the hospital expects to realize more timely payments from the private insurance companies.

Two other techniques for speeding the collection of accounts receivable from private insurance companies also are being studied by the hospital. The first involves granting a discount to private insurance companies for payments within a specified period of time. However, this technique probably will not be adopted because a discount of at least three percent would be necessary to offset the typical 120-day payment delay of private insurance companies. If the third party payers currently making PIP payments took advantage of this three percent discount, which they would, the net effect would be a substantial cash loss for the hospital.

The second approach to speed payment relies on the use of a collection intermediary. A trial program which uses a collection service managed by a former insurance company executive has reduced the average age of accounts receivable in a random sample of accounts. The agent's strong personal ties in the insurance industry aid in the success of this collection service. However, the trial program will be continued until the hospital can ascertain if a permanent improvement has occurred in the collection of accounts receivable from private insurance companies and if the improvement justifies the cost of the collection service.

Figure 2–2 Opportunity Loss Caused by Unanticipated Cost Inflation

Assume that the average rate of inflation in the hospital's health care delivery costs was 12 percent in fiscal 19X1–X2.[a] Further assume that the third party payors base current reimbursements rates on the average cost in the preceding quarter. Given these assumptions, in fiscal 19X1–X2 the hospital would have incurred a chronic underpayment equal to three percent (12 percent/4) of the total actual costs, assuming that this amount would be paid to the hospital at the end of the fiscal year.

For example, assuming a uniform inflation rate of 12 percent and an average of ten Medicare and Medicaid patients per quarter, the following cost and cash flows would occur:

Quarter/fiscal year	Actual costs per patient day at beginning of quarter	Reimbursement per patient day	Patient days	Total reimbursement	Total actual costs	Difference
4/19X0–X1	$ 91.00	—	—	—	—	—
1/19X1–X2	94.00	$ 92.50	10	$ 925	$ 955	$ 30
2/19X1–X2	97.00	95.50	10	955	985	30
3/19X1–X2	100.00	98.50	10	985	1,015	30
4/19X1–X2	103.00	101.50	10	1,015	1,045	30
Lump sum payment at year end	—	—	—	120	—	—
				$4,000	$4,000	$120.

Hence, the underpayment is three percent ($120/$4000) of the total costs actually incurred during the year. The opportunity loss that would result from this underpayment would be a function of the investment opportunities foregone as a result of not having the $120 paid on a more timely basis.

[a] The rate of inflation is calculated as

$$\sum_{i=1}^{4} \frac{EA_i - BA_i}{TA_i} PD_i,$$

where i represents a particular quarter, EA_i is the actual cost per patient day at the end of the ith quarter, BA_i represents the actual cost per patient day at the beginning of the ith quarter, PD_i represents the number of patient days in the ith quarter, and TA_i represents the total actual costs in the ith quarter.

Figure 2–3 One-Time Benefit Possible from Converting Medicaid to PIP

Given: Medicaid payments are currently on a net 120-day basis.
Total Medicaid Revenue Calculation:

Total inpatient revenue	$70,649,303	
Percentage Medicaid	12.73	
Inpatient Medicaid Revenue		$ 8,993,656
Total outpatient revenue	$ 3,927,461	
Percentage Medicaid	40.00	
Outpatient Medicaid Revenue		1,570,984
Total Medicaid Revenue		$10,564,640.

For purposes of estimation, assume that Medicaid revenue is received in equal amounts at equal intervals throughout the year. Therefore:

$$\text{Average Medicaid Receivable} = (120 \text{ days}/365 \text{ days}) \times \$10,564,640$$
$$= \$3,473,306.$$

PIP should theoretically reduce the average age of Medicaid receivables to seven days. However, procedural delays might result in a lesser benefit. The following table gives the one-time benefit of reducing the average age of Medicaid receivables.

Age Reduction (in days)	Average Age of Receivable	Benefit (Reduction in Average Medicaid Receivable)
113	7	$3,270,697
90	30	2,604,980
60	60	1,736,653
30	90	868,327

Finally, the two percent of inpatients who have no insurance have a 50 percent default rate. This default rate resulted in the writeoff of approximately $700,000 of accounts receivable in fiscal 19X1–X2. One solution to this problem is to refuse service to patients who are not covered by insurance and who are clearly incapable of paying the estimated charges. However, management has avoided this course of action for a variety of reasons (see Question 2–6).

Outpatient Accounts

Outpatient revenue, like inpatient revenue, is derived primarily through the creation of accounts receivable. This revenue comprises approximately five percent of total hospital revenue and is derived from services administered in the hospital's 29 outpatient clinics and the emergency room. An important dichotomy exists between the quality of the accounts receivable from patients who are referred to the clinics and the quality of the accounts receivable from unreferred clinic patients and from emergency room patients. The default rate of accounts receivable from referred clinic patients is approximately four percent, while the default rate of accounts receivable from unreferred clinic patients and emergency room patients is so high that it increases the overall percentage of outpatient bad debts to 50 percent. These bad debts result from treating uninsured patients who do not have sufficient funds to pay the hospital charges. Management has been unable to take any action that would increase the collectibility of these accounts.

However, in an attempt to increase outpatient revenue, the hospital has recently reorganized the operations of the outpatient clinics from hospital facilities to physicians' offices. Medicare and Medicaid currently allow private physicians' clinics to collect $9 per patient visit, while hospital clinics are only reimbursed $6 per patient visit. Therefore, the Medicare and Medicaid reimbursement funds flow to the physicians who then are charged by the hospital for office space and for supplies. Hence, although the change is largely organizational, the net result is an increase in the physicians' revenues and an increase in the hospital's outpatient revenues.

Cash Collection

Most of the hospital's cash is collected after the billing of accounts receivable. However, in an attempt to speed the collection of cash and to minimize the probability of bad debts, the hospital makes a collection effort (1) prior to patient admission, (2) at the time of patient admission, (3) during the patient's hospitalization, (4) at the time of the patient's discharge, and (5) after the patient has been billed. This collection cycle is diagrammed in Figure 2-4.

Preadmission Collection Effort. During the preadmission process, the business office collects the information needed to complete the admitting forms (e.g., personal data and insurance coverage) and attempts to verify commercial insurance coverages. Since 90 percent of all scheduled patients and 50 percent of all nonscheduled patients are preadmitted, a patient's

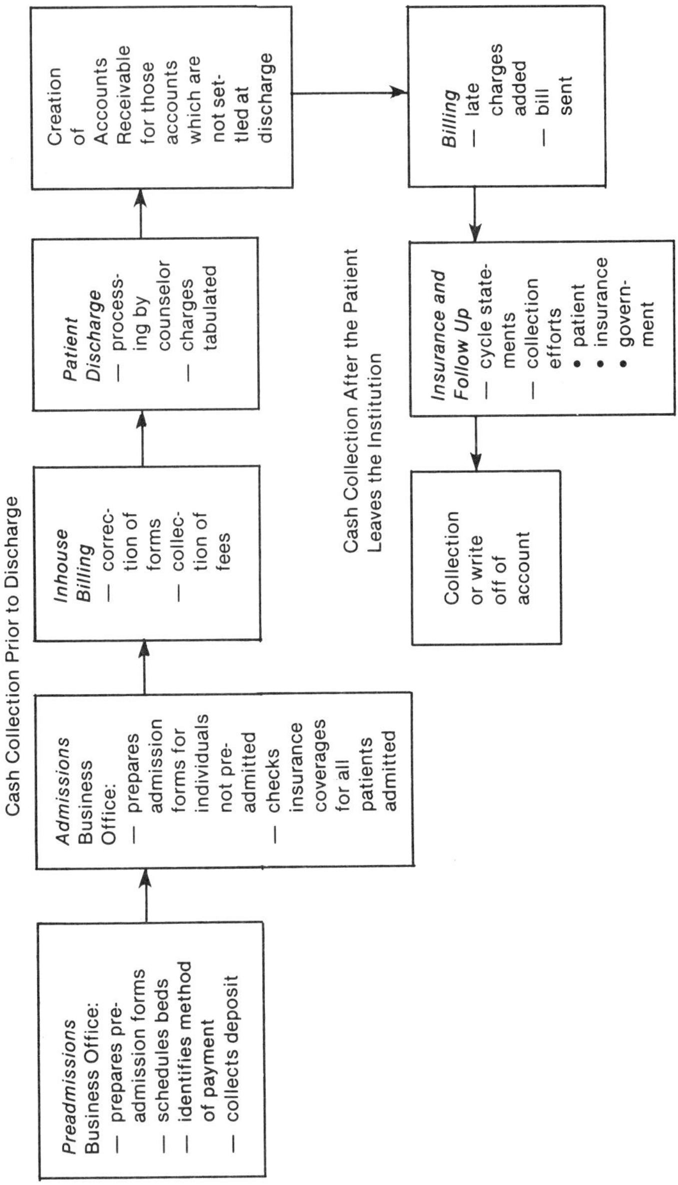

Figure 2–4 The Cash Collection Cycle

ability to pay is usually known prior to admission. The hospital then can plan collection strategies.

Admission Collection Effort. "Urgent" and "emergency" patients enter the hospital without being preadmitted. Therefore, the spouse or a relative of the patient must complete the appropriate admitting forms. All forms, including those filled out during preadmission, are screened by the business office after admission to identify any incomplete or incorrect forms. The business office also sends for approval forms from Medicare, Blue Cross, and Medicaid if the patient is covered by any of these insurers. Medicare approval forms are ordered on the day of admission and orders for Blue Cross approval forms are sent the day after admission; Medicaid approval forms are ordered only twice each week.

Inhouse Billing. The hospital estimates the portion of the patient's bill for which the patient is responsible so that a deposit or prepayment can be obtained. The room and service per diem charge is estimated to be $400 for deposit and prepayment purposes. For example, Medicare patient copayments and deductibles usually amount to $125 per day. Therefore, to calculate a Medicare patient's deposit, the business office multiplies the patient's expected length of stay by $125. For patients who have commercial insurance coverage, the hospital generally tries to collect a deposit equal to 20 percent of the per diem charge multiplied by the expected length of stay. However, if the commercial insurance coverage is comprehensive and has no copayment provisions, then no deposit is required. If a patient is not insured, the deposit is equal to the $400 per diem rate multiplied by the expected length of stay. If the patient has been preadmitted, the hospital tries to collect the deposit between 24 and 48 hours before admission. Otherwise, the patient or the patient's relatives are notified of the required deposit upon admission. However, the hospital's policy is to deny neither service nor admission if adequate deposits are not collected.

Collection at the Time of Discharge. Ideally, the hospital should present the patient with a final bill, including any possible late charges, and determine a payment schedule at the time of discharge. Unfortunately, all efforts to have bills current at the time of discharge have failed because, although the business office only requires one day to prepare the patient's charges, 95 percent of the time the doctors fail to give early notification of discharges to the business office. In addition, even if the bills were current at the time of discharge, the hospital is large and the security is so lax that 30 percent of the patients leave the hospital without seeing either the cashier or one of the business office counselors. These procedural failures cause problems in an otherwise effective inhouse revenue collection process.

Billing of Accounts Receivable. Once a patient leaves the hospital without paying the final bill, an account receivable must be created. The hospital's policy is to wait seven days before preparing the final bill so that all late charges will be listed on it. Since the invoices are printed by a computer at a remote site, another three days go by before the patient receives the bill.

Monthly bills are sent to patients until the account is either collected or written off. After three months, a separate dunning letter is sent to the patient. The business office counselors and the collection manager also review delinquent accounts receivable on a monthly basis. When both the counselor in charge of a particular account and the collection manager agree that the account cannot be collected routinely, increased collection efforts are extended. The accounts of patients who were under the care of private physicians and who have account balances greater than $100 are referred to the hospital's attorney. All other accounts are sent to a collection agency. The results of these extended collection efforts (in millions of dollars) for a seven year period ending in 19X1 were:

	Attorneys	Collection Agency
Accounts referred	$3,160	$4,276
Collections	847	579
Commissions	313	212
Net return	534	367
Percentage return	16.9%	8.6%

If the hospital attorney or the collection agent cannot collect an account, that account is written off.

Analysis of the Satisfaction of Accounts Payable

Most of the hospital's accounts payable are labor related. More than 60 percent of the hospital's operating budget consists of wages, salaries, payroll taxes, and employee benefits. For the purposes of cash management, the payroll and related expenses are viewed as a fixed, biweekly expense of approximately $1 million. These costs are controlled by requiring each department to estimate overtime, insisting that all overtime be authorized by the department head, and vigorously investigating all unfavorable overtime variances. Hence, aside from reducing staff, little opportunity exists to improve the management of this aspect of the cash conversion.

Other cash expenditures occur when inventory and services are purchased. These purchases are controlled primarily through inventory management (see Chapter 4). Quantity discount opportunities are analyzed individually with respect to the hospital's estimated 25 percent inventory carrying cost. In addition, during the low census periods (summer and holidays), purchases are postponed and inventory levels are systematically reduced.

Cash disbursements for supplies and services are controlled in order to take advantage of all available time discounts. Payables not offering discounts are paid within 60 days even though these payments could be delayed from 120 to 180 days. This timely payment policy has produced a cooperative relationship between the hospital and its suppliers. One benefit of this rapport is that the hospital purchasing department has been able to bargain successfully with vendors for postponement of purchase payments during reduced revenue seasons.

The remaining accounts payable of the hospital are created for capital expenditures. The hospital controls these cash disbursements with a comprehensive capital budget (see Chapter 9).

Forecasting and Developing the Cash Budget

The hospital currently uses a manual system to forecast revenues and expenses and develop both the capital and the operating expense budgets, which together form the basis of the cash budget. However, this process is expected to be converted to a computer system in the near future. The current forecasting process involves estimating the revenues and expenses for the coming fiscal year (July/June), collecting budgets from the hospital cost centers, and developing the cash budget.

Forecasting Revenues and Expenses

The revenue and expense forecasts take into account expected patient volume and anticipated inflation. Patient volume estimates are developed from past trends in patient volume, while inflation estimates are based on national trends in various hospital expense categories. The Health Care Index component of the Consumer Price Index is the primary source for these estimates, but inflation figures published in *Hospital Week* also are used.

The hospital's revenue and expense estimates have been fairly accurate in the past. The predictability of patient volume and inflation and the fairly consistent revenue and expense classifications contribute to the accuracy of the revenue and expense estimates. For example, the primary source of revenue is patient revenue which can be accurately forecasted because most patient revenue is derived from Blue Cross, Medicare, and Medicaid. Similarly, the primary hospital expense category is payroll, which does not vary substantially from $1 million every two weeks. The annual variances in supplies and other operating expenses usually are not substantial. Hence, the hospital's revenue and expense forecasts can be quite accurate.

Cost Centers' Proposed Budgets

Once the revenue and expense forecasts have been formulated, the comptroller's office requests a proposed budget from each cost center. These budget proposals are reviewed individually and in the aggregate. Then the appropriate budget adjustments are made so that the total sources and uses of cash in the cost center budgets are coordinated with the forecasts. All cost center budgets for the ensuing fiscal year receive final approval by the end of April.

Preparation of the Cash Budget

The cost center budgets are used to develop the capital budget and the operating expense budget. These two budgets, in conjunction with historical monthly data, are used to develop the final cash budget shown in Figure 2-5. In preparing this budget, noncash transactions are eliminated from both the capital budget and the operating expense budget and the effect of changes in accounts receivable and accounts payable are considered (see Chapter 6).

The cash budget illustrated in Figure 2-5 has been in use for six months during the current fiscal year. Hence, the "Actual" columns have been completed for the months of July through December. Note the continuous updating of the beginning cash balance in the expired portion of the budget. The "Total" column is updated continuously also, so that at year end the actual total sources and total uses of cash are known. The variance between the budgeted and the actual sources and uses of cash provides important information useful in future cash planning activities.

Banking Relationships

The hospital's banking relationships can be an important aspect of cash management. For example, certain banking services may be able to improve the hospital's cash management system. In fact, most banks offer two services which could benefit the hospital: a lock box service and a service that provides information to the hospital regarding anticipated changes in the banking industry which may affect the hospital's cash management system. Of course, the costs and benefits of these services must be evaluated before the hospital elects to use them.

Figure 2–5 19X2–X3 Cash Budget ($000s)

	Total	July to October Actual	Nov Budget	Nov Actual	Dec Budget	Dec Actual
Cash—Beginning Balance	$ 263	$ 263	$ 290	$ 290	$ 611	$ 611
Add: Cash Receipts						
Medicare	13,349	4,511	946	946	1,307	1,307
Blue Cross	17,528	4,909	1,408	1,508	1,500	1,540
Medical Assistance	6,879	2,767	371	518	500	392
Patient Cash	2,508	729		311	174	382
Other Insurance	11,648	2,714	1,307	962	1,007	764
Private Outpatient	2,782	896		272	175	213
Clinic Cash	2,275	810	180	205	180	145
Total Accounts Receivable	$56,969	$17,336	$4,212	$4,722	$4,843	$4,743
Third Party Payments (Prior Years)	$ 1,695	$ 711	$ —	$ 169	$ 155	$ 155
School of Nursing	138	63	2	1	22	1
Cafeteria Sales	553	192	45	49	40	47
Research Overhead	190	—	—	—	—	—
Utilization Review	100	29	8	9	9	—
Miscellaneous Operating	5,302	1,784	262	500	385	706
Restricted Contributions	762	104	35	13	4	—
Endowments	686	285	55	1	55	6
University Loan	200	200	—	—	—	—
Total Receipts	$66,595	$20,704	$4,619	$5,464	$5,513	$5,658
Less: Cash Disbursements						
Payroll	$23,592	$ 7,525	$1,535	$1,745	$2,316	$2,446
Employee Benefits	11,065	3,691	814	947	1,296	1,173
Accounts Payable	21,360	7,905	1,815	1,855	1,657	1,640
Interest	101	34	—	—	34	34
Equipment	1,585	97	55	53	158	42
Alterations and Improvements (A & I)	890	200	93	48	116	123
Prior Year Equipment & A & I	412	237	132	9	22	14
Long-Term Debt	151	26	9	—	65	72
Third Party Payments	1,090	—	—	—	—	—
University Comptroller						
Accounts Payable	3,823	760	357	396	381	25
Working Capital	700	100	—	—	—	—
Overhead (Prior Year)	817	96	90	90	90	90
Equipment Advance	76	6	9	—	18	8
Total Disbursements	$65,662	$20,677	$4,909	$5,143	$6,153	$5,667
Net Increase or (Decrease)	$ 933	$ 27	$ (290)	$ 321	$ (640)	$ (9)
Cash Ending Balance	1,196	290	—	611	(29)	602

Figure 2–5—Continued

	Jan Budget	Jan Actual	Feb Budget	Feb Actual	March Budget	March Actual	April Budget	April Actual	May Budget	May Actual	June Budget	June Actual
Cash—Beginning Balance	$ 602		$ 703		$ 198		$ (90)		$1,469		$1,319	
Add: Cash Receipts												
Medicare	1,013		1,013		1,013		1,520		1,013		1,013	
Blue Cross	2,806		1,230		1,230		1,845		1,230		1,230	
Medical Assistance	530		498		544		509		583		538	
Patient Cash	156		149		168		189		188		236	
Other Insurance	1,182		1,197		1,124		1,233		1,153		1,319	
Private Outpatient	200		201		214		279		244		263	
Clinic Cash	180		180		215		180		180		180	
Total Accounts Receivable	$6,067		$4,468		$4,508		$5,755		$4,591		$4,779	
Third Party Payments (Prior Yrs.)	$ —		$ 160		$ —		$ 400		$ —		$ 100	
School of Nursing	56		4		1		9		3		—	
Cafeteria Sales	45		45		45		45		40		45	
Research Overhead	—		—		—		—		180		10	
Utilization Review	10		10		11		10		10		11	
Miscellaneous Operating	385		386		385		385		385		386	
Restricted Contributions	14		10		130		47		206		238	
Endowments	80		63		63		63		63		62	
University Loan	—		—		—		—		—		—	
Total Receipts	$6,657		$5,146		$5,143		$6,714		$5,478		$5,631	
Less: Cash Disbursements												
Payroll	$2,227		$1,930		$1,930		$1,930		$1,929		$1,930	
Employee Benefits	980		849		849		849		864		863	
Accounts Payable	1,674		1,657		1,657		1,657		1,657		1,658	
Interest	—		—		—		—		—		33	
Equipment	128		219		208		152		285		401	
A & I	111		108		101		52		80		67	
Prior Year Equipment & A & I	25		48		21		25		22		11	
Long-Term Debt	9		9		9		9		9		8	
Third Party Payments	565		350		175		—		—		—	
University Comptroller												
Accts. Payable	737		381		381		381		381		381	
Working Capital	—		—		—		—		300		300	
Overhead (Prior Year)	90		90		90		90		90		91	
Equipment Advance	10		10		10		10		11		11	
Total Disbursements	$6,556		$5,651		$5,431		$5,155		$5,628		$5,754	
Net Increase or (Decrease)	$ 101		$ (505)		$ (288)		$1,559		$ (150)		$ (123)	
Cash Ending Balance	703		198		(90)		1,469		1,319		1,196	

Lock Box Service

A lock box arrangement permits the hospital to maintain a special mail depositor box, called a lock box, at a post office. The hospital's cash receipts are mailed to that lock box and collected by the bank at which the hospital maintains cash accounts. The bank immediately credits these receipts to the hospital's account and mails the results of the transaction to the hospital for posting to the hospital's records. The advantages of a lock box are that the mail float is reduced by several days and the clerical effort needed to process cash receipts is eliminated, which reduces the possibility of cash misappropriations.

These lock box benefits must be quantified and evaluated against the associated costs before the hospital decides to purchase a lock box. While the cost of maintaining a lock box varies among banks, the usual monthly charge is $100 for 1,000 transactions or less and 35¢ for each transaction in excess of 1,000. Usually, the reduced clerical effort and the reduced possibility of a misappropriation of cash receipts rationalize the purchase of a lock box (see Problem 2-8).

The hospital currently maintains one lock box in the city in which it operates. The fact that Medicare and Blue Cross mail their reimbursement checks from the same city was a contributing factor in selecting the location of the lock box. However, the hospital also receives reimbursement checks from Medicaid that are mailed from a city 200 miles away, so the administration currently is evaluating the costs and benefits of maintaining a lock box in that city.

Other Banking Services

Other banking services that aid hospital cash management also may be available. For example, the bank may, upon request and without charge, provide the hospital with an activity analysis of the hospital's cash account. In addition, the bank may counsel the hospital when banking changes could affect the hospital's cash management system. For example, a number of recent developments in electronic fund transfers among banks may be able to reduce the hospital's accounts receivable mail float significantly. Undoubtedly, the bank could provide the hospital with a good deal of valuable information about the possible effects of electronic fund transfers on the hospital's cash management system. However, to date the hospital has not taken the necessary steps to open channels of communication with the banking community.

Recommendations to the Hospital

The cash management system of this hospital could be improved in three general areas. First, the cash flows from some of the third party payers could be improved; second, the billing process could be made more effective; third, the hospital's banking relationships could be strengthened. The appropriate management actions in these areas could enhance cash management and increase cash control.

Payments from Third Party Payers

Prompt payments from Medicaid and private insurance companies, could improve the hospital's cash flows significantly. Currently, these insurers withhold payments from 120 to 180 days. Therefore, the hospital should be fined or otherwise penalized. For example, departments that submit late charges could only be credited with a portion of the late The hospital also should continue to study the possible economic and legal consequences of offering discounts to private insurance companies in order to improve the cash flow from these third party payers.

Patient Billing

Prompt billing of patients should enhance the collectibility of accounts receivable. All patients should be billed at the time of discharge. To insure that each patient's bill is current when the patient is discharged, departments that do not give the business office early notification of discharge should be fined or otherwise penalized. For example, departments that submit late charges could only be credited with a portion of the late charges. Billing at the time of discharge would be facilitated further if an orderly were to escort patients from their beds to either the cashier or a counselor in the business office.

Banking Relationships

The hospital may also be able to improve the effectiveness of the cash management system by strengthening its banking relationships. The first step in this process is to initiate a channel of communication between the hospital's management and the banking community. This communication channel could be used to make management aware of those banking services which may be useful in improving the institution's cash management system.

NOTES

1. The recording procedures required to account for cash are included in Appendix A.
2. This voucher payable will be presented to the cash disbursements clerk. The journal entry to record the cash disbursement will be:

Voucher Payable	$87.00	
Cash		$87.00.

In subsequent sections of this text, the intermediate control step of recording the voucher payable will be eliminated. This is done only to facilitate the exposition. However, all credit entries to cash must be controlled by valid vouchers.

3. Parentheses are used to denote cash outflows or negative amounts.
4. The recording and interpretation of accounts receivable accounting information are discussed in Chapter 3.
5. Another possible interpretation of this discount contract would be that the additional discount applies only to the units purchased in excess of 300. This is not the usual interpretation.
6. The notation (·) means that this transaction information is also recorded in a subsidiary ledger (see Appendix A).

Questions and Problems

Question 2-1. Using the figure on page 9 as the basis of discussion, what are some of the behavioral problems which may interfere with the effective operation of the voucher system in a nonproprietary teaching hospital?

Question 2-2. What are the control disadvantages of using a petty cash fund? Why use the fund if these disadvantages exist?

Question 2-3. What is the principal advantage of using the proof of cash for verifying changes in cash? How frequently should a proof of cash be performed?

Question 2-4. Under what circumstances would a manager want to bypass the opportunity to take a trade discount? A time discount?

Question 2-5. What is the principal control disadvantage of using the gross price method to record purchase discounts?

Question 2-6. List and defend five reasons why denial of service to reduce the uninsured patient account default rate is not the best managerial action (see page 30).

Question 2-7. Construct a diagram which specifies the various interrelationships required to maintain an effective cash management system.

Question 2-8. Assume that an institution attempts to pay current liabilities on the last day within the discount period. Indicate how the information required to effect this policy may be abstracted from the accounting system. Also suggest any cost/benefit considerations regarding the payment of current liabilities in this manner.

Question 2-9. Throughout the management section of this chapter various procedures were suggested to make the management of cash effective. What is the difference between effective cash management and efficient cash management?

Question 2-10. Is there any economic motivation for the third party payers to make periodic interim payments? If not, why do they make them?

Problem 2-1. Prepare a bank reconciliation and the appropriate adjusting entry, given the following information of the Memorial Hospital on July 31, 19X1.

Bank records:	Ending cash balance:		$6,180.00
Hospital records:	Ending cash balance:		$5,451.00
Outstanding checks:	#511:	$58.00	
	#512:	$72.00	
Bank service charge:		$12.00	
NSF check:		$10.00	

Hospital error: Payroll check written for $23.00 was recorded on the books as $32.00.

A 12 percent note outstanding since February 1, 19X1, was collected by the bank on July 31, 19X1. The principal of the note was $600.
Deposit in transit at the end of the period was $42.00.
Bank error: payroll check written for $64.00 was recorded as $46.00.

Problem 2-2. The Erving Clinic's cash transactions for December as reported by the bank are:

Bank Balance 12/1/19X1 $14,384.14

Checks Paid

Number	Amount
437	$193.41
519	34.97
603	123.27
604	497.77
605	4.83

Number	Amount
606	16.17
607	249.73
609	1,000.00
610	41.19

Deposits	
12/6/19X1	$1,397.41
12/13/19X1	2,897.77
12/23/19X1	1,387.99
12/28/19X1	2,677.21

Additional Transactions		
1. Service charge	$ 97.01	
2. Collection of Note 377A	1,949.27	
3. NSF checks	196.80	
Balance 12/31/19X1		$22,238.64

Additional Cash Information

1. The note (377A) collected was a 180-day, 18 percent note. The proceeds recorded by the bank are the principal plus interest less a collection charge of $121.73.
2. The deposit of $1,397.41 was in transit on November 30, 19X1.
3. Collections received by the clinic on 12/29/19X1 were $234.01. They were recorded on the books but were not sent to the bank because they were misplaced (they were sent on January 15, 19X2).
4. Collections received and recorded on 12/30/19X1 and 12/31/19X1 were $697.43. On January 1, these deposits were in the clinic safe. The intention was to send them to the bank with the receipts of the 1st, 2nd, and 3rd of January.
5. The check register of the clinic indicated the following activity for December:

601	$3,921.41	606	$ 17.16
602	627.49	607	249.73
603	123.27	608	28.27
604	497.77	609	1,000.00
605	4.83	610	41.19
		611	397.73.

6. Outstanding checks on 11/30/19X1 were $749.31.
7. Service charges for November were $63.41.
8. A noninterest bearing note for $982.00 was collected on 11/28/19X1.
9. Check 606 was for miscellaneous expense and was correctly charged by the bank.
10. Two checks were returned by the bank during December:

F. Carter, insufficient funds	$127.43
C. Lee, no account	$ 69.37

11. The cash balance on the clinic's books at the end of the month of December was $16,017.80.

Required:

a. A bank reconciliation, 12/31/19X1
b. The appropriate adjusting entry on 12/31/19X1
c. A proof of cash for the month of December.

Problem 2-3. The cash records for the Cedars HMO reflect the following activity for the month of July 19X1:

Cash Receipts		Cash Disbursements		
Date	Amount	Date	Check No.	Amount
7/01	$450	7/01	118	$180
7/06	350	7/05	119	520
7/08	600	7/08	120	120
7/13	540	7/12	121	360
7/15	560	7/15	122	690
7/20	610	7/18	123	230
7/22	300	7/22	124	450
7/27	240	7/25	125	250
7/29	210	7/28	126	400
		7/29	127	440

The balance in the cash account was $1,630 on July 1.
The bank statement for the month of July is shown below:

Balance 6/30/19X1	Credits	Debits	Balance 7/31/19X1
$2,000	$5,030	$3,650	$3,380

Check No.	Date	Amount	Date	Deposits
112	7/01	$130	7/01	$300
115	7/05	400	7/05	450
118	7/05	180	7/07	350
119	7/18	520	7/11	600
120	7/15	120	7/14	540
121	7/15	360	7/18	560
122	7/22	690	7/21	610
124	7/25	540	7/25	300
125	7/28	250	7/28	240
126	7/29	400	7/29	1,080 CM
	7/29	10 SC		
	7/29	50 NSF		

SC = Service charge
NSF = Insufficient funds check
CM = Credit memo (proceeds of collection on a 120-day, $1,000, 24 percent note)

Deposits in transit at the end of June amounted to $300.
Outstanding checks at that time amounted to $670.

Required: a. Prepare a bank reconciliation for the month of July.
b. Make the journal entries to adjust the cash balance recorded on the HMO's books.

Problem 2-4. Garrow Memorial Hospital establishes a petty cash fund for $200.00. During the first six weeks of operation, the following vouchers are drawn on the petty cash fund:

1. Postage	$19.73
2. Certified letter	2.93
3. Purchase special stationery	31.42
4. New typewriter ribbons	6.73
5. IOU from E. Greene	40.00
6. Employee's personal check	80.00

The fund is replenished.

Required:

a. Give the entries to set up and replenish the petty cash fund.
b. Comment on the propriety of items 5 and 6. How should item 6 be handled?

Problem 2-5. The following bank reconciliation was prepared by the accountant of a prepaid medical group on December 31, 19X1. No adjusting entries have been made.

Book balance		$3,754.30
ADD: Outstanding checks	$1,437.18	
Book error in recording wages	18.81	
Note collected by the bank	1,700.00	3,155.99
		$6,910.29
DEDUCT: Deposit in transit		156.72
Service charge		118.73
Balance		$6,634.84

Bank balance	$6,497.30
NSF checks	137.54
Balance	$6,634.84

Required:

Recast the above bank reconciliation in proper form and journalize the adjusting entry.

Problem 2-6. Consider the following purchase transactions for a hospital:

January 3, 19X1 Purchased from Smith Supply, Inc., 183 units of Supply A.

List Price $49.83 per unit. Terms: 5, 1/10, 30; n/45.

January 7, 19X1 Purchased 190 units of Supply B from Smith Supply.

List Price $193.50 per unit. Terms n/30. (Trade Discounts: 3.5 percent if the purchase is 200 units or greater.)

January 8, 19X1 Returned 11 units of Supply A because they did not perform as required.

January 10, 19X1 Paid for the goods purchased on January 7.

January 12, 19X1 Made a partial payment of $1,000 to Smith Supply, Inc.

January 18, 19X1 Made a second partial payment of $2,000 to Smith Supply, Inc.

February 27, 19X1 Paid Smith Supply, Inc., the balance owed.

Required:

a. Make the entries required under the net and gross price methods of recording purchases.

b. Comment on the financial management of the cash disbursements.
c. What was the minimum amount of cash, given the facts above, required to satisfy the payable obligations? Contrast this with the actual cash paid.
d. (i) From a short-term cash flow perspective, was it wise to fail to purchase enough of Supply B to qualify for the trade discount?
   (ii) Would your answer differ if you adopt a more comprehensive view? Assume in six months the hospital must purchase 238 units of Supply B and no additional storage or obsolescence costs are incurred.

Problem 2-7. The hospital administrator of a 400-bed, urban teaching hospital is considering installing a voucher system. You are asked to prepare a report detailing the benefits and anticipated additional costs of installing and operating a voucher system. The administrator also is interested in your suggestions for evaluating the performance of the voucher system over time.

Required:
Prepare the requested report.

Problem 2-8. Riverside Hospital is considering a lock box arrangement for its cash payments. A study conducted by the hospital indicated that the one-time cash flow increase from the use of a lock box would be $183,450. The lock box fee schedule is $150 per month, plus 22.5¢ for every transaction over 175. The hospital cash receipts volume averages 390 transactions per month. The medical director is interested in knowing how much theft or misappropriation would have to occur to make the lock box pay for itself. The medical director also asks you to submit a plan to ascertain how much theft or misappropriation exists currently.

Required:
Make the required calculations and submit your plan to the medical director.

Problem 2-9. The director of nursing in a large urban visiting nursing society is confused about the difference between a bank reconciliation and a proof of cash. The director does not understand what is gained by preparing a proof of cash when bank reconciliations are prepared monthly. Explain which errors or misappropriations will be identified by a proof of cash but not discovered by monthly bank reconciliations.

Problem 2-10. The potential of the accounting system to provide relevant cash management information was illustrated for the payment of accounts payable. Prepare a similar analysis for the collection of cash for services rendered (or accounts receivable collected). Your illustration should provide an indication of the nature of information to be derived from the accounts and how this information is likely to be useful in cash management.

Chapter 3

Accounts Receivable

He that loses 5^{s}, not only loses that sum, but all the advantage that might be made by turning it in dealing, which by the time that a young man becomes old, amounts to a comfortable bag of money.

B. Franklin

In the recent past, patient accounts receivable were not considered an important element in an institution's financial management program. This attitude was a carryover from the days of prompt 100 percent retrospective reimbursement and comprehensive third party coverages. However, given current economic conditions, patient accounts receivable are becoming increasingly difficult to collect. This chapter focuses on the accounting for patient accounts receivable and examines the management of these receivables.[1] Then, a case is presented to illustrate various aspects of patient accounts receivable management.

THE ACCOUNTS RECEIVABLE CYCLE

The accounts receivable cycle begins with the delivery of service for credit (creation of an account receivable) and extends to receiving cash for services rendered (collection), estimating accounts which may not be collected (adjusting), and recognizing that a particular account is not collectable (write off). Each of these economic events affects the accounting system.

Creation of Patient Accounts Receivable

Patient accounts receivable may arise because patients receive services which (1) are not covered by a third party payment plan or (2) are covered by a health insurance plan that provides for copayments by the third party payer and the insuree. The accounting journal entry to record the creation of a patient account receivable of $500 is:

Patient Accounts Receivable (·)	$500	
Service Revenue—(D)		$500.

The first part of this entry, Patient Accounts Receivable (·), denotes that an entry for $500 is made to the control account (Patient Accounts Receivable) and to the patient account (recorded by patient name and number) in the accounts receivable subsidiary ledger (see Appendix A). All of the accounts receivable activity is recorded both in the control account and in the subsidiary ledgers. The balance in the control account must agree with the sum of the balances in the subsidiary ledgers at all times. The second part of the above entry, Service Revenue—(D), denotes that revenue is being recognized and credited to the particular department, D, which performed the service.

Collection of Accounts Receivable: Cash Generation

The collection of an account receivable is recognized whenever a payment is received from the patient. The entry to record the collection of $50 due on a patient account receivable is:

Cash	$50	
Patient Accounts Receivable (·)		$50.

This entry records the $50 increase in cash and the decrease in both the patient accounts receivable control account and the individual patient's account in the subsidiary ledger.

Patient Accounts Receivable Adjustment

Whenever services are rendered on a credit basis, the institution must recognize that some accounts will never be collected. To match the revenues and expenses of a given period, some provision must be made to record the amount of patient accounts that will not be collected. For example, suppose Department A earned revenue of $100,000, as follows:

Cash Payment for Services	$75,000
Patient Accounts Receivable	25,000
Total Revenue	$100,000.

The revenue contribution to income is composed of $75,000 of cash collected for services rendered during the period, plus the anticipated revenue contribution of $25,000 × ∂; where: $0 \leq \partial \leq 1$ and ∂ represents the percentage of credit accounts ultimately converted into cash. Therefore, if revenues and expenses are to be matched properly, an estimate must be made of the percentage of accounts that will not be collected $(1 - \partial)$. This estimate forms the basis for an adjustment to both the period's expense and the accounts receivable to be converted into cash in future periods.

The adjusting journal entry to record anticipated uncollectables of $2,500 is:

Bad Debt Expense	$2,500	
Allowance for Bad Debts		$2,500.

The Bad Debt Expense account increases the expense of the period and matches the expense of the uncollectable accounts with the corresponding service revenue. The Allowance for Bad Debts account is a contra-account to Patient Accounts Receivable. It reflects that portion of patient accounts which are expected to be written off in future periods. (See Appendix A for further discussion of the matching principle and for a more detailed description of contra-accounts.)

The process of estimating the percentage of uncollectable accounts usually is based on past institutional experience. Two methods commonly used to estimate the percentage of accounts receivable that will not be collected are the percentage of some related account method and the aging method.

The Percentage of Some Related Account Method

The percentage of some related account method assumes that a consistent relationship exists between the accounts receivable for a period that are ultimately written off and the activity in some other account. This relationship is established by comparisons between the historic trend in the accounts written off and the historic trends in other accounts. Accounts which vary proportionally with the accounts written off are assumed to be reasonable predictors of future uncollectable accounts. For example, historically, accounts written off may be proportional to gross service revenue, total accounts receivable, accounts receivable at year-end, or total Medicare accounts receivable, to mention a few. In other words, the percentage of some related account method relies on an established historical relationship between accounts written off and any other account which seems to be a reasonable predictor of subsequent collection problems, and is related to the creation of patient accounts receivable.

Suppose an analysis of past operations shows that a consistent relationship exists between the accounts receivable generated in a period which are written off in future periods and the total accounts receivable created during that period. If the most recent review of the bad debts shows that accounts receivable of $5,678 generated during 19X1 ultimately were written off while the total accounts receivable created during 19X1 amounted to $137,411, then the percentage used to estimate bad debts would be $\beta =$ .0413 (i.e., $5,678/$137,411). Therefore, if the total accounts receivable created during 19X3 are $197,432, the adjusting entry to record the allowance for uncollectable accounts for 19X3 will be:

Bad Debt Expense	$8,153.94	
Allowance for Bad Debts		$8,153.94

To record the estimated uncollectable patient accounts receivable. The anticipated expense is $197,432.00 × .0413 = $8,153.94.

Since this percentage relationship is only a means of estimating uncollectable accounts, other accounts also may vary proportionally with accounts ultimately written off. For example, the accounts receivable generated during 19X1 that ultimately are written off in subsequent periods also could be compared to the accounts receivable that are outstanding at the end of 19X1. If the most recent review of the bad debts shows that accounts receivable of $5,678 ultimately were written off in periods subsequent to 19X1 while the accounts receivable outstanding at the end of 19X1 amounted to $39,918, then $\beta = .14224$. If the accounts receivable outstanding at the end of 19X3 amount to $61,403, the estimated allowance for uncollectable accounts for 19X3 would be $8,733.96. This estimate compares favorably with the estimate of $8,153.94 generated by using total accounts receivable created to develop β. Hence, a decision rule should be formulated to determine which account relationships are superior to others in adjusting the patient accounts receivable to their net realizable value.

The decision rule should dictate that if a logical causal relationship exists between the accounts ultimately written off and more than one of the proposed predictor accounts, the proposed predictor account which exhibits the highest correlation with the accounts written off should be selected (see Question 3-7). Suppose, for example, that over the last few years the correlation between the dollar value of the accounts written off and the dollar value of the accounts receivable created was .87, while the correlation between the dollar value of the accounts written off and the accounts receivable outstanding at year-end was .31. In this case, although both the accounts receivable created and the accounts receivable outstanding at year-end bear a logical causal relationship to the accounts written off, the accounts receivable created would be selected as the predictor account because it is more highly correlated (i.e., a strong linear association; see Appendix B) with accounts written off (see Question 3-10).

The percentage of some related account method is a simple means of estimating uncollectable accounts. Under this method, the total estimate of uncollectable accounts is credited to the Allowance for Bad Debts account each year regardless of the activity in that account for the year (see Problem 3-2). Hence, a change in the collectability of patient accounts or a change in the activity of the predictor account could cause a disproportionate balance in the Allowance for Bad Debts account. Therefore, the bad debt estimates must always be compared with the patient accounts actually written off to insure that the assumed relationship still exists.

Although the percentage of some related account method generally is a simple and accurate means of estimating bad debts, a logical causal relationship exhibiting a high degree of correlation cannot always be drawn between patient accounts that ultimately are uncollectable and the activity in another account. In this case, another more systematic method of estimating uncollectable accounts must be used. This method is called the aging method.

The Aging Method

Generally, the chance of writing off an account receivable increases as the length of time the account is outstanding increases. The aging method assumes that the relationship between the age of an account and the chance of writing off the account is fairly constant over time. Therefore, historical data can be used to develop percentage relationships between accounts receivable of a particular age and the number of those accounts that ultimately are written off. These percentages can be used to approximate the probability of writing off accounts in each age category, and hence form a basis for estimating uncollectable accounts.

The following format provides a useful means of developing the information required to estimate the uncollectability of outstanding accounts under the aging method:

Patient Accounts Receivable (Subsidiary)	Current 0 to t_1 days	(Age Categories) t_1 to t_2, · · ·,	Delinquent $>t_m$ days
A_1 ($) →	A_1 ($)		
A_2 ($) →		A_2 ($)	
A_3 ($) →	A_3 ($)		
A_k ($) →			A_k ($)
A_n ($) →		A_n ($)	
Total $ Agrees with Patient Accounts Receivable Control	Sum of Current	Sum of t_1 to t_2, · · ·,	Sum of $>t_m$

This format segments accounts receivable by age and gives a total for each age category.[2] Then the probability of writing off accounts of each age can be applied to the balance in each age category. The sum of these products yields an estimate of uncollectable accounts. The aging method computation is represented by the equation

$$\text{BUC} = \sum_{i=1}^{m} \lambda_i \sum_{j=1}^{k_i} A_j^i \text{ (\$)} \tag{3-1}$$

where: BUC represents the balance which should be in the Allowance for Bad Debts account after adjustment;
m represents the number of age categories;
λ_i represents the probability that an account in the ith age category will be uncollectable (note: $\lambda_i = 1 - \partial_i$);
k_i represents the number of accounts in the ith age category;
A_j^i ($) represents the dollar balance of the jth individual's account in ith age category.

The estimate for uncollectable accounts (BUC) is the amount that should appear as the balance in the Allowance for Bad Debts account. Therefore, the current balance in the Allowance for Bad Debts account must be known. For example, if the BUC is $3,962 and the Allowance for Bad Debts account has a credit balance of $1,732, the adjusting entry would be:

Bad Debt Expense	$2,230.00	
Allowance for Bad Debts		$2,230.00.

This entry brings the balance in the Allowance for Bad Debts account to $3,962, the institution's best estimate of uncollectable accounts at the time of adjustment.

Under the aging method, the dollar amount of the adjusting entry made to the Allowance for Bad Debts account (i.e., the bad debt expense for the period) will equal the BUC only when the balance in the Allowance for Bad Debts account is zero prior to adjustment (see Problem 3-2). When the Allowance for Bad Debts account has a credit balance prior to adjustment, the dollar amount of the adjusting entry will be equal to the BUC *less* the balance already in the Allowance for Bad Debts account (e.g., in the case above, $3,962 − $1,732). On the other hand, when the Allowance for Bad Debts account has a debit balance prior to adjustment, the dollar amount of the adjusting entry will be equal to the BUC *plus* the additional credit necessary to remove the debit balance already in the account. For example, if the Allowance for Bad Debts account had a debit balance of $2,288 and the BUC was $3,962, the adjusting entry would be:

Bad Debt Expense	$6,250.00	
Allowance for Bad Debts		$6,250.00.

This entry eliminates the debit balance of $2,288 which was already in the Allowance for Bad Debts account and leaves a credit balance of $3,962 in the account.

Since the BUC is an estimate of the dollar amount of both the past and current accounts receivable that will not be collected, the increment to the Allowance for Bad Debts account (the Bad Debt Expense) probably will be less than the BUC because the Bad Debt Expense should reflect only the portion of uncollectable accounts applicable to the current period's activity. Hence, in most cases, a credit balance should be in the Allowance for Bad Debts account prior to adjustment. However, the number of accounts written off during the period may leave a debit balance in the Allowance for Bad Debts account at the end of the period. In this case, an error was made in estimating uncollectable accounts in prior periods. Because this is an accounting estimate, it does not qualify as a retroactive adjustment and must be recognized in the period in which the error is discovered.[3] Consequently, the increment to the Allowance for Bad Debts account, and thus the Bad Debt Expense, will be greater than the BUC because this increment reflects the portion of uncollectable accounts applicable to the current period plus the correction of the estimate from a prior period. However, as in the percentage of some related account method, substantial or persistent estimation errors require a review and possible update of the probability estimates of the aged accounts.

Writing Off Uncollectable Accounts

The entry to write off an uncollectable account of $120.00 is:

Allowance for Bad Debts	$120.00	
Patient Accounts Receivable (·)		$120.00.

This entry reduces Accounts Receivable by $120 and reduces the Allowance for Bad Debts account by $120. However, writing off an account has no effect on the Bad Debt Expense account.

Whenever a specific account is ascertained to be uncollectable, an accounting entry is made to write off the account. At that time the patient's account is removed from the accounts receivable subsidiary ledger and placed in an accounts written off file. This account information should be communicated to the department or attending physician so that the appropriate actions may be taken.

Writing off uncollectable accounts is the final step in the accounts receivable cycle. Each step in the cycle has been analyzed in detail. These steps can now be synthesized into a comprehensive example of the accounts receivable cycle.

Extended Example of the Accounts Receivable Cycle

The balances in the Patient Accounts Receivable account and in the Allowance for Bad Debts account of the R. Stones Memorial Hospital on November 29, 19X1 are:

Patient Accounts Receivable		Allowance for Bad Debts	
$2,212,513			$30,544.

The hospital uses the aging method for estimating uncollectable accounts. The subsidiary ledger that separates accounts receivable by age shows the following balances on November 29, 19X1.

Age Category	(1) Current	(2) 31-60 days	(3) 61-90 days	(4) 91-120 days	(5) 121 days-1 year	(6) More than 1 year
Amount	$1,213,067	$516,231	$278,932	$99,656	$69,426	$35,201
Probability of bad debt	.01	.025	.05	.1	.7	.9

All bills for services rendered are sent out on the last day of the month. On November 30, 19X1, invoices for services rendered during the month of November, amounting to $2,846,229, are sent to patients. The entry to record this billing is:

11/30/X1	Patient Accounts Receivable (·)	$2,846,229	
	Service Revenue—(D)		$2,846,229.

Each invoice is also entered in the accounts receivable subsidiary ledger which separates patient accounts receivable by individual. As a result of the November billing, the following changes occur in the subsidiary ledger that separates accounts receivable by age.

Age Category	(1) Current	(2) 31-60 days	(3) 61-90 days	(4) 90-120 days	(5) 121 days-1 year	(6) More than 1 year
Amount	$2,846,229	$1,213,067	$516,231	$278,932	$163,151	$41,132*
Probability of bad debt	.01	.025	.05	.1	.7	.9

*Note that only $5,931 of the outstanding accounts have passed the one-year age limit and have moved from age category (5) to (6).

During the month of December, the following payments are made on accounts in the indicated age categories.

Week Ending	Dollar Amount	Age Category	Total
Dec. 3	$214,609	(2)	
	135,445	(3)	
	126,388	(4)	
	30,320	(5)	
	1,426	(6)	$508,188
Dec. 10	$222,156	(1)	
	139,427	(2)	
	86,793	(3)	
	72,534	(4)	
	20,256	(5)	
	1,573	(6)	$542,739

Week Ending	Dollar Amount	Age Category	Total
Dec. 17	$306,372	(1)	
	101,617	(2)	
	37,921	(3)	
	36,392	(4)	
	18,651	(5)	
	1,316	(6)	$502,269
Dec. 24	$318,789	(1)	
	156,318	(2)	
	18,628	(3)	
	18,396	(4)	
	16,993	(5)	
	1,015	(6)	$530,139
Dec. 31	$275,562	(1)	
	118,939	(2)	
	11,437	(3)	
	12,682	(4)	
	11,535	(5)	
	937	(6)	$431,092

Payments on patient accounts receivable are posted at the end of each week. These payments reduce Patient Accounts Receivable (the control account), the individual patient accounts receivable, and the aged patient accounts receivable. The weekly entries to record the payments listed above are as follows.

12/3/X1	Cash	$508,188	
	Patient Accounts Receivable (·)		$508,188
12/10/X1	Cash	542,739	
	Patient Accounts Receivable (·)		542,739
12/17/X1	Cash	502,269	
	Patient Accounts Receivable (·)		502,269
12/24/X1	Cash	530,139	
	Patient Accounts Receivable (·)		530,139
12/31/X1	Cash	431,092	
	Patient Accounts Receivable (·)		431,092

During December the following information is gathered regarding accounts receivable outstanding:

Dec. 15: M. L. Adams, whose account of $4,050 has been outstanding since May 31, 19X1, declared bankruptcy on December 13, 19X1.

Dec. 22: S. Corleone, whose account of $3,998 has been outstanding since October 31, 19X0, died on December 11, 19X1 and left no estate. His survivors are not responsible for his debts.

The entries to write off these accounts are:

12/15/X1	Allowance for Bad Debts	$4,050	
	Patient Accounts Receivable (M. L. Adams)		$4,050
12/22/X1	Allowance for Bad Debts	3,998	
	Patient Accounts Receivable (S. Corleone)		3,998

On December 31, another monthly billing is prepared. The total invoices for December amount to $1,996,524. The entry to record this billing is:

12/31/X1	Patient Accounts Receivable (·)	$1,996,524	
	Service Revenue—D		$1,996,524.

These entries leave the following balances in Patient Accounts Receivable and in the Allowance for Bad Debts accounts.

Patient Accounts Receivable		Allowance for Bad Debts	
$4,532,791			$22,496

After posting the entries in the aged accounts receivable subsidiary ledger, the balances in each age category are:

Age Category	(1) Current	(2) 31-60 days	(3) 61-90 days	(4) 91-120 days	(5) 121 days-1 year	(6) More than 1 year
Amount	$1,996,524	$1,723,350	$482,157	$226,007	$67,758	$36,995*
Probability of bad debt	.01	.025	.05	.1	.7	.9

*$6,128 of the outstanding accounts have been transferred from age category (5) to age category (6).

Since the accounting period of the R. Stones Memorial Hospital is the calendar year, an estimate of uncollectable accounts must be made on December 31. By applying the appropriate bad debt probability to the balance in each age category and summing the products, the estimate of uncollectable accounts can be calculated as follows:

$$\begin{aligned} BUC &= .01\ (\$1{,}996{,}524) + .025\ (\$1{,}723{,}350) + .05\ (\$482{,}157) \\ &\quad + .1\ (\$226{,}007) + .7\ (\$67{,}758) + .9\ (\$36{,}995) \\ &= \underline{\underline{\$190{,}484.}} \end{aligned}$$

Hence, $190,484 is the amount that should appear in the Allowance for Bad Debts account on the hospital's balance sheet. Since this account already has a credit balance of $22,496, the accounts receivable adjusting entry is:

12/31/X1	Bad Debt Expense	$167,988	
	Allowance for Bad Debts		$167,988.

If the R. Stones Memorial Hospital used the percentage of some related account method for estimating uncollectable accounts, all entries would have been identical to those given above, except the final adjusting entry. For instance, suppose that the hospital uses the dollar amount of total services rendered on credit as the basis for estimating uncollectable accounts. Further suppose that over the past five years uncollectable accounts were approximately one percent of services rendered on credit during the year ($\beta = .01$). If total services rendered on credit for 19X1 amounted to $23,782,193, then one percent of this amount, or $237,822, should be entered as the Bad Debt Expense for 19X1. The entry to record this estimate would be:

12/31/X1	Bad Debt Expense	$237,822	
	Allowance for Bad Debts		$237,822.

This entry would bring the total balance in the Allowance for Bad Debts account to $260,318 on December 31, 19X1. The balance in Patient Accounts Receivable would be $4,532,791, as it was when the aging method was used to estimate uncollectable accounts.

Collection of Accounts Written Off

The above example examined the accounts receivable cycle from the creation of patient accounts receivable through the eventual writing off of uncollectable accounts. Although the example included all of the ordinary transactions in the accounts receivable cycle, one more transaction that affects accounts receivable may occur—an account that previously was written off may be collected.

Recall that whenever a patient account is collected, the entry to record the collection is:

Cash	***	
Patient Accounts Receivable (·)		***.

This results in an increase in cash and a decrease in both the patient accounts receivable control account and a reduction in the subsidiary ledger. If cash is collected on a patient account that was previously written off, prima facie evidence exists that the account was not a bad debt. Therefore, given that the usual entry was made to record the cash collected for the account previously written off, the entry that was made to write off the account should be reversed as follows:

Patient Accounts Receivable (·)	***	
Allowance for Bad Debts		***

This entry records the reinstatement of an account that was previously written off.[4] After the cash collection entry and the reversal of the write-off entry are posted to the control account and subsidiary ledger, the accounts will be stated properly, i.e., cash will be increased and accounts receivable decreased.

Internal Control of Accounts Receivable

Proper internal control should be exercised over accounts receivable because the accounts receivable cycle involves the handling of cash. Tasks should be separated so that one person opens the mail and lists the checks received, another makes the bank deposit and records the cash receipts, and a third records accounts receivable transactions. Separating these duties reduces the potential for cash misappropriations.

For example, suppose the same person is responsible for both cash receipts and accounts receivable. As payments are received, the clerk records the cash receipts in both the cash receipts journal and the accounts receivable subsidiary ledger. If a payment is received on an account that previously was written off, the clerk will not find the account in the accounts receivable subsidiary ledger. If the clerk pockets this receipt, both cash and the allowance for bad debts will be understated, but the balance in accounts receivable will be correct. The understatement of both cash and the allowance for bad debts will be undetectable unless the patient later demands an audit of the account. If these clerical duties were separated, however, collusion would be necessary for misappropriations to occur.

Another example of the misappropriation of cash receipts is called stepping. Stepping is the process whereby a portion of each day's cash receipts is withheld and a portion of the next day's cash receipts is applied to the patient accounts from which receipts were withheld the previous day. Consequently, the only change that occurs in accounts receivable is the one-day increase in the time lag between the patient remittance and the recording of the receipt. Usually, stepping is undetectable unless another clerk takes charge of the duties of the regular clerk. This form of misappropriation may occur if one person opens the mail, makes the bank deposits, and records the cash receipts, or if one person records both cash receipts and accounts receivable transactions. However, if the clerical duties are separated, collusion would be necessary to withhold cash through stepping (see Problem 3-6).

These examples emphasize the importance of adequate internal control over accounts receivable. No one individual should both have control of assets and be responsible for recording transactions affecting those assets. Although this rule will not stop misappropriation, it should reduce its incidence.

THE MANAGEMENT OF ACCOUNTS RECEIVABLE

Managing accounts receivable is a complex and often misunderstood process. The following conversation between the "manager" of accounts receivable in a large hospital and one of the authors, pursuant to a consulting engagement, illustrates how confusing the management of accounts receivable can be:

Consultant: What is your write-off policy regarding patient accounts receivable?

Manager: Huh? What's a write-off policy?

Consultant: I am not sure what you may call it. What I want to know is when do you remove a patient's account from the active accounts receivable and put that account into an inactive file?

Manager: Why would I do that?

Consultant: Huh?

Manager: Accounts receivable are assets. Why would I write them off? I never say die, pardon the pun. There is always an outside

> chance that an account will be collected. When I came to this hospital, the accounts receivable were only around $280,000. Since I have been here, I have built them up to what they are now (around $640,000). Besides, if I write them off, it may make someone look bad . . . like my boss.

Even in the face of traditionally infused misunderstanding, however, the problem of managing an institution's accounts receivable may be considered in a complex but logical framework.

Patient Accounts Receivable: A Policy Question

By rendering health services on credit and thereby creating accounts receivable, an institution can generate additional revenues that would have to be foregone under a payment for service policy. However, accounts receivable (1) delay payments from patients who otherwise would have paid when the services were rendered, (2) give rise to additional expenses as the institution tries to collect patient accounts, and (3) usually give rise to accounts that are never collected. Hence, while a policy which permits the creation of accounts receivable will expand institutional revenue, it will also increase institutional expenses. Therefore, two factors should be considered in formulating an institution's accounts receivable policy:

1. The effect that a change in the credit terms of service would have on both patient demand for services and the institution's cash flow; and
2. The costs associated with creating and maintaining accounts receivable.

Effects of Credit Terms of Service on Patient Demand and on Institutional Cash Flows

The effect that a change in an institution's credit policy would have on demand and on cash collection is represented in Figure 3-1. The graph at the left shows the demand for services, under both a payment for service policy (curve D_1) and a permissive credit policy (curve D_2). Under the payment for service policy, patients must pay for all, or most, services as they are rendered. Hence, if a patient cannot currently afford to pay for the needed health services, these services must be sought where credit is available. However, under the permissive credit policy, nearly all services are rendered on credit. Therefore, the patient who cannot currently afford to pay for the health services needed, as well as the patients who can afford to pay, can receive the needed services for a promise to pay. Consequently, given price P_1, only Q_1 units of service would be demanded under the pay-

Figure 3-1 Demand and Account Relationships under Strict Payment for Service and Permissive Credit Policies

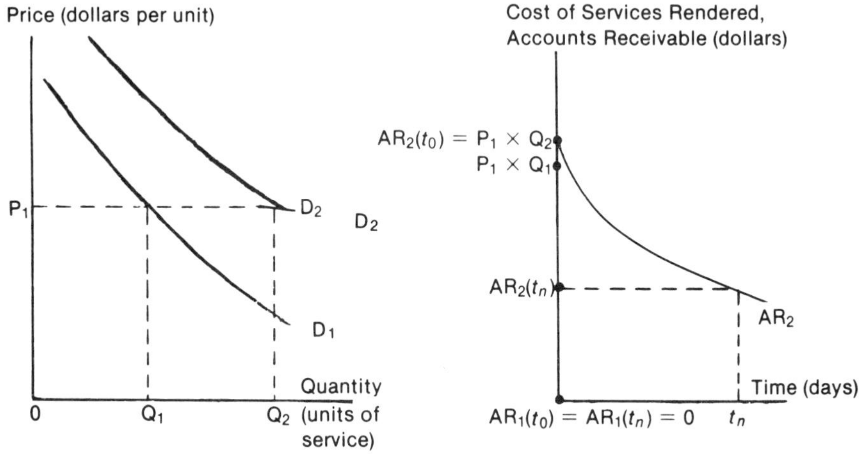

ment for service policy, while Q_2 units of service would be demanded under the permissive credit policy.

The graph at the right illustrates the simplest case of the accounts receivable created on a given day as a result of rendering the services demanded in the graph at the left. In this case, under the payment for service policy, patients are assumed to pay for all services as they are rendered, and, under the permissive credit policy, *all* services are assumed to be rendered on a credit basis. Therefore, patient accounts receivable are nonexistent over time under the payment for service policy. The curve representing accounts receivable under this policy (AR_1) is zero over time, i.e., it lies on the time axis. Under the permissive credit policy, however, accounts receivable at time t_0 are equal to the total services rendered on the given day, $P_1 \times Q_2$. The curve representing accounts receivable under this policy (AR_2) slopes downward to the right, illustrating the decline in accounts receivable as collections are made. If all of the accounts created on the given day are collected by time t_n, AR_2 will intersect the time axis at t_n. If accounts outstanding at time t_n are written off, AR_2 will kink at t_n and drop to the time axis. The graph illustrates the case in which accounts are outstanding at time t_n and have not been written off. The dollar value of these accounts is represented by $AR_2(t_n)$.

The total cash collection under each policy may be calculated as follows.

Total Cash Collection = Cash for Service + Collections of Accounts

$$\text{Payment for Service: } C_1 = [P_1 \times Q_1 - AR_1(t_0)] + [AR_1(t_0) - AR_1(t_n)]$$
$$= [P_1 \times Q_1 - 0] + [0 - 0]$$
$$= P_1 \times Q_1$$

$$\text{Permissive Credit: } C_2 = [P_1 \times Q_2 - AR_2(t_0)] + [AR_2(t_0) - AR_2(t_n)]$$
$$= [P_1 \times Q_2 - P_1 \times Q_2] + [AR_2(t_0) - AR_2(t_n)]$$
$$= AR_2(t_0) - AR_2(t_n)$$

Note that C_2 may be greater than, less than, or equal to C_1, depending on the relative magnitudes of Q_1, Q_2, and $AR_2(t_n)$.

A more complex and realistic example incorporates the fact that some services are assumed to be rendered on a credit basis under the payment for service policy and others are assumed to be rendered on a payment for service basis under the permissive credit policy. Figure 3-2 illustrates the effect of these changes.

The demand curves in Figure 3-2 are the same as those in Figure 3-1. However, $AR_2(t_0)$ is less than $P_1 \times Q_2$ because some of the accounts

Figure 3-2 Demand and Account Relationships under Mixed Credit Policies

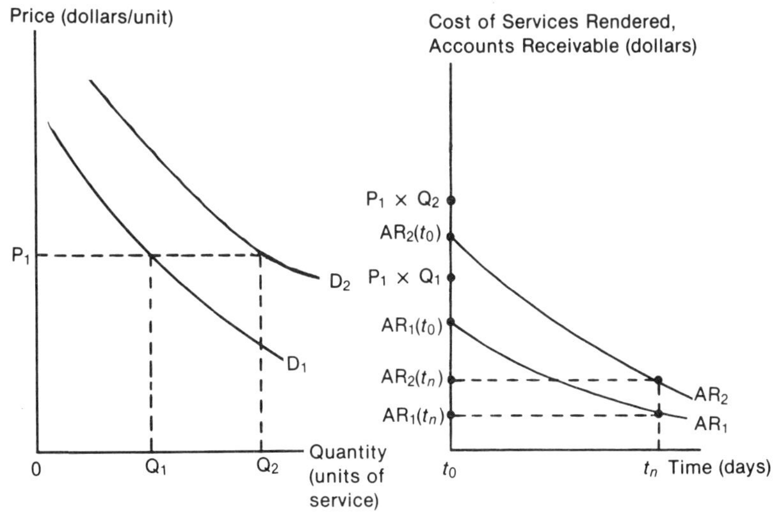

under the permissive credit policy are collected when services are rendered. In addition, AR_1 (t_0) is greater than zero because some of the services under the payment for service policy are rendered on credit. The graph on the right also shows that any accounts still outstanding at time t_n have not been written off. These accounts are AR_1 (t_n) under the payment for service policy and AR_2 (t_n) under the permissive credit policy. The graph shows that $AR_2(t_n) > AR_1(t_n)$, but $AR_2(t_n) \leq AR_1(t_n)$ is also a possibility.

Again, the total cash collection under each policy may be calculated as follows.

Total Cash Collection = Cash for Service + Collections of Accounts

$$\text{Payment for Service: } C_1 = [P_1 \times Q_1 - AR_1(t_0)] + [AR_1(t_0) - AR_1(t_n)]$$
$$= [P_1 \times Q_1] - [AR_1(t_n)]$$

$$\text{Permissive Credit: } C_2 = [P_1 \times Q_2 - AR_2(t_0)] + [AR_2(t_0) - AR_2(t_n)]$$
$$= [P_1 \times Q_2] - [AR_2(t_n)]$$

To evaluate the effect of the different credit policies, these cash collections should be compared to the difference between 1) interest revenue earned, if any, as a result of investing the cash collected and 2) expenses incurred as a result of creating and maintaining accounts receivable.

Costs of Holding Accounts Receivable

The major costs of maintaining numerous accounts receivable created under a permissive credit policy are:

1. Writing off delinquent accounts which would have been collected if cash had been demanded when the services were rendered, and
2. Supplies, equipment, and personnel required to process information on the creation, collection, rebilling, and write off of accounts receivable.

The cost of maintaining one uncollected account receivable is shown graphically in Figure 3-3.

Figure 3-3 indicates that the costs of maintaining one account receivable increase, probably at an increasing rate, until time t_k, when the account is written off. The increasing slope reflects the increased collection effort required to convert noncurrent accounts receivable. At time t_k, when the account is written off, the entire account balance becomes a cost as reflected by the vertical increase at t_k (see Question 3-8). Of course, as the number

Figure 3-3 Cost of Maintaining an Account Receivable

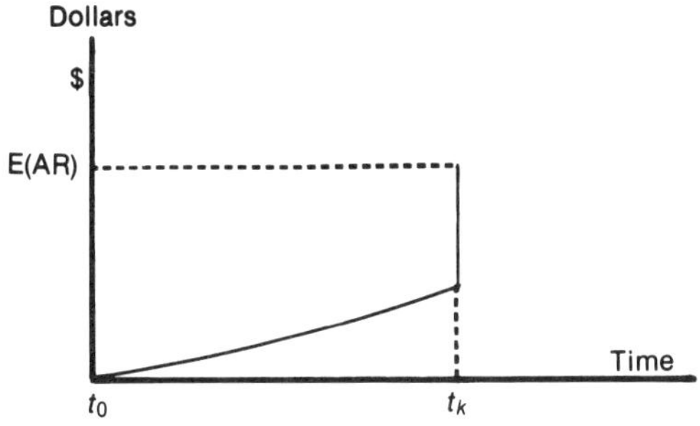

of uncollected accounts increases, the total cost of maintaining uncollected accounts increases.

Interest Earned on Cash Invested

In some cases, a change in the institution's credit policy will result in excess cash which could be invested temporarily. The interest earned as a result of investing cash collections is dependent on the initial cash differential:

$$P_1 \times Q_1 - AR_1(t_0) \geq P_1 \times Q_2 - AR_2(t_0), \text{ or}$$

$$P_1 \times Q_1 - AR_1(t_0) \leq P_1 \times Q_2 - AR_2(t_0).$$

If a greater amount of cash is generated initially, a greater amount of interest revenue can be earned on investing that cash.

The simplest case, illustrated in Figure 3-1, shows

$$P_1 \times Q_1 - AR_1(t_0) > P_1 \times Q_2 - AR_2(t_0)$$

because $AR_1(t_0) = 0$ and $AR_2(t_0) = P_1 \times Q_2$. This relationship occurs because cash payments ($P_1 \times Q_1$) for all services rendered are collected immediately under the payment for service policy, while no cash is collected under the permissive credit policy until the patients are billed. Hence, in this case, clearly more interest revenue could be earned under the payment for service policy.

The more complex case illustrated in Figure 3-2 shows that the difference between $P_1 \times Q_1 - AR_1(t_0)$ and $P_1 \times Q_2 - AR_2(t_0)$ is quite small. Although $P_1 \times Q_1 - AR_1(t_0)$ is still greater than $P_1 \times Q_2 - AR_2(t_0)$, a minor shrinkage in either $P_1 \times Q_1$ or $AR_2(t_0)$ or both could change this relationship. Similarly, increases in $P_1 \times Q_2$ or $AR_1\,(t_0)$ or both might make $P_1 \times Q_2 - AR_2(t_0) > P_1 \times Q_1 - AR_1(t_0)$. Consequently, it is not clear which policy will yield a greater amount of immediate cash and, subsequently, greater interest revenue. Therefore, estimates must be made regarding patient demand and payment schedules so that the costs and benefits associated with various credit policies can be approximated.

Example of the Effects of a Credit Policy Change

Assume that a clinic has an annual visitation rate of 26,487 patients and that payments are made primarily through third party payers. Further assume that the charge for each visit is $12.73 and that costs in excess of $12.73 per visit will not be reimbursed. Such excess costs, in addition to various copayments and excluded services, must be paid by the patients. Given fixed costs of $159,853.79, variable costs of $4.79 per visit, accounts receivable billing costs of $16,093.18 and written off accounts of $25,738.81, the excess of revenue over cost for the period may be computed as follows.

Gross Revenue (26,487 × $12.73)		$337,179.51
Service Costs:		
Fixed Costs	$159,853.79	
Variable Costs (26,487 × $4.79)	126,872.73	
Total Service Costs		$286,726.52
Gross Profit		50,452.99
Less: Cost of Accounts Receivable Maintenance		
Accounts Written Off	$25,738.81	
Billing Costs	16,093.18	
Total Cost of Accounts Receivable Maintenance		41,831.99
Net Revenue in Excess of Cost		$ 8,621.00

If the clinic administrator is distressed over the adverse effect that the large number of accounts receivable and uncollectable accounts have on profitability, the administrator may decide to change the payment policy and require immediate payment for services not covered by third party payers.

Assume that this change will reduce billing costs by 80 percent and will reduce written off accounts by 90 percent. If demand is estimated to dissipate by 12 percent and any additional cash from immediate payments, estimated to be $38,418 in this case, is expected to be invested at 7.5 percent, the expected financial performance can be computed as follows.

Gross Revenue (26,487) × (1 − .12) × ($12.73)		$296,717.97
Service Costs:		
Fixed Costs	$159,853.79	
Variable Costs		
(26,487) × (1 − .12) × ($4.79)	111,648.00	
Total Service Costs		271,501.79
Gross Profit		25,216.18
Less: Other Costs and Revenues		
Cost of Accounts Receivable Maintenance		
Accounts Written Off		
($25,738.81) × (1 − .90)	$2,573.88	
Billing Costs		
($16,093.18) × (1 − .80)	3,218.64	
Revenue from Cash Investment		
$38,418 × .075	(2,881.35)	
Net Other Costs and Revenues		2,911.17
Net Revenue in Excess of Cost		$ 22,305.01

In this case, the policy to restrict credit would be economically favorable, providing that the estimates are accurate.

The most critical estimate is usually the dissipation of demand because as demand shrinks, the fixed cost included in each visit increases (see Question 3-5). For example, prior to the anticipated policy change, the fixed cost per visit is $6.04 ($159,853.79/26,487), while under the proposed policy change, the fixed cost per visit is $6.86 ($159,853.79/23,309). Although the total cost per visit under the proposed policy change compares favorably with the reimbursement ceiling:

Gross Profit per Visit	=	Reimbursement	−	(Fixed Costs	+	Variable Costs)
$1.08	=	$12.73	−	($6.86	+	$4.79)

and even though modifying the organization's credit policy is economically desirable, the reduction in demand causes a reduction in the gross profit per visit.

In addition, a change to a restrictive credit policy could dissipate demand materially overtime. As indicated in this example, as patient demand shrinks, a larger portion of fixed operating cost is included in the cost of each visit. If these higher costs per visit exceed the reimbursement ceiling, the unreimbursed excesses must be shifted to the patients, thereby further raising costs and possibly again diminishing demand (see Question 3-9).

This example illustrates the various elements necessary to make a decision regarding an institution's credit policy. Unfortunately, in most institutions little, if any, thought is given to the effect that the credit policy will have on cash collections, the cost of accounts receivable management, and patient demand. These aspects will be considered further in the case study presented in this chapter.

Factors Affecting Management of Patient Accounts Receivable

Generally, the problems associated with managing accounts receivable are directly related to the size and type of accounts created in the institution. Many factors may give rise to credit problems and, eventually, to problems in accounts receivable. Some of these factors are:

- Often the medical staff is not interested in the economics of effective medical care delivery.
- The bookkeeping aspects of accounting for accounts receivable are complex and most health care information systems fail to provide timely information to physicians about the delinquent accounts of various patients.
- Even when physicians are aware of patient payment delinquency, it is doubtful that this information is used to deny service.
- Traditionally, accounts receivable management in health care institutions has been neglected due to the 100 percent reimbursement policies of third party payers, and these traditions are not easily changed.
- Most health care institutions do not have the management expertise to develop the information necessary to measure the savings and costs involved in adopting a payment for service policy. Therefore, managers in health care institutions often rely upon the advice of data management services or computer consulting firms. Because these groups often sell patient billing packages as part of their software line, they usually advise that the institution's receivables problems can be solved or minimized by their system (see Appendix C).

Even though these factors often constrain management's attempts to abate accounts receivable mismanagement, four systems procedures, (1) collection at the time of discharge, (2) review of aged accounts, (3) delinquencies reports, and (4) interest penalties, should aid in coping with the myriad patient accounts receivable management problems fostered by the factors discussed above.

Collection at the Time of Discharge

To collect accounts receivable from patients at the time of discharge, most health care institutions would have to make a number of policy changes (also see Chapter 2). Four such policy changes would involve having access to an information system that could generate the data needed to prepare the patient bill before the patient leaves the institution, collecting insurance information before the patient is admitted for service, employing an individual familiar with the copayment and service coverage arrangements of the major third party payers, and informing patients of the payment for service policy as appointments are made.

After the services have been rendered, the individual familiar with the insurance coverage arrangements of the major third party payers could analyze the billing and insurance information and apportion each patient's bill into (1) the amount due from the third party payer and (2) the amount due from the patient. The self-pay portion of the bill could be prepared and given to the patient at the time of discharge. At this time, the patient who was informed of the payment for service policy when the appointment was made could write a check for the amount due or arrange to make a number of periodic payments to satisfy the bill.

Unfortunately, these policy changes may be difficult to implement given the current health care environment. Therefore, accounts receivable may have to be created. In this case, three other procedures—review of aged accounts, delinquency reports, and interest penalties—can promote the timely conversion of accounts receivable.

Review of Aged Accounts

Regardless of the credit policy, the overriding consideration in managing accounts receivable is to collect the receivable. A periodic review of the accounts by age can aid in achieving this objective. Aged accounts indicate the magnitude of delinquent accounts. If many accounts are delinquent, either more information is needed from patients before services are rendered on credit, or a credit policy change is necessary.

The age groupings should cover neither too small nor too great a period. Generally, creating the following two polar groupings is useful.

Current	Accounts to Be Written Off
$(0 - t_1)$	$(>t_m)$

The number of age divisions between the poles is determined by the collection actions taken between each age grouping. For example, if a group administrator ascertains that the best cash flow from receivables occurs when requests for payment are sent on a monthly basis for three months after the first bill is sent, the age categories for that group will be as follows.

Current	First Notice	Second Notice	Third Notice	Write Off
$(0 - t_1)$	$(t_1 - t_2)$	$(t_2 - t_3)$	$(t_3 - t_4)$	$(>t_5)$

Note that the movement of an account from one age category to another is synchronized with managerial actions intended to convert that account. This synchronization yields a two-part principle for aging accounts receivable:

> The aging segmentations are too narrow if an account can move from one category to another without eliciting a management collection action.
>
> The aging segmentations encompass too great a time span if an account moving from one category to another elicits a drastic management action. For example, if an account goes from current to write off status, the aging segmentations are too encompassing.

If an account is still outstanding after all collection efforts have been attempted, the account may be retained in accounts receivable (accounts which have received a third notice but are not yet written off). However, once the account reaches an age at which historically less than five or ten percent of the outstanding accounts ultimately are collected, then the account should be written off.

Whenever an account is written off, a decision must be made whether or not to inform the patient of the write off action. Some people believe that informing individuals that their account has been written off eliminates any chance of future payments on those accounts. Others feel that future bad debts may be diminished and payments on such accounts may be forthcoming if individuals are informed that their accounts have been written off and no future services will be delivered until they have tendered all monies owed. In either case, once an account is written off, it should be maintained in an accounts written off file so that if payments are made, the account can be reinstated and recorded as paid.

Delinquencies Reports

Physicians providing service should receive a report regarding the delinquent accounts of their patients. In addition, a copy of the patient delinquency report should be included in the patient file. Then, if service subsequently is rendered to patients whose accounts are delinquent, an exception report should be issued to the chief of staff or to the medical director.

Interest Penalties

An interest penalty could be charged on accounts that are delinquent from the time they become delinquent until they are paid (see Problem 3-7). The maximum size of this interest penalty is fixed by law, depending upon the jurisdiction. Although few health care institutions employ this procedure to improve the conversion of patient receivables, interest penalties could improve the cash flow from patient accounts receivable.

MANAGEMENT OF PATIENT ACCOUNTS RECEIVABLE: A GROUP PRACTICE

This case examines the management of patient accounts receivable (self and third party pay) for a group practice. Under the management policies instituted by the group, the accounts receivable balance is equal to approximately one year's billing and the average age of 60 percent of these accounts is 18 months. As a result, the group is now experiencing serious cash flow problems. Members of the group charged with investigating this problem have concluded that more timely conversion of accounts receivable is necessary; however, they are fearful that requiring patients to pay for services as they are rendered may cause a significant number of patients to seek care at other institutions. In order to examine the important aspects of these problems, the following will be considered: description of the present system, problems evidenced in the present system, proposed changes, and attendant policy changes.

Present System: Accounts Receivable Information Collection—Outpatient Care

The information required for billing outpatient care is obtained from the visit record and the patient's registration form. The patient's registration form is completed by the patient on the first appointment. This form contains all of the personal information required for billing, including insurance information and special billing instructions from the physician, such as "bill insurance only," "reduce charges," or "professional courtesy." The visit record has a number of sections that are filled out at various stages of the visit. The personal information section, which provides space for the patient's name, address, date of visit, and general type of service to be received, is completed by the group's receptionist. The record then accompanies the patient throughout the visit so that the actual services provided can be noted on the record.

At the completion of the visit, the patient is given the option of paying for the visit immediately or of being billed. If the patient does not insist on paying at this time, the clerk assumes that the patient wishes to be billed. On those rare occasions when a patient elects to pay, the receptionist directs the person to the cashier, who reviews the visit record to determine the charges. Since the fees charged by the physicians for different types of service vary, the cashier also must check the section of the patient's registration form where the physician has noted any deviation from the published fee schedule. The cashier then totals the charges, collects the cash, issues a receipt, and indicates on a separate form attached to the visit record those charges to be billed to third party payers. The third party payers' invoices are prepared from these forms, and a carbon copy of the information on each receipt appears in the cash receipts journal. Unfortunately, the cashier rarely computes the charges properly, necessitating a good deal of paper work for both the clerical staff of the group and the third party payers.

In most cases, patients prefer to be billed. Accordingly, the billing copy of the visit record and the registration form are filed with the other records for the day. These records are collected and processed later by the outpatient billing clerk.

Processing of Charges: Creation of Patient Accounts Receivable

The outpatient billing clerk collects the visit records of patients preferring to be billed and patients who have paid a portion of their bill but require further billing to a third party payer. Using information contained on the visit record and on the patient's registration form, the clerk calculates the charges for the visit and determines whether to bill the patient directly or to bill a third party payer. While only Medicare will pay for office visits, Blue Shield and most private insurance plans will pay for certain laboratory work. In the experience of the clinic, only about 35 percent of all outpatient charges must be processed for submission to third party payers. After the appropriate claim forms have been completed, the clerk enters the results of the transaction in the outpatient accounts receivable journal. The patient's account ledger is placed under the journal as the entry is made, and a carbon copy of the entry is made on the ledger. This entry constitutes the recording in the accounts receivable control account and the accounts receivable subsidiary ledger.

At the end of the month, the ledgers are reviewed. Accounts with other than a zero balance are pulled and sorted according to the number of notices for payment that have been sent out on each account. Accounts which previously have been sent a third notice are not pulled. Once the appropriate ledgers have been pulled and separated, they are sent to a private contractor who photocopies the ledger and mails the copy to the patient with a request for payment. Accounts which have been sent a third notice are considered a collection problem. The group administrator has an assistant who is responsible for following up on these delinquent accounts.

Problem Areas Within the Present System

An attempt has been made to quantify the effect of major problem areas on the revenue generated by the medical group. The two major failings deal with the lack of management action to convert patient accounts receivable in a timely manner and the impact of inefficiencies in the present system of recording and billing patient accounts receivable. Possible increases in revenue from the more timely conversion of patient accounts receivable in excess of $65,000 per year, or nearly ten percent of annual group revenue, have been isolated, while the cumulative effect of inefficiencies within the present system has been estimated to account for revenue loss of $80,000–$100,000 per year. The details of these problem areas are described below.

Services Rendered But Not Recorded as Accounts Receivable

To ascertain the magnitude of services rendered but not recorded as patient accounts receivable, the records of all patients appearing for outpatient care during randomly selected test weeks in 19X1 were examined. A total of 612 patients were provided $12,600 in services during those weeks. Of these services, $1,146, or approximately nine percent of the total, collectable from 72 patients, were not recorded by the system. A projection of this sum yields an annual revenue loss of approximately $15,000. The sources of these omissions were (1) improper completion of the visit record by the receptionist and (2) errors in the entries made on the visit records by the physician, resulting in incorrect assumptions by the outpatient billing clerk. In some cases, for instance, the receptionist failed to check the block on the form indicating that the patient was to see a physician and the physician failed to enter the services performed. Consequently, the billing clerk assumed that only laboratory work was performed and the bills were prepared accordingly. During the test weeks, $780 in charges were omitted in this way. In other cases, the receptionist checked the physician block, but the physician failed to make the appropriate entry. Although normal procedure dictates that the billing office should call the physician to verify what services were provided, a number of these cases slip by the billing clerk and are never billed. This type of error, amounting to $420 during the test weeks, may result in either a reduction in group income due to unbilled services or delay in processing other bills while the billing office tries to verify services actually performed.

In addition to these errors, certain types of incomplete entries were noted on the visit records. The most common of these was the entry of "revisit." A "revisit" entry indicates to the billing office that the visit was an intermediate revisit, and the patient is billed $15. However, a review of these entries with the physicians involved indicated that in three of the five cases marked in this way, the actual entry should have been "brief revisit," and the charge should have been $10.

Reduced Charges

The policy for offering reduced charges is very flexible. The amount charged each patient is determined by each physician, resulting in a range of charges for the same service. The study of the visit records has indicated that the magnitude of reduced charges for outpatient care during the study weeks amounted to $800, or more than six percent of the total charges for services performed. The cumulative effect of both these reduced charges and the errors in completing the visit records were over 15 percent of the charges for services performed during the test weeks.

Cashier Collections

The Group Practice Committee has stated that its payment policy is to encourage cash payments at time of service. However, less than 25 percent of the outpatients seen by the Medical Group pay the cashier. The group paying at the time service is delivered consists of people receiving immunizations (who are required to pay the cashier on the day of service), people paying bills mailed to their homes, and people receiving care that day. Less than five percent of the people seeing a physician or a lab technician pay the cashier on the day of service. The reason for this low percentage is that patients are not encouraged by the receptionist to pay their bill when service is received.

Errors in Processing Claims for Third Party Payment

A study of a random sample of outpatient ledgers was conducted to analyze the aging of the group's accounts receivable. One of the byproducts of this study was the isolation of a number of claims for third party payment for services actually performed and reported to the billing office, but not submitted for reimbursement. Bills for outpatient care of $588 have not been submitted to third party payers.

Delay in Processing Claims to Third Party Payers

The accounts receivable collection system seems to have reached a state of equilibrium where charges for services performed on a particular day are processed by the accounts receivable department approximately 37 days later. During the interim, the billing department is busy requesting signatures on forms from physicians and patients. Billing clerks also spend time obtaining correct insurance information and private insurance forms for accounts that already have begun to be processed. The actual completion of the claim requires very little time once the signatures, coverage numbers, and coverage dates have been obtained.

Delay in Billing Patients Directly

Usually a patient is billed only after a notice of charges disallowed or a payment is received from the third party payer. Therefore, patients actually receive their bills between one and five months after the service is performed, depending on how long it takes the third party payer to process the bill. Consequently, the values in the aging distribution of accounts receivable remain relatively constant through the fourth month after processing and then decrease in the fifth month when patients first receive their bills. In addition, the delay in processing patient accounts helps to explain the difficulty with converting overdue accounts, since as suggested, the older an account is, the more difficult it is to collect.

Mailing Process to Bill Accounts Receivable

The actual billing process requires three or four days work from both the inpatient and outpatient billing clerks who manually review each account and pull each patient account ledger with other than a zero balance which has not been sent a third notice. Then these clerks must separate the ledgers into first, second, and third notice categories and refile them once they have been photocopied. This process not only delays the normal work of these clerks, which is processing bills, but also disrupts the work flow of others in the department who require the patient's ledger.

Form of the Bill

During the weeks after mailing, the processing of other bills is delayed further with numerous calls from patients inquiring about their bills. Not only are bills hand written, but poor photocopying sometimes makes the bills difficult to read. The form of the bill also makes it difficult to understand. Minor omissions, such as an indication to "disregard the notice if payment has already been made," result in further calls to the billing department from confused patients.

Collection of Delinquent Accounts

Once a patient has been sent a third notice, the billing department takes no further action. However, a copy of the patient's bill is sent to the group administrator, who is supposed to discuss each account with the appropriate physician and then write the account off or send the patient a series of physician-signed letters.

This procedure has not been followed for the last four years. Patients who have been sent third notices during this period have received no more notices from the billing department, no letters from the physician, and no visits from collection agency personnel; but their accounts also have not been written off.

Review of Claims for Third Party Payment

Third party payment claims are currently reviewed as time allows. During the study, the unanswered claims sent to Medicare prior to 19X1 were reviewed and a total of approximately $15,000 in charges were found. The study of the aging of accounts receivable indicates that sizeable amounts also exist in unanswered claims sent to Blue Shield and private insurance plans.

Account Review and Control

The billing department must devote all of its time to processing bills in order to keep up with the constant inflow of visit records. Consequently, no time is left for instituting any account review and control procedures.

Internal Control

The bookkeeping assistant verifies that the amount of cash turned over for deposit each day agrees with the total shown in the payments section of the cash receipts journal, but no controls insure that all cash collections have been entered in the journal. For example, no internal controls exist for cash collections received by physicians' secretaries. Although evidence of misdealings are not apparent at this time, considerable misappropriations could occur.

In addition to the lack of control over cash collections, no controls exist to insure that the visit record for each patient actually is received by the billing office. In fact, the current system is so lax that the visit record could be misplaced during the week as it awaits pick up by the billing clerk, or the patient could walk out of the office with it. In either case, the billing office would have no indication that services had been performed.

Proposed Policy and Systems Changes

Given the problems identified with the current system, three policies should be instituted:

1. All patients should be informed at the time of their appointment that they are required to pay for services not covered by their third party insurance plan before they leave the office.
2. All delinquent account information should be provided routinely to the group physician of record. If that physician continues to deliver service, a listing of the services provided and their cost should be given to the physician in charge of the group.
3. All reduced charge information should be summarized and reported to the physician in charge of the group.

To implement these policy changes, a new position, patient accounts supervisor, should be created. The job description of this new position is stated as follows:

> The patient accounts supervisor must be knowledgeable regarding (1) the myriad ways various third party payers qualify and exclude services, and (2) the various copayment arrangements which make the patient responsible for a portion of the cost of services rendered. The patient accounts supervisor will have a station in the group. Individuals will be routed to this station prior to leaving service.

None of these changes necessitates an upgrading of the group's computer facility, hardware, or software (except for some minor reprogramming), and no additional billing personnel are required. In addition, even if patient volume increases by 30 to 40 percent over the next few years, no additional full time personnel should be required. The net benefit of these changes is estimated to be $75,000–$100,000 if patient volume remains fairly constant.[5]

NOTES

1. The accounting for accounts receivable from third party payers is identical to the accounting for accounts receivable from patients. The important considerations regarding the

management of accounts receivable from third party payers were extensively discussed in Chapter 2.
2. The aging of the accounts receivable assumes that each patient charge will be aged separately. For example, if a particular patient has two charges, one for $830 which is 183 days old and one for $73.50 which is 11 days old, each of the charges would be aged separately. An alternative method would be to select the age category of the largest charge. In this case, the entire patient account of $903.50 would be categorized as if it were 183 days old. This alternative method is not recommended.
3. See Accounting Principles Board (APB) Opinion #20, paragraph 31.
4. These two entries may be combined into the following entry:

Cash	***	
Allowance for Bad Debts		***.

5. The dissipation of demand was tested by telephoning a number of patients and asking them if the elimination of credit would affect their utilization of the group. Eighty-five percent indicated that a "pay as you go" policy for those charges not covered by a third party would be acceptable. The status of the medical group's system was investigated one year after the proposed changes were instituted. At that time, in spite of the payment for service policy, patient volume had increased. Further, the realized net monetary benefits were slightly greater than had been estimated.

Questions and Problems

Question 3-1. What are the advantages of the aging method of estimating the allowance for bad debts? Under what conditions will the aging method give the same results as the percentage of some related account method?

Question 3-2. How can the percentage of some related account method be used to generate control information which will enable management to isolate ineffective accounts receivable management?

Question 3-3. Assume you are the administrator of a small group practice. You employ three full time employees. The group collects a substantial amount of cash from patients as well as third party payers. The accounts receivable of the group average 30 percent of revenue. Prepare a statement of the job responsibilities of the three individuals regarding handling of cash, opening the mail, preparing bank reconciliations, preparing the proof of cash, writing off accounts receivable, billing third parties and patients, writing checks, delivering cash receipts to the bank at the end of the day, posting to the accounts receivable control accounts, and posting to the accounts receivable subsidiary ledgers.

Question 3-4. Why should patient accounts receivable written off be segregated from current patient accounts receivable?

Question 3-5. How would you ascertain the possible effect of a change in credit policy on the patient demand of:

a. an urban prepaid group practice;
b. a large urban teaching hospital; and
c. a rural group practice?

Question 3-6. Why is it important to establish a policy regarding the coordination of an accounts receivable collection action with a change in an account's age classification?

Question 3-7. Assume that the dollar value of accounts written off is highly correlated with both the value of the ending inventory and total revenue. Discuss the relative merits of estimating the allowance for bad debts using (a) the value of the ending inventory or (b) the total revenue.

Question 3-8. Considering Figure 3-3, is there any economic relationship between the size of the vertical shift at t_k and the point at which collection efforts should stop? What are the managerial implications of this relationship?

Question 3-9. Given the analysis on page 69, suggest where these self-perpetuating rounds of cost increases and demand decreases will stop. Is there an economic stopping point short of cessation of service? What managerial actions can stop this downward spiral?

Question 3-10.

a. Assume that cash collections are used to estimate the Allowance for Bad Debts. In most circumstances cash collections and the dollar value of accounts receivable which are written off would be inversely correlated. (The sign of the correlation coefficient is negative.) Does this mean that there are no circumstances when cash collections would increase and more accounts would be written off?
b. Given a negatively correlated predictor relationship, formulate a means of estimating the Allowance for Bad Debts.
c. Is it possible that an account which is correlated .31 with accounts written off could be a perfect predictor of bad debts (i.e., $S_e = 0$)? If this could occur, why is the correlation coefficient of any use in selecting an account to estimate future uncollectables?

Question 3-11. Figures 3-1 and 3-2 examine accounts receivable created on a particular day. Modify these figures to reflect the activity in the accounts receivable control account over a number of days.

Problem 3-1. The Free Clinic of South Philadelphia experiences the following economic events during 19X1 and 19X2:

a. C. Jones receives service on July 6, 19X1. He is billed $173.50.
b. On July 29, 19X1, Jones disputes his bill. He points out that two charges for K. C. Jones erroneously have been recorded on his bill. These charges are for $19.49 and $27.28.
c. At the end of the year, 12/31/19X1, the aging of the accounts receivable indicates that eight percent of the current accounts (accounts less than 30 days old) are expected to be uncollectable.) The total noncurrent accounts receivable which will be uncollectable is estimated to be 3.5 times the current accounts receivable that are expected to be uncollectable. The current accounts receivable at year-end amount to $29,434.81. Assume the balance in the Allowance for Bad Debts account on 12/31/19X1, prior to adjustment, is $2,526.52.
d. On January 8, 19X2, after repeated collection attempts, C. Jones' account is written off.
e. C. Jones, who requires semiannual treatment, is denied service on January 13, 19X2. As a result, on January 15, 19X2, he sends in the balance owed, which has been increased by three percent to recoup collection costs.

Required: Make the appropriate journal entries.

Problem 3-2. The balance in the Allowance for Bad Debts account at Memorial Hospital before the adjusting entries are prepared on 12/31/19X1 is $489.22 DR. Based upon the aging of accounts receivable, a total of $8,677.84 should be in the Allowance for Bad Debts account on 12/31/19X1. During 19X2, patient accounts receivable increase through operations by $187,247.31. Cash collections on accounts receivable during 19X2 amount to $205,170.16, and cash collections at the time services are rendered amount to $8,427.04. During 19X2, $6,397.21 in patient accounts receivable are written off. The hospital administration estimates that 2.65 percent of total patient revenue is a fair estimate of the accounts which will be uncollectable subsequent to 12/31/19X2.

Required: Make the appropriate journal entries from 12/13/19X1 through 12/31/19X2.

Problem 3-3. The hospital administrator is concerned about the number of patient accounts receivable which are uncollectable. This problem is having an important detrimental effect on cash flow, as well as profitability. Therefore, the administrator is considering instituting a payment for service policy. To evaluate that decision, the following information is collected:

Patient revenue during the next year is estimated to be $685,000. If the credit policy is changed to a payment for service policy, patient revenue is expected to decrease by eight percent. Under the current credit policy, the following is estimated: (1) bad checks from patients will average 15 percent of average accounts receivable, (2) short-term financing requirements will be $30,000, which must be borrowed at 9.35 percent, (3) collection costs will be one percent of patient revenue, (4) accounts written off will be eight percent of average accounts receivable, and (5) average accounts receivable will be 27 percent of patient revenue. Under a payment for service policy, the following is estimated: (1) bad checks will be ten percent of average accounts receivable, (2) collection costs will be $1,000, (3) accounts written off will be nine percent of average accounts receivable, and (4) average accounts receivable will be ten percent of patient revenue.

Required:

a. How much would other costs (administrative and delivery) have to decrease under the payment for service policy to make the administrator indifferent to chosing between the two credit policies?
b. Discuss the likelihood that administrative or delivery costs would decrease under a payment for services policy.

Problem 3-4 Assume you are the manager of the hospital's accounts receivable department. Your primary management problem is with physicians who continually deliver service without the slightest concern for the patient's ability to pay.

a. How would you effect a change in the physicians' attitude toward the collection of patient accounts receivable?
b. Assume your best efforts fail to change the physicians' attitude. The physicians remain adamant about their policy of not concerning themselves with the collection of patient receivables. Develop a proposal for a patient accounts receivable system which,

recognizing the physicians' attitude, provides for effective management of patient accounts receivable.

Problem 3-5. How should the hospital administrator decide:

a. At what intervals request for payment notices should be sent to patients?
b. How many payment request notices should be sent?
c. When should a particular patient's account be written off?
d. Who should participate in the decision to write off delinquent patient accounts?

Problem 3-6. You are a part time employee. You are temporarily taking the place of an accounts receivable posting clerk whose duties include opening the mail. The clerk has been with the institution for 11 years. You are replacing the clerk due to illness. Your first task is to send out monthly statements to patients who have positive balances. Two days after the bills have been sent, a number of irate patients call indicating they have paid their accounts. The hospital administrator, fielding most of these calls, is upset with you, feeling that you have not been doing your job properly.

Assuming you are not a nitwit, what may be the reason for the phone calls received by the hospital administrator? What corrective action would eliminate the problems you identified?

Problem 3-7. Assume a hospital charges an interest penalty of three percent on all accounts outstanding 90 days or longer after the third billing. Further assume that an aging of the accounts on 12/31/19X1 shows that $193,000 in patient accounts receivable are outstanding 90 days or longer after the third billing.

a. If the hospital's accounting period is the calendar year, what adjusting entry should be made on 12/31/19X1?
b. What accounting entry would be made on 1/30/19X2 if $93,000 of these accounts, plus the interest owed, are collected?
c. What accounting entry would be made on 2/12/19X2 if an additional $75,000 of these accounts, plus 20 percent of the interest owed, are collected? It is determined that the remaining interest owed will not be collected.
d. What accounting entry would be made on 3/1/19X2 if the remaining $25,000 is collected and no interest is paid? It is ascertained that 50 percent of that interest eventually will be collected.

Problem 3-8. The KJCM Clinic maintains an accounts receivable control account and the appropriate subsidiary ledger. On December 31, 19X1 the Patient Accounts Receivable balance is $191,411.38.

Subsidiary Ledgers

Current	Group I	Group II	Group III	Delinquent
0-30 days	31-60 days	61-90 days	91-180 days	≥ 181 days
\$89,412.63	\$41,621.77	\$24,600.11	\$10,899.14	

The clinic manager informs you that 10.4 percent of the ending balance of patient accounts receivable is a reasonable estimate of the bad debts expense for 19X1. After some investigation, you ascertain that the percentage of delinquent accounts which are collected during subsequent periods is equal to the ratio of the delinquent accounts to the nondelinquent accounts. You further discover that the percentage of accounts in Groups III, II, I, and the Current accounts which are written off decreases by a factor of ½ as follows.

Group III: $\lambda_{III} = \frac{1}{2} \times \lambda_{delinquent}$
Group II: $\lambda_{II} = \frac{1}{2} \times \lambda_{III}$
Group I: $\lambda_{I} = \frac{1}{2} \times \lambda_{II}$
Current: $\lambda_{C} = \frac{1}{2} \times \lambda_{I}$

Required:

a. Determine the dollar amount of accounts which have been outstanding 181 days or longer.
b. Assuming the credit balance in the Allowance for Bad Debts account is \$26,004.97, what is the adjusting journal entry on December 31, 19X1 under (i) the aging method and (ii) the percentage of some related account method?
c. If the administrator wishes to maximize reimbursement, which method of estimating future bad debts should be selected?
d. Comment on the size of the credit balance in the Allowance for Bad Debts account.

Chapter 4

Inventory: Accounting and Control Aspects

Waste not; want not.

Anonymous

Inventory accounting and inventory management are important aspects of institutional cost control. Because a number of alternative accounting methods are available for associating particular inventory costs with service revenue, an understanding of the economic implications of selecting a particular costing alternative is important. Management of the institution's inventory, on the other hand, is important in conserving and efficiently utilizing this costly resource. Hence, accounting for the use of inventory and inventory management should be integral parts of the institution's management program.

ACCOUNTING FOR THE FLOW OF INVENTORY COSTS

The physical flow of inventory items and the flow of inventory costs do not necessarily share the same temporal movement. Given *n* homogeneous inventory items having *n* different costs, any of these *n* costs may be assigned to any of the *n* items, as long as each cost is only assigned once. The assignment of particular costs to particular items is a product of management's choice regarding the physical flow of inventory and the flow of inventory costs.

Physical Inventory Flows

The physical flow of inventory items may be random, first-in, first-out (FIFO) or last-in, first-out (LIFO). A random outflow of inventory items is not a systematic means of managing physical inventory flows. Under the random method, any item may be used to fill a requisition, regardless of when the item was purchased. On the contrary, FIFO and LIFO are systematic methods of managing physical inventory flows. Under the FIFO method, the oldest items in the inventory, those that were purchased first, are the first items to leave inventory when a requisition is received. Under the LIFO method, on the other hand, the newest items in the inventory, those that were purchased last, are the first items selected to fill requisitions. The most reasonable of these three methods of managing physical inventory flows is FIFO because it minimizes the chance of obsolescence and spoilage.

Inventory Costing Methods

Coupled with these three methods of managing physical inventory flows are four systematic methods of accounting for the flow of inventory costs. The four methods of costing inventory are (1) specific identification, (2) weighted average, (3) first-in, first-out (FIFO), and (4) last-in, first-out (LIFO). Any one of these costing methods may be used in conjunction with any one of the methods of managing the physical inventory flow.

Specific Identification

Under the specific identification method, each item in the inventory is costed at the price paid for that specific item. To accomplish this costing, each item must be tagged with its cost. As items in inventory are used, the tags are removed. Summing the costs marked on the tags yields the total cost of the inventory items used. Similarly, summing the costs marked on the tags of the items remaining in inventory at any point in time yields the total value of the inventory at that point in time.

Weighted Average

The weighted average method spreads the individual costs in the inventory and assigns one weighted average cost to all items. To calculate the weighted average cost of the inventory initially, multiply each cost in the inventory by the number of items at that cost, sum the products and divide by the total number of items in the inventory. This calculation may be represented as follows:

(4-1)
$$\bar{C} = \frac{\sum_{i=1}^{k} C_i n_i}{\sum_{i=1}^{k} n_i}$$

where: $\bar{C}$ represents the weighted average cost per unit;
k represents the number of different costs in the inventory;
C_i represents the cost of items in the ith cost category;
n_i represents the number of items in the ith cost category.

Once the weighted average cost has been calculated, this $\bar{C}$ becomes associated with all items that were in inventory at the time of the calculation. Consequently, unless the average unit cost of items currently entering the inventory is equal to the weighted average cost already assigned to the inventory items, every purchase will change the weighted average cost. As new purchases are made and the weighted average cost is updated, this update cost $\hat{C}$ becomes associated with all items in inventory. The cost of inventory items used can be calculated by multiplying the weighted average cost by the number of items used; the value of the items remaining in inventory at any point in time can be calculated by applying the weighted average cost to the number of items in the inventory at that point in time.

FIFO

Under both the FIFO and the LIFO methods of inventory costing, the time sequence of inventory purchases is important. Records must be kept of the date, quantity, and cost of inventory purchases. As in the two costing methods described above, the physical flow of inventory items does not affect these costing methods.

Regardless of the order of the physical flow of inventory items, the FIFO costing method requires that the first item leaving the inventory be costed at the oldest cost in the inventory and that all subsequent flows from inventory be costed at the oldest price remaining in inventory. For example, if 20 units of a new item X were purchased at $70 per unit on May 1, 19X1 and an additional 10 units of item X were purchased at $75 per unit on May 3, 19X1, then the first 10 units of item X leaving the inventory must be costed at $70 per unit, the next 10 at $70 per unit, and the last 10 at $75 per unit. In other words, the first costs to enter the inventory are the first costs to leave. In a sense inventory cost layers are created, and costs cannot flow from any layer until all prior cost layers have been depleted. Consequently, the value of the inventory at any point is determined by applying the most recent costs to the appropriate number of items.

LIFO

Under the LIFO costing method, the flow of costs is reversed. Given the inventory cost layers, costs cannot flow from any layer until all more recently acquired layers have been depleted. If the 30 units of item *X* in the example above were purchased and costed under the LIFO method, the first 10 units leaving the inventory would be costed at $75 per unit, the next 10 at $70 per unit, and the last 10 at $70 per unit. In other words, the first item leaving the inventory must be costed at the most recent cost in the inventory, and all subsequent items leaving inventory must be costed at the remaining most recent cost.

Illustrative Example

The following example may further clarify these four costing methods. The inventory purchasing pattern for the Riverside Health Maintenance Organization (HMO) during 19X0 is as follows.

		Number of Units	Unit Cost	Total
Jan. 1, 19X0	Beginning Inventory	20	$2.00	$40.00
May 1, 19X0	First Purchase	10	$3.00	$30.00
Dec. 1, 19X0	Second Purchase	5	$4.00	$20.00
		35		$90.00

A total of 35 units with 35 individual prices are available for use during 19X0. Assume that during the year, 17 of these units are used in the operations of the HMO. Of the 17 units used, 12 units were purchased at $2.00 per unit, 4 at $3.00 per unit, and 1 at $4.00 per unit.

To determine the cost of the goods used in operations, one of the four costing methods described above must be selected. The costing methods are outlined below, and the cost of the 17 units is calculated under each method.

I. Specific Identification

Rule: Ascertain the actual cost of each inventory item used and sum these costs to determine the cost of goods used.

In this case, the 17 items used would be costed as follows.

12 items at $2.00 =	$24.00	
4 items at $3.00 =	12.00	
1 item at $4.00 =	4.00	$40.00

II. Weighted Average

Rule: Given the individual costs of the units available for use during the period, calculate the weighted average cost of these units. Then cost each of the items used at this weighted average cost.

In this case, the individual costs of the 35 units available for use during the year are given above. The total cost of these 35 units is $90.00. Hence, the weighted average cost of each unit would be:

$$\frac{\text{Total Cost}}{\text{Total Units}} = \frac{\$90}{35} = \$2.5714$$

and the cost of 17 units used during 19X0 would be:

17 items at $2.5714 = $43.71.

III. FIFO

Rule: Given the stratified cost layers of the units available for use during the period and the number of units actually used, select costs for the units used during the period beginning with the oldest cost and proceeding through the cost layers to the more recent costs.

In this case, the stratified cost layers of the units available for use during the year are given above. Since 17 units are used during the year, the cost of goods used would be computed as follows:

17 items at $2.00 = $34.00.

IV. LIFO

Rule: Given the stratified cost layers of the units available for use during the period and the number of units actually used, select costs for the units used during the period beginning with the most recent cost and proceeding through the cost layers to the older costs.

In this case, the stratified cost layers of the units available for use during the year are given above. Hence, the 17 units used during the year would be costed as follows:

5 items at $4.00 =	$20.00	
10 items at $3.00 =	30.00	
2 items at $2.00 =	4.00	$54.00.

Inventory Identities

Since these four inventory costing rules assign a value to the total goods used during the period, they simultaneously assign a value to the ending inventory. The following identities help to elucidate this fact.

(4-2) Units in Beginning Inventory + Units Purchased
≡ Units Available for Use

(4-3) Units Available for Use − Units Used
≡ Units in Ending Inventory

These unit relationships are intuitive. The cost relationships that indicate how the value of the ending inventory is associated with the cost of goods used during the period are logical extensions of these unit relationships.

The cost of the goods available for use during the period is obtained by assigning costs to the units in relation (4-2). The cost assigned to the units in the beginning inventory is equal to the cost assigned to the previous period's ending inventory. The cost assigned to the units purchased during the period is equal to the amount that must be paid to vendors to obtain the items purchased. Hence, the first cost relationship is as follows:

(4-4) Cost of Beginning Inventory + Cost of Purchases
≡ Cost of Goods Available for Use

The cost of goods available for use during the period may be defined as the sum of all costs available to be assigned to items leaving inventory during the period. Assigning costs to items leaving inventory gives value to the units used and reduces the pool of costs available for future assignment. The pool of costs remaining after costs have been assigned to all items leaving the inventory during the period is equal to the value of the ending inventory. Hence, the value of the ending inventory may be calculated by applying the unassigned costs to the units in the ending inventory or by subtracting the cost of goods used from the costs of goods available for use. This latter relationship is represented as follows.

(4-5) Cost of Goods Available for Use — Cost of Goods Used
≡ Cost of Ending Inventory

The inventory costing cycle is presented schematically in Figure 4-1.

Figure 4-1 Inventory Costing Cycle

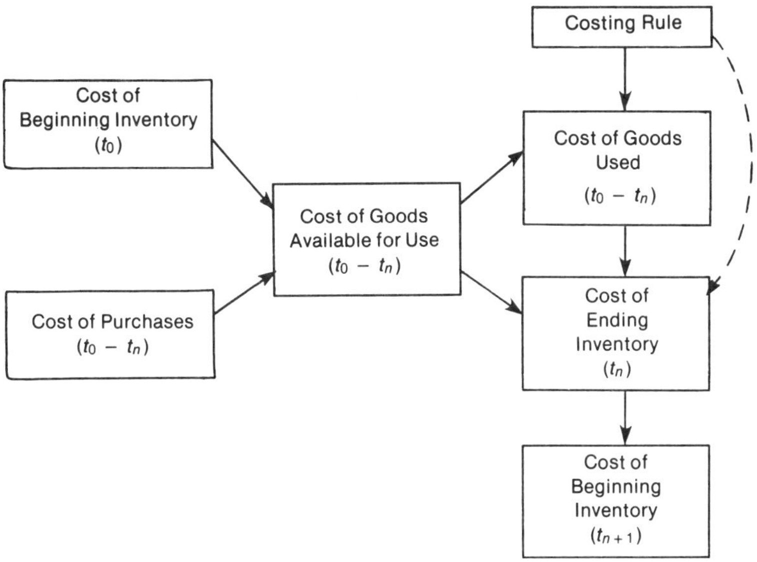

Systems of Accounting for Inventory Costs: Perpetual and Periodic

Once a systematic method of costing inventory items has been chosen, management must decide when to cost the items leaving inventory. Two alternatives are available.

1. Assign a cost to each item leaving inventory at the time the item leaves the inventory, or
2. Assign costs to all items that leave inventory during the year at year-end when the physical inventory is counted.

The first alternative is called the perpetual accounting system; the second is the periodic accounting system.

The Perpetual Accounting System

Under the perpetual accounting system, each time an item is requisitioned from inventory, a cost is assigned to the requisitioned item according to one of the four inventory costing methods. The assignment of a cost to an inventory item constitutes an economic transaction affecting the institution. Hence, an accounting entry must be made to record the cost assigned to each item leaving inventory. This entry increases the Cost of Goods Used account and decreases the Inventory control account. Consequently, under the perpetual accounting system, the value of the Inventory control account should be identical to the cost of the physical inventory. The following example shows the accounting entries that must be made under the perpetual accounting system.

Consider the following acquisition and issuance information for Riverside HMO.

Date	Transaction	Units	Cost per Unit
Jan. 1, 19X0	Beginning Inventory	20	$2.00
May 1, 19X0	First Purchase	10	3.00
June 1, 19X0	First Issuance	15	
Dec. 1, 19X0	Second Purchase	5	4.00
Dec. 2, 19X0	Second Issuance	2	

If the LIFO costing method is used to cost items leaving inventory and the perpetual system is used to account for the cost of goods used, then the following accounting entries would be made during the year.

5/1/X0	Inventory	$30.00	
	Accounts Payable (·)		$30.00
	To record the purchase of 10 inventory items at $3.00 per unit.		
6/1/X0	Cost of Goods Used	$40.00	
	Inventory		$40.00
	To record the use of 15 inventory items, 10 costed at $3.00 per unit and 5 costed at $2.00 per unit.		
12/1/X0	Inventory	$20.00	
	Accounts Payable (·)		$20.00
	To record the purchase of 5 inventory items at $4.00 per unit.		
12/2/X0	Cost of Goods Used	$ 8.00	
	Inventory		$ 8.00
	To record the use of 2 inventory items costed at $4.00 per unit.		

These entries affect the Cost of Goods Used account and the Inventory control account as follows.

Cost of Goods Used

(✓)	$ -0-		
6/1	40.00		
12/2	8.00		
	$48.00		

Inventory

(✓)	$40.00	6/1	$40.00
5/1	30.00	12/2	8.00
12/1	20.00		
	$42.00		

The $48.00 balance in the Cost of Goods Used account arose from

First Issuance:	10 units at $3.00 =	$30.00	
	5 units at $2.00 =	10.00	
Second Issuance:	2 units at $4.00 =	8.00	$48.00

and the $42.00 balance remaining in the ending inventory is composed of

15 units at $2.00 =	$30.00	
3 units at $4.00 =	12.00	$42.00.

This system of accounting for the cost of goods used requires a considerable amount of bookkeeping. However, it provides continuous information regarding the cost of goods used to date and the value of the inventory. In addition, if a discrepancy exists between the value in the Inventory account and the value assigned to the physical inventory after it has been counted, an adjusting entry will be required under the perpetual accounting system. This adjusting entry isolates the losses due to theft, spoilage, spillage, or obsolescence.

The Periodic Accounting System

Under the periodic accounting system, the assignment of cost to items leaving inventory during the year occurs at the end of the institution's fiscal year, when the physical inventory is counted. During the year, as new items are purchased and stored in inventory, the costs associated with these purchases are recorded in a temporary account called Inventory Purchases.[1] The date, the number of units purchased and the dollar value of each unit is recorded in a subsidiary ledger. Inventory usage, on the other hand, is recorded by date and number of units used in another subsidiary ledger. However, the amount recorded in the Inventory control account remains constant during the year at the value of the beginning inventory.

At the end of the fiscal year, the number of items in the ending inventory is ascertained by a physical inventory count. The cost of goods used is then calculated by:

1. applying the appropriate costing rule to the units in the ending inventory and then subtracting the cost of the ending inventory from the cost of goods available for use (cost of goods available for use ≡ cost of beginning inventory + cost of purchases), or
2. subtracting the units in the ending inventory from the total units available for use (units available for use ≡ units beginning inventory + units purchased) and then applying the appropriate costing rule to the units used.

Once the cost of goods used or the value of the ending inventory is known, a journal entry is made to close the Purchases account to the Inventory control account and to close the appropriate inventory costs to the Cost of Goods Used account. The following example illustrates the entries and the calculations necessary under the periodic accounting system.

Again, consider the purchasing pattern for Riverside HMO.

Date	Transaction	Units	Cost per Unit
Jan. 1, 19X0	Beginning Inventory	20	$2.00
May 1, 19X0	First Purchase	10	3.00
Dec. 1, 19X0	Second Purchase	5	4.00

The entries to record these purchases would be as follows.

5/1/X0	Purchases	$30.00	
	Accounts Payable (·)		$30.00
	To record the purchase of 10 inventory items at $3.00 per unit.		
12/1/X0	Purchases	$20.00	
	Accounts Payable (·)		$20.00
	To record the purchase of 5 inventory items at $4.00 per unit.		

Assume that when the physical inventory is counted on December 31, 19X0, 18 units are in the inventory. Since the LIFO method is used to cost items leaving inventory during the year, the costs assigned to the items remaining in inventory on December 31 should be the oldest costs in the inventory. Therefore, each of the 18 items remaining in inventory on December 31, 19X0 should be costed at $2.00 per unit. Hence, the value of the ending inventory would be:

18 items at $2.00 per unit = $36.00.

Since the value of the beginning inventory was $40.00, the Inventory control account must be reduced by $4.00. In addition, the Purchases account must be closed (reduced to zero). The following entry makes these adjustments and simultaneously determines the cost of goods used.

12/31/X0	Cost of Goods Used	$54.00	
	Purchases		$50.00
	Inventory		4.00

To record the use of 17 inventory items, 5 items costed at $4.00 per unit, 10 items costed at $3.00 per unit, and 2 items costed at $2.00 per units, and to state the balance in the Inventory account properly.

This same entry would have been made if costs had been assigned to the inventory units used. For example, if 35 units were available for use during the year and 18 units remain in inventory on December 31, 17 units were used during the year. Applying the LIFO costing method, the cost of these 17 items would be:

5 items at $4.00 =	$20.00	
10 items at $3.00 =	$30.00	
2 items at $2.00 =	$ 4.00	$54.00.

In this case, the amount to be debited to the Cost of Goods Used account and the amount to be credited to the Purchases account are known. The balancing entry is the $4.00 credit to the Inventory control account.

The periodic accounting system requires considerably less bookkeeping than the perpetual accounting system. Under periodic accounting, no adjustment is needed to record the losses due to theft, spoilage, spillage, or obsolescence because these losses are included in the cost of goods used. Hence, some useful information regarding these cost may be hidden under this system. Nevertheless, if proper internal control is exercised over the requisition system and over the physical flow of inventory (FIFO physical flow), such losses will be minimal and need not be highlighted. Still, the costs and benefits of the periodic system must be weighed against the cost and benefits of the perpetual system before a decision can be made regarding the inventory accounting system to be used by the institution.

Extended Example

The following information is available regarding the medical supplies inventory of the South Street Medical Center on July 1, 19X1.

Medical Supply A
1,060 units; cost: $9.18 per unit
Total cost: $9,730.80
Medical Supply B
381 units; cost: $37.50 per unit
Total cost: $14,287.50

Hence, the total value of the medical supplies beginning inventory is $24,018.30. The activity for the year July 1, 19X1, to June 30, 19X2, is given below:

Inventory Purchases

Date	Supply Type	Units Purchased	Cost Per Unit
July 10	B	43	$42.75
October 1	A	234	$14.73
December 13	A	497	$21.18
May 11	B	73	$49.72

Inventory Issuances

Date	Supply Type	Units Used
July 3	A	197
August 10	B	211
September 21	A	432
October 9	B	62
December 3	A	361
January 9	A	218
April 6	B	39
May 8	B	101
June 30	A	18

In the following paragraphs, the cost of goods used and the value of the ending inventory are calculated under the weighted average, FIFO and LIFO costing methods, for both the perpetual and periodic accounting systems.

Weighted Average

The average cost of each item in the beginning inventory is equal to the unit price given above. Therefore, under the perpetual accounting system, the entry to record the issuance of 197 units of Medical Supply A on July 3, 19X1, would be as follows.

7/3/X1	Cost of Goods Used (A)	$1,808.46	
	Inventory (A)		$1,808.46

To record the issuance of 197 units of Medical Supply A at $9.18 per unit.

The next entry would be made on July 10, when 43 units of Medical Supply B are purchased.

7/10/X1	Inventory (B)	$1,838.25	
	Accounts Payable (·)		$1,838.25

To record the purchase of 43 units of Medical Supply B at $42.75 per unit.

This purchase changes the average cost of each of the 424 units of Medical Supply B as follows:

$$\text{Average Cost}_B = \frac{(381 \times \$37.50) + (43 \times \$42.75)}{381 + 43}$$

$$= \$38.032429 \text{ per unit.}$$

Hence, the following entry would be made to record the issuance of 211 units of Medical Supply B on August 10.

8/10/X1	Cost of Goods Used (B)	$8,024.84	
	Inventory (B)		$8,024.84

To record the issuance of 211 units of Medical Supply B at $38.032429 per unit.

The entries to record the issuance of 432 units of Medical Supply A on September 21 and to record the purchase of 234 units of Medical Supply A on October 1 are shown below.

9/21/X1	Cost of Goods Used (A)	$3,965.76	
	Inventory (A)		$3,965.76

To record the issuance of 432 units of Medical Supply A at $9.18 per unit.

10/1/X1	Inventory (A)	$3,446.82	
	Accounts Payable (·)		$3,446.82

To record the purchase of 234 units of Medical Supply A at $14.73 per unit.

This purchase changes the average cost of Medical Supply A as follows.

$$\text{Average Cost}_{\text{A}} = \frac{(431 \times \$9.18) + (234 \times \$14.73)}{431 + 234}$$

$$= \$11.132932 \text{ per unit.}$$

Prior to the purchase, 431 units of Medical Supply A remain in inventory. After the purchase, however, 665 units of Medical Supply A, costed at $11.132932 per unit, are in inventory.

If the entries are made for the remainder of the fiscal year, with the average cost being recomputed after each purchase, the total amount recorded in the Cost of Goods Used (A) account will be $13,891.79, and the total amount recorded in the Cost of Goods Used (B) account will be $15,707.39. Since a total of $29,599.18 of Medical Supply A and Medical Supply B are used during the year, the value of the ending inventory will be $13,860.21. This amount will be distributed between Medical Supply A and Medical Supply B as follows:

Medical Supply A
565 units; cost: $17.366881 per unit
Total value: $9,812.29
Medical Supply B
84 units; cost: $48.189485 per unit
Total value: $4,047.92

Under the periodic accounting system, on the other hand, the calculation of the cost of goods used is quite simple because the average cost of the inventory items is calculated only once, at the end of the fiscal year. In addition, the only journal entries required during the year are the entries to record the purchases of inventory items. These entries are listed.

7/10/X1	Purchases (B)	$1,838.25	
	Accounts Payable (·)		$1,838.25

To record the purchase of 43 units of Medical Supply B at $42.75 per unit.

10/1/X1	Purchases (A)	$3,446.82	
	Accounts Payable (·)		$3,446.82

To record the purchase of 234 units of Medical Supply A at $14.73 per unit.

12/13/X1	Purchases (A)	$10,526.46	
	Accounts Payable (·)		$10,526.46

To record the purchase of 497 units of Medical Supply A at $21.18 per unit.

5/11/X2	Purchases (B)	$ 3,629.56	
	Accounts Payable (·)		$ 3,629.56

To record the purchase of 73 units of Medical Supply B at $49.72 per unit.

On June 30, 19X2, the end of the fiscal year, the average cost of the items in each of the inventories would be calculated by dividing the cost of goods available for use during the year by the total number of units available for use during the year. The results of these calculations are as follows.

$$\text{Average Cost}_A = \frac{(1060 \times \$9.18) + (234 \times \$14.73) + (497 \times \$21.18)}{1060 + 234 + 497}$$

$$= \$13.235109 \text{ per unit}$$

$$\text{Average Cost}_B = \frac{(381 \times \$37.50) + (43 \times \$42.75) + (73 \times \$49.72)}{381 + 43 + 73}$$

$$= \$39.749115 \text{ per unit}$$

Of the 1,791 units of Medical Supply A available for use during the period, 565 units remain in the inventory on June 30, 19X2. Each of these items is costed at $13.235109, as are each of the 1,226 units of Medical Supply A used during the year. Consequently, the following entry would be made on June 30, 19X2.

6/30/X2	Cost of Goods Used (A)	$16,226.24	
	Purchases (A)		$13,973.28
	Inventory (A)		2,252.96

To record the use of 1,226 units of Medical Supply A, costed at $13.235109 per unit, and to adjust the balance in the Inventory (A) account to the proper value.

Similarly, of the 497 units of Medical Supply B available for use during the year, 84 units remain in inventory on June 30, 19X2. Each of these items and each of the 413 units used during the year are costed at $39.749115. The following entry would be made to record these amounts.

6/30/X2	Cost of Goods Used (B)	$16,416.38	
	Purchases (B)		$ 5,467.81
	Inventory (B)		10,948.57

To record the use of 413 units of Medical Supply B costed at $39.749115 per unit and to adjust the balance in the Inventory (B) account to the proper value.

Therefore, under the periodic accounting system and the weighted average costing method, a total of $16,226.24 of Medical Supply A and $16,416.38 of Medical Supply B are used during the year. Hence, the total cost of goods used during the year is $32,642.62 and the value of the ending inventory is $10,816.77. This amount is distributed between Medical Supply A and Medical Supply B as follows.

Medical Supply A
565 units; cost: $13.235109 per unit
Total value: $7,477.84

Medical Supply B
84 units; cost: $39.749115 per unit
Total value: $3,338.93

FIFO

When the FIFO costing method is used, the cost of goods used during the year is the same under both the perpetual and the periodic accounting systems (see Question 4-2). The same cost of goods used results under each accounting system because under the FIFO costing method, the oldest costs in the inventory are the first costs to be assigned to items leaving inventory. Since the costs of subsequent purchases are always the last costs to be assigned, the order of the flow of costs never changes, regardless of when the institution accounts for these costs. However, as illustrated below, the accounting entries under each system are slightly different.

Under the perpetual accounting system, each time an inventory item is purchased or requisitioned, a journal entry must be made. The following entries are exemplary of the entries required during the year.

7/1/X1	Cost of Goods Used (A)	$1,808.46	
	Inventory (A)		$1,808.46
	To record the issuance of 197 units of Medical Supply A costed at $9.18 per unit.		
7/10/X1	Inventory (B)	$1,838.25	
	Accounts Payable (·)		$1,838.25
	To record the purchase of 43 units of Medical Supply B at $42.75 per unit.		
8/10/X1	Cost of Goods Used (B)	$7,912.50	
	Inventory (B)		$7,912.50
	To record the issuance of 211 units of Medical Supply B costed at 37.50 per unit.		

If the entries were made for the remainder of the fiscal year, the total cost of goods used during the year would be $27,831.48. This total consists of $12,175.98 attributable to the use of Medical Supply A and $15,655.50 attributable to the use of Medical Supply B. Hence, the 565 units of Medical Supply A and the 84 units of Medical Supply B remaining in inventory would be valued at $11,528.10 and $4,099.81, respectively, and the total value of the ending inventory would be $15,627.91.

The same values would be assigned to the cost of goods used and the ending inventory under the periodic accounting system. However, the only entries that would be made during the period would be the entries to record the purchases of inventory (see pp. 100–101).

At the end of the fiscal year, the physical inventory would be counted. A total of 565 units of Medical Supply A and 84 units of Medical Supply B would remain in inventory. The following calculations would be necessary to ascertain the value of this ending inventory.

Medical Supply A — 565 units			
497 units	costed at $21.18	=	$10,526.46
68 units	costed at $14.73	=	1,001.64
565 units	Total value	=	$11,528.10

Medical Supply B — 84 units			
73 units	costed at $49.72	=	$3,629.56
11 units	costed at $42.75	=	470.25
84 units	Total Value	=	$4,099.81

Therefore, the adjusting entries on June 30, 19X2 would include the following.

6/30/X2	Cost of Goods Used (A)	$12,175.98	
	Inventory (A)	$ 1,797.30	
	Purchases (A)		$13,973.28
	Cost of Goods Used (B)	$15,655.50	
	Purchases (B)		$ 5,467.81
	Inventory (B)		$10,187.69

As expected, the cost of goods used and the value of the ending inventory are $27,831.48 and $15,627.91, respectively. Also, note that the amounts closed out of the Purchases accounts are identical to those amounts closed out under the periodic accounting system for the weighted average costing method.

LIFO

Unlike the FIFO costing method, amounts assigned to the cost of goods used and to the ending inventory may vary under the LIFO costing method, depending on whether the perpetual or the periodic accounting system is used. The LIFO costing method assigns costs to items leaving inventory, beginning with the most recent cost and proceeding through the costs toward the oldest cost. Thus, every purchase of inventory items changes the order of the costs not yet assigned to inventory items.

The journal entries for perpetual accounting and for periodic accounting under the LIFO costing method are similar to those illustrated above for the respective accounting systems. The calculation of the cost of goods sold and the value of the ending inventory under the perpetual accounting system are summarized in Tables 4-1 and 4-2.

Table 4-1 Inventory Costs: Medical Supply A, LIFO Perpetual

		Goods Purchased			Goods Used			Goods in Inventory (oldest to most recent costs)		
Date	Transaction	Units	Cost/Unit	Total Cost	Units	Cost/Unit	Total Cost	Units	Cost/Unit	Total Cost
7/1/X1	Beginning Inventory							1,060	$ 9.18	$ 9,730.80
7/3/X1	Issuance				197	$ 9.18	$ 1,808.46	863	9.18	7,922.34
9/21/X1	Issuance				432	9.18	3,965.76	431	9.18	3,956.58
10/1/X1	Purchase	234	$14.73	$ 3,446.82				431 234	9.18 14.73	7,403.40
12/3/X1	Issuance				234 127	14.73 9.18	4,612.68	304	9.18	2,790.72
12/31/X1	Purchase	497	21.18	10,526.46				304 497	9.18 21.18	13,317.18
1/9/X2	Issuance				218	21.18	4,617.24	304 279	9.18 21.18	8,699.94
6/30/X2	Issuance				18	21.18	381.24	304 261	9.18 21.18	$ 8,318.70
	Totals	731		$13,973.28	1,226		$15,385.38			

Table 4-2 Inventory Costs: Medical Supply B, LIFO Perpetual

		Goods Purchased			Goods Used			Goods in Inventory (oldest to most recent costs)		
Date	Transaction	Units	Cost/Unit	Total Cost	Units	Cost/Unit	Total Cost	Units	Cost/Unit	Total Cost
7/1/X1	Beginning Inventory							381	$37.50	$14,287.50
7/10/X1	Purchase	43	$42.75	$1,838.25				381 43	37.50 42.75	16,125.75
8/10/X1	Issuance				43 168	$42.75 37.50	$ 8,138.25	213	37.50	7,987,50
10/9/X1	Issuance				62	37.50	2,325.00	151	37.50	5,662.50
4/16/X2	Issuance				39	37.50	1,462.50	112	37.50	4,200.00
5/8/X2	Issuance				101	37.50	3,787.50	11	37.50	412.50
5/11/X2	Purchase	73	49.72	3,629.56				11 73	37.50 49.72	$ 4,042.06
	Totals	116		$5,467.81	413		$15,713.25			

Under LIFO costing and perpetual accounting, the total cost of goods used is $31,098.63 ($15,385.38 of Medical Supply A and $15,713.25 of Medical Supply B) and the value of the ending inventory is $12,360.76 ($8,318.70 of Medical Supply A and $4,042.06 of Medical Supply B).

Under a periodic accounting system, on the other hand, the value of the beginning inventory and the purchases information is compiled on June 30, 19X2, so that the goods available for use during the year can be calculated as follows.

	Medical Supply A		
	Units	Unit Cost	Total Cost
Beginning Inventory	1,060	$ 9.18	$ 9,730.80
10/1/X1 Purchase	234	14.73	3,446.82
12/13/X1 Purchase	497	21.18	10,526.46
Goods Available for Use	1,791		$23,704.08

	Medical Supply B		
	Units	Unit Cost	Total Cost
Beginning Inventory	381	$37.50	$14,287.50
7/10/X1 Purchase	43	42.75	1,838.25
5/11/X2 Purchase	73	49.72	3,629.56
Goods Available for Use	497		$19,755.31

When the physical inventory is counted on June 30, 19X2, a total of 565 units of Medical Supply A and 84 units of Medical Supply B will be in the inventory. Under the LIFO method, these units are costed at the oldest costs in inventory during the year. Hence, $5,186.70 of Medical Supply A and $3,150.00 of Medical Supply B constitute the ending inventory. Then, using the identity Cost of Goods Available for Use—Cost of Goods Used ≡ Cost of Ending Inventory, the cost of goods used during the period can be calculated.

Medical Supply A	$23,704.08—Cost of Goods Used (A) =	$ 5,186.70
	Cost of Goods Used (A) =	$18,517.38
Medical Supply B	$19,755.31—Cost of Goods Used (B) =	$ 3,150.00
	Cost of Goods Used (B) =	$16,605.31

Therefore, the total cost of goods used is $35,122.69 and the total value of the ending inventory is $8,336.70.

Conclusion

The values assigned to the cost of goods used and to the ending inventory can vary substantially, depending on the costing method and accounting system used. Predicting the ranges of these values and the relative magnitudes of the values occuring under the various combinations of costing methods and accounting systems is important in selecting an accounting system and a costing method. Even though developing comprehensive rules for ascertaining inventory and cost valuations is complex, general rules may be formulated which enable management to predict relative magnitudes. For example, in general when purchase prices of inventory items are rising (falling), the cost of goods used computed under the LIFO costing method will be greater (less) than the cost of goods used computed under the FIFO costing method, and the cost of goods used developed under the weighted average method will be greater (less) than the FIFO value, but less (greater) than the LIFO value, regardless of the accounting system used. Furthermore, the largest (smallest) value for the cost of goods used, given rising (falling) prices, will occur under LIFO costing used in conjunction with a periodic accounting system.

Consideration in Selecting a Costing Method and an Inventory Accounting System

Bookkeeping costs and the generation of information are other important factors in selecting an inventory accounting system and a costing method. Guidelines for selecting between timely information with high bookkeeping costs and less timely information with modest bookkeeping costs are outlined in the following paragraphs.

Direct Costs

Inventory items used in the direct care of patients or requisitioned on a specific case basis should be controlled by a perpetual accounting system. The rationale underlying this guideline is that accumulating total cost information in a timely fashion is important for billing purposes (see the case discussed in Chapter 1). In addition, the departmental designation associated with the perpetual accounting system facilitates the accumulation of costs on a departmental or functional area basis. This information is necessary for evaluation purposes.

Allocated Costs

A periodic accounting system should be used for inventory items which are not directly chargeable to a patient or to a particular department. Supporting this view is the fact that indirect costs are allocated to departments at year-end on some objective basis that yields an approximation of annual departmental usage. For example, the total cost of floor cleaning solution used during a particular year may be allocated by square footage per department. Since a periodic accounting system accounts for the total cost of inventory items not directly chargeable to a patient or a department at year-end and since the cost of operating a periodic accounting system is less than the cost of operating a perpetual accounting system, a periodic accounting system is preferred to a perpetual accounting system to account for indirect costs.

Inflation and Technological Innovation

LIFO costing in conjunction with a periodic accounting system generates the largest cost figures in a market of rising prices. Therefore, this combination should be used when inflation and technological innovation cause the purchase prices of inventory items to rise. The rationale underlying this guideline is twofold. First, most health care institutions are dependent on cost for reimbursement, whether the reimbursement system is retrospective or prospective. Therefore, accounting rules which develop the highest costs will yield the largest reimbursement. Second, if an institution or group is organized as a tax-paying entity, accounting rules which develop high costs reduce taxable income and thus reduce the income taxes that must be paid.

Electing LIFO: A Possible Risk

The LIFO costing method was devised originally to increase the expense deducted from revenue in profit oriented organizations and thus reduce taxable income and tax payments. However, most health care institutions are interested in LIFO costing because this method increases reimbursable costs. Unfortunately, a latent risk lies in electing the LIFO method in an inflationary economy.

Because the LIFO method assigns the most recent costs (which are also the highest costs in an inflationary economy) to the items leaving inventory, the oldest (and lowest) costs remain in the ending inventory. After several periods, the old costs that remain in inventory may be significantly lower than the costs assigned to items currently leaving inventory. In this case, if the inventory must be depleted, the old costs will be assigned to items leaving inventory and the costs of goods used may be significantly lower than expected.

For example, assume that the following information is available regarding the inventory of Supply Q at the Winkler Hospital on December 31, 19X5.

Date of Purchase	Units	Unit Cost	Total Cost
1/9/X1	11	$19.72	$ 216.92
1/3/X2	190	28.40	5,396.00
1/29/X3	49	43.80	2,146.20
2/2/X4	27	68.40	1,846.80
1/15/X5	13	93.81	1,219.53
Total	290		$10,825.45

Further assume that for prospective reimbursement purposes, the administrator at the Winkler Hospital estimates that the cost per unit of Supply Q during 19X6 will be $112.46 (the unit cost from the last invoice). If during 19X6, 185 units of Supply Q are used and, due to a market shortage, no purchases are made, the actual LIFO usage cost of Supply Q will be $7,938.93, while the reimbursement, based on the administrator's estimate, will be $20,805.10. The $12,866.17 difference between the estimated cost and the actual cost will be a source for a reimbursement adjustment at the appropriate audit time. Similarly, if Winkler Hospital were a tax-paying entity, the tax payments in 19X6 would be $\alpha \times$ $12,866.17 (where α is the tax rate) greater than expected.

Hence, inventory management is very important under LIFO costing. Purchases must be managed so that old inventory costs are not assigned to items leaving inventory. In addition, excess purchases, which increase inventory carrying costs by causing the accumulation of additional inventory layers that cannot be used in future periods, also must be avoided. In summary, inventory must be managed so that the number of units in the ending inventory each period falls within a reasonable range.

Inventory Cost Adjustments

In preceding sections, the unit purchase prices of inventory items were used to cost the inventory. Although unit purchase prices may be a basis for assigning inventory costs in some cases, other situations may require adjustments to the purchase prices before inventory costs are assigned. For example, the shipping costs paid by the institution in acquiring the inventory and the cost savings from purchase discounts have an effect on the total amount of cash disbursed to acquire inventory. Therefore, these costs and cost savings should be apportioned among the appropriate units to adjust the inventory purchase prices before costs are assigned to the inventory.

Under a perpetual accounting system, these apportionments should be made each time the institution pays inventory shipping costs and each time a purchase discount transaction occurs (i.e., when discounts are taken under the gross price method or when discounts are lost under the net price method). Under a periodic accounting system, on the other hand, these apportionments should be made at year-end with the appropriate costs and cost savings being apportioned between the cost of goods used and the items remaining in inventory at year-end. In either case, the computations and bookkeeping necessary to apportion these costs and cost savings are considerable (see Problem 4-6).

A simpler and more economical means of handling the costs and cost savings that affect the unit purchase prices of inventory items is to record them in separate accounts and to treat them as a period adjustment to the cost of goods used. Under this method, shipping costs are debited to a Transporation-In account, a Purchase Discounts Taken account is credited for the amount of the discount taken when payments are made within the discount period under the gross price method, and a Purchase Discounts Lost account is debited for the amount of the discount lost when payments are made after the discount period has expired under the net price method. At year-end, the amount recorded in each of these accounts is closed to the Cost of Goods Used account. Hence, all shipping costs incurred, all discounts taken, and all discounts lost during a period adjust the expenses of that period.

This policy of expensing costs in the period in which they are incurred is directly contrary to the accrual method of accounting[2] and usually will cause a misstatement of the cost of goods used during the period. However, any misstatement that occurs as a result of expensing these costs usually is insignificant because the number of items in ending inventory is relatively constant over time and the costs or cost savings that would be apportioned to those items do not change substantially from one accounting period to the next. Hence, the costs or cost savings that would be apportioned to the goods used are well estimated by the shipping costs incurred and the discounts taken or lost during the period

The Lower of Cost or Replacement Cost Rule

Another adjustment to inventory unit costs is needed when the utility of the inventory items, as reflected in the market price, falls below the recorded unit cost. This reduction in utility may be caused by physical deterioration, obsolescence, or a reduction in the replacement cost. In these cases, the value of the inventory should be written down to coincide with the replacement cost. This adjustment recognizes the inventory shrinkage loss in the period in which it is realized and results in an accurate matching of revenues and cost of goods used in future periods.

The rule for making this adjustment is often called the lower of cost or replacement cost rule.[3] "Cost" is defined as the amount at which the inventory items currently are recorded on the institution's books. "Replacement cost," is defined as the current market price of the inventory items. However, in making the adjustment to the lower of cost or replacement cost, replacement cost can neither be greater than the net realizable value (the estimated price to be charged to the patient less the estimated costs of implementing the inventory items), nor less than the net realizable value less the normal profit (where applicable). The process of selecting the appropriate valuation for the inventory is diagrammed in Figure 4-2.

Consider the following example for medical supplies D, E, F, and G.

Medical Supply	Number of Units	Cost	Replacement Cost	Estimated Patient Charge	Implementation Costs	Normal Profit
D	500	$10.29	$12.50	$12.50	$2.48	$3.20
E	600	15.98	9.80	13.00	1.98	3.98
F	600	9.50	15.58	18.75	1.50	1.50
G	400	8.40	7.33	10.30	1.03	1.29

The first step in calculating the correct inventory value for these supplies is to calculate the net realizable value (estimated patient charge less implementation costs) for each medical supply. The net realizable values for each medical supply in this case are as follows: D, $10.02; E, $11.02; F, $17.25; G, $9.27.

For supply D, the replacement cost of $12.50 is greater than the net realizable value of $10.02. Hence, replacement cost should be revalued at $10.02. Then this revalued replacement cost is then compared with the $10.29 recorded cost so that medical supply D can be recorded at the lower of the two costs. In this case, the inventory value of each unit of medical supply D should be equal to the net realizable value $10.02, or the recorded cost of each unit should be reduced by $.27. Hence, the following adjustment would be necessary.

Inventory Shrinkage	$135	
Inventory (D)		$135

To adjust the cost of 500 units of medical supply D from $10.29 per unit to the replacement cost of $10.02 per unit.

Figure 4-2 Valuation of Inventory

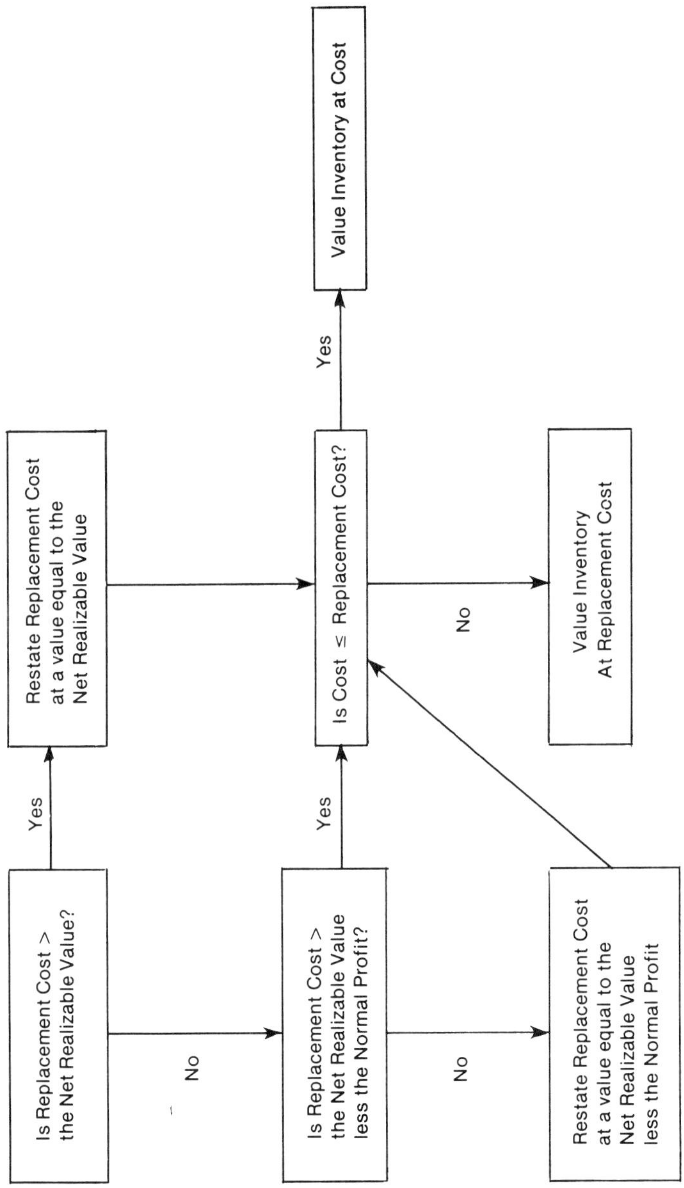

This process should be followed for medical supplies E, F, and G also. Table 4-3 shows the results of the lower of cost or replacement cost analysis for these supplies. The relevant data for selecting the appropriate costs are also given.

Table 4-3 Lower of Cost or Replacement Cost for Inventory Items E, F, and G

Medical Supply	Replacement Cost	Net Realizable Value	Net Realizable Value Less Normal Profit	Cost	Selected Cost
E	$ 9.80	$11.02	$ 7.04	$15.98	$9.80
F	15.58	17.25	15.75	9.50	9.50
G	7.33	9.27	7.98	8.40	7.98

The adjusting entry that would correct the inventory balances for these medical supplies is as follows.

Inventory Shrinkage	$3,876.00	
Inventory (E)		$3,708.00
Inventory (G)		168.00

To adjust the costs of 600 units of medical supply E and 400 units of medical supply C from $15.98 per unit and $8.40 per unit, respectively, to the replacement costs of $9.80 per unit and $7.98 per unit, respectively.

Of course, these adjustments should be made only if the total inventory shrinkage is significant.

In this example, the lower of cost or replacement cost rule is applied to each group of medical supplies. The items within each group in this case can be considered together because all of these items have the same recorded cost. If, however, the items within each group had varying costs, some higher and some lower than replacement cost, each item might have to be considered individually. Management must decide whether present and future income will be more accurately reflected by applying the lower of cost or replacement cost rule to individual inventory items or by applying the rule to groups of inventory items.

Similarly, the lower of cost or replacement cost rule may be applied simultaneously to two or more related inventory groups. For instance, if medical supplies E and F are always used together and patients are billed \$31.75 (\$13.00 + 18.75) for the use of these supplies, then the lower of cost or replacement cost rule could be applied to the combined costs of these two groups. If this were done, the recorded unit cost of supplies E and F would be \$25.48 (\$15.98 + 9.50) and the unit replacement cost of these supplies would be \$25.38 (\$9.80 + 15.58). In this case, the increase in the replacement cost of medical supply F has offset the decrease in the replacement cost of medical supply E. Hence, each of these supplies could be stated at cost.

The lower of cost or replacement cost adjustment is important in the health care field because third party payers often impose reimbursement ceilings. Hence, if the inventory costs are not adjusted when replacement costs are less than recorded costs, then, in subsequent periods, service costs may exceed the reimbursement ceiling of specific third party payers. However, if the adjustment is made, the Inventory Shrinkage account will increase general and administrative expenses in the current period and thus increase the costs of revenue-producing departments receiving cost stepdowns. Therefore, an estimate of expected inventory shrinkage should be included in the cost budget so that these costs can be included in service charges as overhead costs.

INVENTORY MANAGEMENT

In the past, inventory management was not an integral part of the institution's management program. Large amounts of inventory routinely were maintained for the convenience of the medical staff and to avoid the chance of being out of a particular medical supply. However, in the current economic environment, excess inventory needlessly restricts cash flows. At the same time, insufficient inventory may result in inadequate patient treatment and severe malpractice consequences. Therefore, an effective management program must safeguard against stockouts while maintaining an inventory level that will not restrict cash flows. Stockout problems can be avoided by ascertaining the size of the safety stock (i.e., the maximum amount of inventory that will be used between the time more inventory is ordered and the time the new order is delivered and ready for use), while cash outflows can be minimized through economic order quantity analysis.

Inventory Management: The Economic Order Quantity (EOQ)

Three costs are associated with acquiring and maintaining inventory: (1) the purchase price of the inventory, net of any appreciable discounts taken, (2) purchase order costs, and (3) inventory carrying costs. Purchase order costs include all the costs associated with processing purchase orders, while inventory carrying costs include the cost of funds committed to maintain inventory and the costs of security, storage, receiving, and dispensing. Given these costs for a specific inventory item and the expected yearly usage of the item and the number of units of inventory in each order, the total cost for inventory procurement and storage may be formulated as:

$$\text{(4-6)} \qquad TC = M \times (1 - D) \times EYU + P \times \left[\frac{EYU}{I}\right] + C \times \left[\frac{I}{2}\right]$$

where: TC represents total inventory maintenance and procurement costs;
M represents the average per unit purchase price of the inventory items;
D represents any discount available on the purchase of inventory items;
EYU represents expected yearly usage (in units);
P represents the purchase order cost per order;
I represents the number of units in each inventory order[4]; and
C represents the per unit inventory carrying cost.

The resources needed to maintain and order inventory can be minimized by finding the value for I that minimizes this total cost function. Equation (4-6) is minimized through the usual calculus methods as follows.

$$\frac{dTC}{dI} = -P \times \left[\frac{EYU}{I^2}\right] + \frac{C}{2} = 0$$

which may be written as:

$$\frac{P \times EYU}{I^2} = \frac{C}{2}$$

and simplified as:

$$\text{(4-7)} \qquad \hat{I} = \left[\frac{2 \times P \times EYU}{C}\right]^{1/2}$$

This value, $\hat{I}$, is called the economic order quantity (EOQ). The EOQ is the number of units of inventory that should be ordered each time inventory reaches the safety stock level because orders of this size will minimize the costs of acquiring and maintaining inventory.

For example, assume that the cost of processing a purchase order is \$1.85 and that the carrying cost for this inventory item is \$.50 per unit. If 10,000 units are expected to be used this year, the EOQ is computed as:

$$\text{(4-8)} \qquad \text{EOQ} = \left[\frac{2 \times \text{P} \times \text{EYU}}{\text{C}}\right]^{1/2}$$

$$= \left[\frac{2 \times \$1.85 \times 10{,}000}{\$.50}\right]^{1/2}$$

$$= 272 \text{ units}$$

and 37 orders (i.e., 10,000/272) should be placed during the year.

Changes in the EOQ will occur with changes in EYU, P, or C. Careful examination of the EOQ function shows that increases in EYU or inceases in P will increase the amount in the numerator of equation (4-8) and, thereby increase the EOQ. Conversely, increases in C will increase the denominator of equation (4-8) and decrease the EOQ. The magnitude of any change in the EOQ resulting from a change in EYU, P, or C can be computed by substituting the new values of EYU, P, or C in equation (4-8) and subtracting the new value of the EOQ from the former value (see Problem 4-3).

The EOQ model provides information useful in efficiently managing inventory and, therefore, may aid in conserving institutional resources. However, in order for the EOQ model to be used effectively, purchase order costs, inventory carrying costs, and expected yearly usage must be defined specifically and measured accurately. Guidelines for assigning useful values to each of these parameters are given below.

Purchase Order Cost Coefficient: P

The cost of processing each purchase order can be computed by summing the expected annual costs of the purchasing department (or the purchasing function, including salaries, equipment, indirect costs, etc.) and then dividing this expected total cost by the total number of purchase orders expected to be processed during the year. The expectations regarding annual costs and the number of purchase orders processed annually usually are derived from historical data. Of course, if a new method of processing purchase orders is anticipated or if demand is expected to change dramatically, the estimates must reflect these changes.

Computing the expected cost of processing each purchase order yields the most objective measure of P. Other approaches attempt to measure the marginal or incremental cost of processing various orders. These approaches are arbitrary, and usually cannot be defended on an objective measure basis (see Question 4-11).

Inventory Carrying Cost Coefficient: C

The cost of holding each unit of inventory can be computed by summing the institutional cost of funds[5], the expected annual costs of the inventory storage area (apportionment of assumed rent), the expected annual salaries or wages of personnel involved in the security, receipt, and issuance of inventory, the expected annual indirect costs associated with inventory storage, etc., and then dividing these expected total storage and issue costs by the average number of units expected to be in inventory during the year. Since the number of units in inventory during the year will range between zero and the total number of units expected to be in each inventory order, the average number of units expected to be in inventory during the year is equal to one-half the total number of units expected to be in each inventory order (see Question 4-9). Again, historical data usually can be used to derive the relevant expected values.

Expected Yearly Usage: EYU

Precisely estimating the expected yearly usage is important because expectations regarding the total units available for use and the number of purchase orders to be processed during the year are dependent on expected yearly usage. However, precise estimations of expected yearly usage often are difficult to make. While sophisticated models have been derived to forecast demand, experience shows that reasonable approximations of yearly usage often can be obtained from individuals responsible for ordering inventory items and from individuals who use the inventory items.

Safety Stock

The safety stock is the amount of inventory that the institution must have on hand when new orders are placed if the chance of a stockout is to be minimized. The size of the safety stock is a function of:

1. the variability of inventory usage;
2. the time lag between ordering and receiving inventory purchases;
3. the importance of the inventory items in medical treatment plans and the quantity of acceptable alternative inventory items commonly available; and
4. the size of the EOQ.

Hence, these four parameters can be used to devise a safety stock heuristic for calculating the size of the safety stock that will reduce the risk of a stockout to a desirable level. The heuristic, outlined below, is a simple and efficient means of calculating the size of the safety stock.

Safety Stock Heuristic

Step 1: Examine the historical data on inventory usage and segment the annual (assuming the control period is one year) statistics into periods of materially different usage. The variability in inventory usage should be fairly constant between years (i.e., heavy usage should occur during the same months each year). The average yearly inventory usage also should be computed from this data as follows:

$$\text{AYU} = \frac{\sum_{j=1}^{m} \text{YU}_j}{m} \tag{4-9}$$

where: AYU represents the average yearly usage computed from the historical data;
YU_j represents the yearly usage in year j; and
m represents the number of years for which relevant data can be collected (see Problem 4-12).

Step 2: Once the periods of varying usage are defined, the mean usage and the standard deviation in usage between the time a purchase order is initiated and the time the ordered goods are available for use (henceforth called the order lag) should be computed for each period (see Problem 4-8). Then the expected yearly usage during the respective order lags in the ensuing year can be computed as follows (see Question 4-15):

$$\text{EU}_i = \frac{\mu_i}{\text{AYU}} \times \text{EYU} \qquad i = 1, \ldots, k \tag{4-10}$$

where: EU_i represents the expected usage during an order lag in period i;

μ_i represents the historical mean usage during an order lag in period i;
AYU represents the average yearly usage as computed from historical data (equation (4-9));
EYU represents the expected yearly usage for the ensuing year; and
k represents the number of periods of materially different usage.

Step 3: Through discussions with the administration and the medical personnel using the inventory, ascertain the maximum acceptable stockout percentage. Then convert this percentage into a distribution measure (e.g., a z-score). For example, if the maximum acceptable stockout percentage is five percent and if the historical usage deviations are distributed normally about the mean, then the distribution measure, or z-score, associated with this stockout percentage is 1.65. (Note: this is a one-tail test value.) Once the density conversion of the maximum stockout percentage is determined, the safety stock level in each period can be computed as:

$$SS_i = EU_i + \frac{\sigma_i}{\mu_i} \times EU_i \times z \tag{4-11}$$

where: SS_i represents the size of the safety stock in period i that will reduce the chance of a stockout to an acceptable level;
EU_i represents the expected usage during an order lag in period i;
σ_i represents the historical standard deviation in usage during an order lag in period i;
μ_i represents the historical mean usage during an order lag in period i; and
z represents the density conversion of the minimum acceptable confidence level regarding the chance of a stockout.

Step 4: If the size of the safety stock computed in Step 3 is less than or equal to the EOQ, then new orders should be placed when the inventory reaches the safety stock level. However, if the size of this computed safety stock is greater than the EOQ, new orders will have to be placed before prior orders are received. Hence, a new safety stock level must be computed. For example, assume that the SS_i computed in Step 3 is 171 units and that the EOQ is 100 units. The expected daily inventory usage can be computed by calculating the historical average daily usage as shown in equation (4-12) and then adjusting this amount to reflect the expected yearly usage in the ensuing year as shown in equation (4-13).

$$\text{(4-12)} \qquad ADU_i = \frac{MU_i}{t_i}$$

where: ADU_i represents the average daily usage computed using historical data;
MU_i represents the historical mean usage in period i; and
t_i represents the number of days in period i.

$$\text{(4-13)} \qquad EDU_i = \frac{ADU_i}{AYU} \times EYU$$

where: EDU_i represents the expected daily usage in period i;
ADU_i represents the historical average daily usage in period i;
AYU represents the historical average yearly usage; and
EYU represents the expected yearly usage in the ensuing year.

If the computed EDU_i is 50 units and the EU_i in Step 2 is 150 units, the expected order lag can be computed as 3 days using equation (4-14).

$$\text{(4-14)} \qquad EOL_i = \frac{EU_i}{EDU_i}$$

where: EOL_i represents the expected order lag during period i;
EU_i represents the expected usage during an order lag in period i; and
EDU_i represents the expected daily usage in period i.

This expected order lag information can be used to compute the maximum expected daily usage during an order lag in period i as shown in the following equation.

$$\text{MEDU}_i = \frac{\text{SS}_i}{\text{EOL}_i} \tag{4-15}$$

where: MEDU_i represents the maximum expected daily usage during an order lag in period i;
SS_i represents the size of the safety stock in period i that will reduce the chance of a stockout to an acceptable level; and
EOL_i represents the expected order lag during period i.

In the given example, the MEDU_i would be computed as follows:

$$\text{MEDU}_i = \frac{\text{SS}_i}{\text{EOL}_i}$$

$$= \frac{171}{3}$$

$$= 57 \text{ units.}$$

Given this information, the size of a new safety stock level that is less than the EOQ can be determined as shown in Table 4-3.

In cases I, II and III, inventory orders are received and ready for usage on March 2, 4, and 5. Since the expected order lag is three days, each of these orders should have been placed three days earlier on April 29, March 1 and March 2, respectively. In case IV, on the other hand, inventory orders are received and ready for usage on March 2, 4, and 6. Each of these orders should have been placed on April 29, March 1 and March 3. Notice that in all of these cases (I, II, III and IV), the number of units remaining in inventory on the inventory order dates is less than 71 units. This pattern indicates that each time the inventory is reduced to 71 units, a new order should be placed. Consequently, the revised safety stock level is 71 units. A more direct means of computing the size of the revised safety stock is represented in equation (4-16).

$$\text{Revised SS}_i = \text{SS}_i - \phi \times \text{EOQ} \tag{4-16}$$

where: ϕ represents the largest integer by which the EOQ can be multiplied while maintaining $\text{SS}_i > \phi \times \text{EOQ}$.

Table 4-3 Inventory Usage and Receiving Patterns

		Number of Units			
Date	Transaction	Case I	Case II	Case III	Case IV
3/1/X0	Beginning Inventory	82	83	84	85
	Maximum Expected Usage	57	57	57	57
3/2/X0	Beginning Inventory	25	26	27	28
	Receive	100	100	100	100
	Available for Use	125	126	127	128
	Maximum Expected Usage	57	57	57	57
3/3/X0	Beginning Inventory	68	69	70	71
	Maximum Expected Usage	57	57	57	57
3/4/X0	Beginning Inventory	11	12	13	14
	Receive	100	100	100	100
	Available for Use	111	112	113	114
	Maximum Expected Usage	57	57	57	57
3/5/X0	Beginning Inventory	54	55	56	57
	Receive	100	100	100	0
	Available for Use	154	155	156	57
	Maximum Expected Usage	57	57	57	57
3/6/X0	Beginning Inventory	97	98	99	0
	Receive	0	0	0	100
	Available for Use	97	98	99	100

This heuristic is a simple and efficient means of calculating the size of the safety stock. An example is given below to illustrate the use of the heuristic.

Example

Assume that the following data has been extracted from the historical inventory usage records of the Cedars Hospital.

	Total Usage				Mean Usage During Order Lag	Standard Deviation
Period	19X3	19X2	19X1	19X0		
Jan.-May	4,896	4,721	4,496	4,347	255.67	40.22
June-Aug.	1,156	1,002	988	954	82.98	13.52
Sept.-Dec.	2,699	2,476	2,380	2,229	178.78	25.74
Total	8,751	8,199	7,864	7,530		

Given this information, the average yearly usage can be computed as follows.

$$\begin{aligned}\text{AYU} &= \frac{8{,}751 + 8{,}199 + 7{,}864 + 7{,}520}{4}\\ &= \frac{32{,}344}{4}\\ &= 8{,}086 \text{ units.}\end{aligned}$$

If the expected usage in 19X4 is 9,400 units, the expected usage during an order lag in each period in 19X4 can be computed as follows.

$$\begin{aligned}\text{EU}_1 &= \frac{255.67}{8{,}086} \times 9{,}400\\ &= 297.22 \text{ units}\\ \text{EU}_2 &= \frac{82.98}{8{,}086} \times 9{,}400\\ &= 96.46 \text{ units}\\ \text{EU}_3 &= \frac{178.78}{8{,}086} \times 9{,}400\\ &= 207.83 \text{ units.}\end{aligned}$$

Assume that discussions between the administration and the medical personnel using the inventory arrive at an acceptable stockout level of one percent. The normal density conversion of this percentage is 2.33. Hence, the safety stock level in each period in 19X4 would be computed as follows:

$$\begin{aligned}\text{SS}_1 &= 297.22 + \frac{40.22}{255.67} \times 297.22 \times 2.33\\ &= 407 \text{ units}\\ \text{SS}_2 &= 96.46 + \frac{13.52}{82.98} \times 96.46 \times 2.33\\ &= 134 \text{ units}\\ \text{SS}_3 &= 207.83 + \frac{25.74}{178.78} \times 207.83 \times 2.33\\ &= 278 \text{ units.}\end{aligned}$$

Note that all fractional units are rounded to the next whole unit. This procedure is necessary to keep stockouts within the one percent acceptable level.

Assume that the size of the EOQ is 314 units. In the first period, the computed safety stock level is greater than the EOQ. Hence, a new safety stock level must be computed for this period as follows:

$$\text{Revised } SS_1 = 407 - 1 \times 314$$

$$= 93 \text{ units.}$$

Therefore, new inventory orders will be placed during the first period when the inventory is reduced to 93 units. During the second and third periods, new inventory orders will be placed when the inventory is reduced to 134 units and 278 units, respectively.[6]

SAFEGUARDING THE INVENTORY

Effective inventory management does not end with minimizing the cash expended for inventory or with controlling the size of the safety stock. Safeguarding the inventory on hand is equally important. A series of steps are outlined below to aid in safeguarding the institution's inventory from theft, loss, spoilage, and obsolescence.

The first step in safeguarding the inventory is to restrict access to inventory storage areas. This requires hiring an inventory clerk who is responsible for filling inventory requisitions. A well-defined job description, incorporating the record keeping procedures necessary for removing items from inventory, should be designed for this position. In addition, procedures must be established for removing items from inventory when the inventory clerk is not on duty (see Question 4-8).

The second step in safeguarding the inventory involves documenting who requested what items from inventory, what department required the inventory items, and why the items are needed. Prenumbered inventory requisition forms aid in gathering this information. These requisition forms should be filled out and signed by the individuals in authority in the department requiring the inventory. Once the requisition is filled, the form should be countersigned by the inventory clerk. If requisitions cannot be filled completely due to stockouts, this information should be noted on the requisition form by the inventory clerk. One copy of this requisition should be sent to the accounting department, a second to the department making the requisition, and a third retained by the inventory clerk.

The third step in inventory protection involves reducing the risk of spoilage and obsolescence. As inventory items are received, they should be inspected and counted to see that the shipment agrees with the number and type of items ordered. In addition, the items should be checked for breakage, spoilage dates, etc. Then, the inventory items should be placed in stock so that the most recently received items will be the last to be used (FIFO physical flow).

Periodic inventory counts and inventory audits are the final step in safeguarding the inventory. Both should be performed at the end of the fiscal year so that the institution's financial statements can be prepared. However, periodic surprise inventory counts and inventory audits also should be performed to assure that the procedures outlined for inventory control are being followed on a regular basis.

Inventory safeguarding is an important aspect of inventory management. The cost savings from taking purchase discounts, from ordering the EOQ, and from minimizing stockouts will never offset inventory losses arising from theft, spoilage, and obsolescence. The costs incurred in safeguarding the inventory usually are dollars well spent in protecting a valuable stock of resources.

NOTES

1. See Appendix A for a discussion of temporary accounts.
2. See Appendix A for a discussion of the accrual method of accounting.
3. See *Accounting Research Bulletin* No. 43 for a detailed discussion of this accounting concept.
4. I/2 is the average number of units in inventory between orders, assuming no "beginning inventory."
5. The institutional cost of funds is the amount of interest that the institution would have to pay, on the average, to borrow money to purchase inventory (see Question 4-13). Hence,

$$C_f = r \times M \times (1 - D) \times I/2$$

where: C_f represents the total cost of funds;
r represents the interest rate charged on borrowed funds;
M represents the average unit price of the inventory items;
D represents any discount available on the inventory items; and
I/2 represents the average number of units in inventory between orders, assuming no beginning inventory.

6. Computing the safety stock required during a transition period, i.e., the end of one period and the beginning of another, must be dealt with as the situation dictates. There are many possibilities which may occur in practice. In general, the lag time, anticipated usage of both periods, and the expected arrival of orders previously placed must be evaluated so that the proper amount of safety stock may be maintained during the transition period.

Questions and Problems

Question 4-1. Which accounting system, perpetual or periodic, would be the simplest to implement in an urban teaching hospital? Which accounting system would provide for the best control over inventory? Which accounting system would facilitate billing patients and third party payers?

Question 4-2. Prove that the inventory value developed under FIFO perpetual always equals the inventory value developed under FIFO periodic.

Question 4-3. If a proprietary hospital is attempting to minimize the income tax it must pay in any particular year, which costing method should be selected if prices are rising: LIFO, FIFO, or Average? Would your answer differ if the sources of inventory were undependable (i.e., if due to work slowdowns and trucking strikes, inventory may not be delivered in a timely manner?

Question 4-4. Will inventory ever have to be revalued to the lower of cost or replacement cost when prices are falling? Does your answer depend on which costing method is used?

Question 4-5. Assume that management's policy is to take time discounts whenever they are offered, regardless of when the invoice is paid. How would this information be incorporated into the inventory total cost equation?

Question 4-6. Assume that inventory storage costs (H(X)) behave according to the following function:

$$H(X)\begin{cases} \$0, & 0 \leq X \leq X_A \\ \$B, & X > X_A \end{cases}$$

where: X is a variable representing the size of an inventory order; X_A is an inventory order of a particular size; and B represents the dollar per unit storage cost.

How would this information affect the economic order quantity?
How should it be incorporated into the economic order formula?

Question 4-7. What information sources would management use to gather information for developing a safety stock algorithm? How would management ascertain the percentage of the time that a stockout would be acceptable? Be specific in answering this question.

Question 4-8. Develop a control system for safeguarding inventory during the late night shift when the inventory storage area officially is closed but can be opened for the needed supplies if an emergency occurs.

Question 4-9. Demonstrate that the value of the inventory carrying cost coefficient is best estimated by the total inventory storage and issue costs divided by one-half the number of units in each inventory order.

Question 4-10. One of the staff physicians recently attended a management seminar on inventory control. This physician asks you to explain the following comment made by one of the speakers:

> When the value of the EOQ is significantly above or below its expected value, the carrying cost (C) and purchase order cost (P) coefficients may have to be adjusted and the EOQ equation resolved.

Question 4-11. In the text, the total costs (fixed and variable) of purchasing, maintaining, and issuing inventory were used to ascertain the economic order quantity. Other options would be to use variable costs or marginal costs to compute the economic order quantity. Discuss the implications of using:

1. average total cost (a full cost approach),
2. variable costs, or
3. marginal costs.

Question 4-12. a. Is it possible that an institution may not have enough space to store the EOQ of its various inventory items?
b. If the inventory space is inadequate, how would this problem be resolved? Evaluate the costs and benefits of each option.

Question 4-13. One measure of the cost of funds is the institution's borrowing rate. Discuss the following alternative measures of the cost of funds on the EOQ model:

a. The weighted average rate of interest on all outstanding debt,
b. The anticipated rate of interest at some time in the future, and
c. The internal rate of return, i.e., the institutional rate of earning on invested assets.

Question 4-14. The safety stock heuristic assumes that the standard deviation is a constant proportion of the mean over specific periods. Graph this assumption where the ordinate represents utilization and the abscissa represents time.

Question 4-15. How would you use regression analysis to estimate EU_i? Discuss the merits of using equation (4-10) to estimate EU_i rather than regression.

Problem 4-1. Consider the following inventory transactions of the Collins Clinic during 19X1:

	Purchases		Usage
	Number of units	Unit cost	Number of units
Jan. 1	106	$8.83	
Jan. 7			43
Feb. 27			41
March 3	34	6.93	
March 10			81
April 1	139	4.97	
June 30			16
June 30*	43	3.75	

*The purchase of June 30 has been recorded on the books but has not been received. When the order was placed on June 30, 19X1, the following entry was made:

Inventory or Purchases	$161.25	
Accounts Payable		$161.25

The beginning inventory on January 1, 19X1 was 48 units at $10.14 per unit.

Required:

a. Assuming the physical count is eight units short, how many units are on hand at 6/30/19X1?

b. Compute the value of the ending inventory, the cost of goods used, and shrinkage valuation for the eight missing units under each of the various costing methods and accounting systems.

c. Assume the following entry is made to reflect the inventory shortage:

Inventory Shrinkage	$81.12	
Inventory		$81.12

How was the price of $81.12 computed for the missing units? Was it proper? Defend your answer.

d. If the administrator wishes to maximize reimbursement, what costing method and inventory system should be selected? Why?

Problem 4-2. The salaries and other direct costs of the purchasing department of the KJCM HMO during 19X1 were $5,548.41. Fixed costs allocated to the purchasing department were $1,953.13. The number of purchase orders processed during 19X1 was 1,475. During 19X2, the volume of purchase orders is expected to increase by 10 percent to reflect the activity of a new research wing. Inflation during 19X1 was 12.5 percent; it is expected to be 12 percent in 19X2. The cost of inventory security and disbursement for 19X1 was $3,550. The average institutional cost of funds in 19X1 was 14 percent; it is expected to be 15 percent in 19X2. The fixed costs allocated for storage space amount to $.12 per cubic foot. There are 16,800 cubic feet of inventory storage available. The demand for inventory item A is expected to be 11,000 units in 19X2. The market price of inventory item A was $8.25 per unit during 19X1. Inventory item A is allocated 715 cubic feet of storage space. Assume that the activity of the purchasing department for particular inventory items is proportional to the ratio of the cubic footage required to store those inventory items to the total available inventory storage space.

a. What is the EOQ for inventory item A for 19X2, assuming the administrator wishes only to consider direct costs?
b. What is the EOQ for inventory item A for 19X2, assuming the administrator wishes to consider all costs?
c. What effect will proportionate cost increases in per unit inventory carrying cost and per unit purchase order cost have on the EOQ?

Problem 4-3. The carrying cost of inventory item Q at Pine Valley Hospital is $1.73 per unit and the purchase order cost is $7.53 per order. The cost of item Q is $5 per unit. No discounts are available for this item. The yearly demand for item Q is estimated to be 480 units.

Required:
a. What is the inventory management cost equation?
b. What is the EOQ? (Do not use the formula; use calculus to compute the answer.)
c. What will the change in the EOQ be for a change in the unit purchase order cost?

Problem 4-4. The hospital administrator of the Memorial Hospital wishes to use the average method of costing inventory usage. The hospital uses the periodic inventory system. The following information has been collected.

	Units	Price
Beginning Inventory	403	$11.00
Purchase 1	79	12.00
Purchase 2	134	8.00
Purchase 3	418	9.00

During the period 937 units were used.
The cost of goods used was computed as:

$$937 \times \$10 = \$9{,}370$$

The ending inventory was computed as:

$$97 \times \$10 = \$970$$

From this information, the cost of goods available for use is computed as $10,340.

Required:

a. How did the administrator compute the average cost?
b. Was this proper? If not, why not?
c. What is the proper average cost per unit?

Problem 4-5. The administrator of the E. Banks Clinic measures the following EOQ parameters.

Estimated Yearly Usage	19,500 units
Per Unit Carrying Cost	$2.19
Processing Costs per Purchase Order	$4.77

The clinic experiences two distinct periods of demand:

P_1: 13,000

P_2: 6,500

The EOQ is computed as:

$$\text{EOQ} = 291 = \left[\frac{2 \times \$4.77 \times 19{,}500}{\$2.19}\right]^{1/2}$$

One of the physicians, in working with the EOQ formula, computes the EOQ for period 1 as:

$$238 = \left[\frac{2 \times \$4.77 \times 13{,}000}{\$2.19}\right]^{1/2}$$

For period 2 the physician computes:

$$168 = \left[\frac{2 \times \$4.77 \times 6{,}500}{\$2.19}\right]^{1/2}$$

Required:
The physician does not understand why the EOQ for both periods 1 and 2 is less than the EOQ computed using the expected yearly usage. Explain why this happened.

Problem 4-6. a. Using the information in Problem 2-6, make the per unit cost adjustments for inventory item Supply A on (1) January 12 and January 18 under the gross price method, and (2) January 13 and February 2 under the net price method. Assume none of Supply A is used until March 1, 19X1, and the organization uses the LIFO costing method and a perpetual accounting system.

b. Make the necessary cost adjustments assuming that 60 percent of the inventory of Supply A is used on January 16, 19X1.

c. Discuss the difference between (1) allocating cost adjustments to specific inventory items, and (2) recognizing all cost adjustments as period costs.

Problem 4-7. The following information is recorded in the medical supplies inventory accounts of Riverside Hospital at the end of the fiscal year, June 30, 19X1.

Medical Supply	Number of Units	Cost
A	528	$ 9.86
B	659	18.53
C	493	5.32

Additional information regarding medical supplies A, B and C follow.

Case	Medical Supply	Replacement Cost	Estimated Patient Charge	Implementation Costs	Normal Profit
I	A	$10.36	$12.17	$ .98	$ .77
	B	17.29	20.22	1.01	1.10
	C	5.47	7.89	.52	1.98
II	A	11.52	13.20	1.60	1.04
	B	19.99	20.22	1.60	.66
	C	5.00	6.55	1.00	.52
III	A	9.86	9.86	.55	.89
	B	18.53	19.21	1.11	.59
	C	5.32	7.63	1.87	.54
IV	A	9.98	10.50	.55	.76
	B	19.51	25.25	2.34	2.30
	C	5.12	6.00	.55	.68

Required: a. Complete the following table by:

i) Computing the value at which each medical supply should be recorded in each case; and

ii) Computing the value at which the medical supplies inventory should be valued if medical supplies A, B, and C are always used together.

b. Give the adjusting entry for each case in part a(i).

	Value of Medical Supply			
Case	A	B	C	Aggregate
I				
II				
III				
IV				

Problem 4-8. Assume the administrator of the Oakdale Hospital collects the following order lag information for years 19X5, 19X6, and 19X7, for the three periods of materially different usage.

Year 19X5: Usage (in units) during an order lag
Period 1: 345, 255, 337, 353, 261, 259, 332, 280
Period 2: 81, 61, 77, 59, 59, 80, 82, 60
Period 3: 173, 131, 124, 123, 170, 169, 138, 177

Year 19X6: Usage (in units) during an order lag
Period 1: 257, 357, 331, 258, 333, 260, 259, 283
Period 2: 86, 83, 67, 63, 64, 84, 87, 65
Period 3: 132, 171, 125, 123, 137, 178, 168, 170

Year 19X7: Usage (in units) during an order lag
Period 1: 253, 250, 328, 351, 252, 252, 329, 280
Period 2: 68, 91, 88, 87, 90, 68, 69, 70
Period 3: 126, 172, 138, 168, 171, 133, 179, 124

The total inventory usage during the periods for years 19X5, 19X6, and 19X7 was

	Total Usage		
	19X7	19X6	19X5
Period 1	3,677	3,754	3,896
Period 2	1,016	964	900
Period 3	3,879	3,887	3,883
Total	8,572	8,605	8,679

The total usage of the inventory item in 19X8 is expected to be 9,100. A one percent stockout percentage is acceptable. The economic order quantity for this inventory item is 195.

Required: Compute the safety stock for each of the three periods.

Problem 4-9. The administrator of a prepaid medical group gathers the following information regarding purchases to be made for medical supply J.

Price of J before quantity discounts:	\$6.00
Unit purchase order cost (P):	2.12
Unit carrying cost (C):	.68
Expected yearly usage (EYU):	12,500 units

Quantity discount schedule:
$100 \leq$ order < 250: 1%
$250 \leq$ order < 400: 2%
$400 \leq$ order < 600: 2.5%

The administrator asks you to compute the EOQ. Is this the most economical order quantity? If not, what is? Defend your answer with computations.

Problem 4-10. The medical director asks you to estimate the amount of inventory theft that occurs during the year. Assuming it is significant, the director wants to take the necessary steps to hold theft to a minimum.

Required:
Prepare a report detailing how you would estimate inventory theft. Assume the dollar value of inventory theft is significant. Suggest the steps necessary to hold theft to a minimum. As part of your report, discuss the cost/benefit aspects of your proposal.

Problem 4-11. There are three transformations which are often used when the mean and variance are correlated as they are assumed to be in the safety stock heuristic. The square root transformation is used if the mean and variance are proportional. When this is the case, each observation is replaced by its square root. The logarithmic transformation is used if the variance is proportional to the square of the mean. When this is the case, each observation is replaced by its natural log. The reciprocal transformation is used if the standard deviation is proportional to the mean. When this is the case, each observation is replaced by its reciprocal. The result of each of these transformations when used appropriately is that changes in the mean are not correlated with changes in the variance or standard deviation.

Required: Assuming that the transformation was used appropriately, what effect would each of these transformations have on the safety stock heuristic?

Problem 4-12. The safety stock heuristic illustrated for the Cedars Hospital used years 19X0–19X3 to develop a projection of the expected usage during 19X4. This implies that all four years contain information useful in making the necessary usage projection.

Required:

a. Assume that at the beginning of 19X3 a new standard of medical care policy was instituted which affected inventory utilization. With this information, develop estimates of the expected usage during 19X4.

b. Suggest guidelines which would aid in ascertaining which years contained relevant information and therefore should be used to develop safety stock information.

Chapter 5

Financing the Organization: A Debt Perspective

Better is half a loaf, than no bread.

Heywood—Proverbs

In recent years, the demand for health care services has grown rapidly. Two major consequences of this increase in demand have been significant advances in medical technology and a serious deterioration of health care facilities. Hence, the need to modernize and improve current health care facilities has arisen. These renovations often require such large capital outlays that the traditional means of financing capital expenditures, including internally generated funds, philanthropic sponsorship, government grants, and ownership contributions, have been exhausted. Therefore, health care institutions have turned to long-term debt obligations as a means of financing capital expenditures (see Question 5-1).

Although many different types of long-term debt obligations are available to health care institutions, similar accounting entries are used to record the various long-term debt arrangements. The first section of this chapter will examine these accounting entries for the specific case of taxable bonds. In the second section of the chapter, the various financing alternatives will be discussed.

ACCOUNTING FOR BONDS

An institution enters into a bond agreement when a buyer is willing to give the institution cash in exchange for a bond indenture. The bond indenture specifies the length of time, called the *term of the bond,* that the institution can retain the buyer's money, the amount of money, called the *face value* of the bond, that the institution will pay to the buyer at the end of the term of the bond, and the interest rate, called the *stated interest rate,* that the institution will pay annually on the face value of the bond. The bond indenture also may have a *call provision* that specifies the conditions under which the institution may retire the bond before the term expires. Usually, the call provision will be exercised when the market rate of interest falls to a point where retiring the current bond issue and issuing a new lower interest bond is more economical than continuing to pay the high rate of interest on the bonds currently outstanding (see Problem 5-4). Further, the bond indenture must specify the conditions of *default.* A bond is considered to be in default when the institution breaches some portion of the bond contract. At the time of default, the face value of the bonds plus the accrued interest payable and any related penalties must be paid to the bondholder immediately.

Depending on the financial risk associated with the institution, the bond indenture also may contain certain restrictions. For example, the institution may be required to make payments to a *sinking fund,* a restricted interest-earning bank account, so that the value of the sinking fund is equal to the face value of the bonds at the end of the term. Furthermore, the institution may be subject to a *pledge of assets* or *financial ratio restrictions.* Under a pledge of assets restriction, a kind of mortgage agreement is established between the institution and the buyer of the bond whereby the buyer retains an ownership interest in the assets purchased with the funds generated from the bonds until the bond has been retired. The financial ratio restrictions, on the other hand, usually require that the institution's current assets always exceed the current liabilities by a specified minimum percentage. The institution's failure to meet any of the specified restrictions constitutes default (see Question 5-2).

An examination of the bond indenture specifications shows that three economic events during the term of the bond affect the financial status of the institution: the sale of the bonds, the payment of interest, and the retirement of the bonds. Each of these events constitutes a transaction that must be entered in the institution's accounting system.

Sale of Bonds

A good deal of time and resources must be devoted to develop the information required to issue a bond. Ordinarily, the institution must have certified financial statements for a number of years prior to the issuance. In addition, if the bonds are to be traded in established securities markets, the formal requirements of the particular exchange also must be satisfied.

An investment banker can aid in preparing an institution for a bond issuance (see Appendix 5-A). The investment banker can advise the institution about the legal requirements of different types of bond issuances and aid in gathering and developing the required preissuance information. In addition, the investment banker can help attract potential institutional investors, as well as ascertain the appropriate face value, term, and stated interest rate of the bonds.

The face value, term, and stated interest rate are crucial elements in the marketability of the bond. Ideally, bonds should sell at a price equal to their face value. However, fluctuations in the market interest rate between the time the bond certificates are printed and the time they are sold, inaccurate speculation, and the idiosyncracies of federal and state policy[1] may cause the stated interest rate to be higher or lower than the market interest rate. If the stated interest rate is higher than the market interest rate, investors will be willing to pay a *premium,* or price greater than the face value of the bond, to obtain the higher rate. If the stated interest rate is lower than the market interest rate, the institution will have to sell the bonds at a *discount,* i.e., reduce the price of the bonds to a value lower than the face value, to attract investors. In any case, the actual price at which the bond is sold generally is decided during negotiations between the investment banker and the investor.

Calculating the Price of the Bond

Calculating the price of the bond is relatively simple. The investor is willing to pay a price that is less than or equal to the present value of the future cash inflows from the bond. The institution, on the other hand, is willing to sell the bond at a price that is greater than or equal to the present value of the future cash outflows of the bond. Hence, the bond must sell for a price that is equal to the future bond cash flows if the institution and the investor are to agree on a price.

For example, suppose the Memorial Hospital is offering a bond with a face value of $100,000, a term of ten years, and a stated interest rate of six percent, interest payable semiannually. The cash flows from this bond issuance will be $3,000 (1/2 × .06 × $100,000) every six months for 20 six-month periods and a final payment of $100,000 at the end of 20 periods. Hence, if the market rate of interest is six percent, the bond issuance should sell for $100,000, calculated as follows:

$$\begin{aligned} \text{Price} &= \text{Present value of future cash flows} \\ &= \$3{,}000 \times 14.877475 + \$100{,}000 \times .55367576 \\ &= \$100{,}000 \end{aligned}$$

where: 14.877475 is the present value of an annuity (equal payments paid at equal intervals) of $1 invested at three percent for 20 periods;[2] and
.55367576 is the present value of $1 invested at three percent for 20 periods.[3]

However, if the market rate of interest is not six percent, the bonds should sell at a premium or at a discount. For example, if the Memorial Hospital bonds are sold when the market rate of interest is eight percent, the price of the bonds should be calculated as:

Price = Present value of future cash flows
= $3,000 × 13.590326 + $100,000 × .45638695
= $86,409.67

where: 13.590326 is the present value of an annuity of $1 invested at four percent for 20 periods; and
.45638695 is the present value of $1 invested at four percent for 20 periods.

In this case, the bonds should sell at a discount of $13,590.33 ($100,000 − $86,409.67). On the other hand, if the bonds are sold when the market rate of interest is four percent, the price of the bonds should be:

Price = Present value of future cash flows
= $3,000 × 16.351433 + $100,000 × .67297134
= $116,351.43

where: 16.351433 is the present value of an annuity of $1 invested at two percent for 20 periods; and
.67297134 is the present value of $1 invested at two percent for 20 periods.

In this case, the market interest rate is less than the stated interest rate and the bonds should sell at a premium of $16,351.43 ($116,351.43 − $100,000).

Journal Entries

Once the bonds have been priced, they can be sold. The sale of the bonds constitute an economic transaction that must be entered in the institution's accounting system. The accounting entry must record the amount of the premium or discount, as well as the amount of cash received and the face value of the bonds sold. The journal entries for the sale of the Memorial Hospital bonds at face value, at a discount, and at a premium are as follows.

Cash	$100,000.00	
6% Bonds Payable		$100,000.00

To record the sale of ten-year, six percent bonds at face value.

Cash	$86,409.67	
Discount on 6% Bonds Payable	13,590.33	
6% Bonds Payable		$100,000.00

To record the sale of ten-year, six percent bonds at a discount of $13,590.33.

Cash	$116,351.43	
Premium on 6% Bonds Payable		$16,351.43
6% Bonds Payable		100,000.00

To record the sale of ten-year, six percent bonds at a premium of $16,351.43.

Note that the value in the 6% Bonds Payable account is the same in every case because, regardless of the amount of cash received for the bond, $100,000 must be paid to the bondholders when the term expires.

Payment of Bond Interest

After the bonds have been sold, periodic interest payments must be made on specified interest payment dates. In all cases, whether the bonds are sold at a discount, at a premium, or at face value, the amount of cash paid to the bondholders on each interest payment date is equal to the product of the face value of the bond and the stated interest rate divided by the number of interest payments made annually. However, the interest expense incurred by the institution on each interest payment date is not necessarily equal to the amount of cash disbursed for interest payments. For example, if the bonds are sold at a discount, the institution ultimately pays the bondholders the difference between the face value of the bond and the amount of cash received for the bonds, as well as the periodic interest payments. Hence, the amount of the discount is like an additional interest payment that must be made at the end of the life of the bond.

To match expenses and revenues properly, this additional bond interest expense should be recognized over the term of the bond. Therefore, if bonds are sold at a discount or a premium, the amount recorded in the discount or premium account must be *amortized* over the term of the bond. As these accounts are amortized, the interest expense account will be appropriately increased or decreased.

Calculating the Bond Interest Expense

Two methods of amortizing bond discounts and bond premiums have been developed: the straight line method and the effective interest rate method. The straight line method apportions equal amounts of the discount or premium to each interest payment period. The effective interest rate method apportions the exact amount of the discount or premium which, in conjunction with the cash interest payment, makes the interest expense equal to the product of the market interest rate at the time the bonds were sold and the net bonds payable (net bonds payable = bonds payable − unamortized bond discount, or bonds payable + unamortized bond premium). Although the straight line method is more simple to use, the effective interest rate method accounts for the time value of money and, hence, reflects periodic interest expenses more accurately.

In the case of the Memorial Hospital bonds sold at a discount, the total discount to be amortized over the life of the bonds is $13,590.33. Under the straight line method of amortization, $679.52 ($13,590.33/20) would be amortized on each of the 20 interest payment dates. Hence, the bond interest expense on each interest payment date would be $3,679.52 ($100,000 × .06/2 + $679.52).

Under the effective interest rate method of amortization, on the other hand, the discount amortization on the first interest payment date would be calculated as follows:[4]

$$CIP + BDA = MIR \times NBP$$

where: CIP represents the cash interest payment;
BDA represents the bond discount amortization;
MIR represents the market interest rate at the time the bonds were sold; and
NBP represents the net bonds payable.

Hence, for the Memorial Hospital bonds sold at a discount, the bond discount amortization would be:

$$\begin{aligned} \text{CIP} + \text{BDA} &= \text{MIR} \times \text{NBP} \\ \$3{,}000 + \text{BDA} &= .04 \times \$86{,}409.67 \\ \text{BDA} &= \$456.39. \end{aligned}$$

Therefore, the bond interest expense on the first interest payment date would be $3,456.39. Similarly, on the second interest payment date, the effective interest rate amortization of the discount would be calculated as:

$$\begin{aligned} \text{CIP} + \text{BDA} &= \text{MIR} \times \text{NBP} \\ \$3{,}000 + \text{BDA} &= .04 \times (\$86{,}409.67 + \$456.39) \\ \text{BDA} &= \$474.64, \end{aligned}$$

and the bond interest expense would be $3,474.64.

Note that under the effective interest rate method of amortization, when bonds have been sold at a discount, the interest expense in the current period is greater than the interest expense in the prior period.[5] This is reasonable because the institution is paying interest on the bondholder's investment, and through the amortization of the bond discount, the bondholder's investment increases each period. Under the straight line method of amortization, however, the interest expense is the same in all periods. Therefore, interest expense is reflected more accurately under the effective interest rate method of amortization.

Of course if bonds are sold at face value, no discount or premium needs to be amortized. Calculating the interest expense in this case is straightforward because the interest expense is equal to the cash payment. In the Memorial Hospital bonds illustration, when the bonds are sold at face value, the interest expense each period is $3,000.

Journal Entries

The payment of interest and the amortization of the bond discount or premium constitute economic transactions that must be recorded in the institution's accounting system. The journal entry to record the payment of interest on the Memorial Hospital bonds sold at face value is:

Bond Interest Expense	$3000.00	
Cash		$3000.00

To record the semiannual interest payment on the ten-year, six percent bonds payable.

When bonds are sold at a discount or a premium, the journal entry to record the amortization of the discount or premium usually is included with the entry to record the cash interest payment. Hence, the cash interest payment and the effective interest rate amortization of the bond discount for the first period of the Memorial Hospital bonds would be recorded as follows:

Bond Interest Expense	$3,456.39	
Discount on 6% Bonds Payable		$ 456.39
Cash		3,000.00

To record the payment of interest and amortization of discount on ten-year, six percent bonds payable sold at a discount of $13,590.33.

Similarly, the entry to record the cash interest payment and the effective interest rate amortization of the bond premium for the first period of the Memorial Hospital bonds[6] would be:

Bond Interest Expense	$2,327.03	
Premium on 6% Bonds Payable	672.97	
Cash		$3,000.00

To record the payment of interest and the amortization of premium on ten-year, six percent bonds payable sold at a premium of $16,351.43.

Note that the cash interest payment is the same, $3,000, in each case, because the cash interest payment is computed from the stated interest rate and the face value of the bond.

Accrued Bond Interest Payable

The foregoing discussion is based on the assumption that one of the semiannual interest payment dates occurs at the end of the institution's fiscal year. However, these dates are not always coincident. For example, Memorial Hospital's fiscal year may end on June 30, while the interest payment dates of the bonds are October 31 and April 30. When this occurs, an adjusting journal entry must be made to recognize the interest expense associated with the portion of the interest payment period preceding the end of the fiscal year.

The concept of accrued interest payable is easily seen through an illustration. Assume that the Memorial Hospital bonds are sold at face value on May 1, 19X0. If the hospital's fiscal year ends on June 30, 19X0, the interest associated with the months of May and June must be recorded in the accounting records. These two months represent two-twelfths of the year; therefore, two-twelfths of the total interest payable for the entire year, or \$1,000 (2/12 × .06 × \$100,000), is associated with this period. Of course, when bonds are sold at face value, the annual interest expense is identical to the annual cash interest payments. Accordingly, the adjusting journal entry to record the bond interest expense for the period May 1, 19X0, to June 30, 19X0 is:

6/30/X0	Bond Interest Expense	\$1,000.00	
	Accrued Bond Interest Payable		\$1,000.00

To record the accrual of interest on ten-year, six percent bonds at 6/30.

A similar analysis can be conducted for the first four months of fiscal 19X0–X1. The interest expense for the months July through October, 19X0, would be \$2,000 (4/12 × .06 × \$100,000). Hence, when the interest is paid on October 31, 19X0, the following journal entry could be made:

10/31/X0	Bond Interest Expense	\$2,000.00	
	Accrued Bond Interest Payable	1,000.00	
	Cash		\$3,000.00

To record the payment of interest on ten-year, six percent bonds payable sold at face value.

Alternatively, a reversing entry[7] could be made in Memorial Hospital's accounting system on July 1, 19X0. Then the normal journal entry could be made to record the payment of bond interest on October 31. These two journal entries would be:

7/1/X0	Accrued Bond Interest Payable	\$1,000.00	
	Bond Interest Expense		\$1,000.00

To reverse the 6/30/X0 accrual of interest on ten-year, six percent bonds payable sold at face value.

10/31/X0	Bond Interest Expense	$3,000.00	
	Cash		$3,000.00

To record the payment of interest on ten-year, six percent bonds payable sold at face value.

Note that these two entries have the same effect as the first entry suggested for October 31, 19X0.

In the case of bonds sold at a discount or at a premium, the accrual of bond interest is more complicated. For example, if the Memorial Hospital bonds are sold on May 1, 19X0, when the market interest rate is eight percent, the accrued interest payable on June 30, 19X0, again will be $1,000. However, the interest expense will be greater than $1,000 due to the amortization of the bond discount. The following calculation must be made to compute the effective interest rate amortization of the bond discount for the period May 1, 19X0, through June 30, 19X0.

$$\text{CIP} + \text{BDA} = \text{MIR} \times \text{NBP}$$

$$\$1{,}000 + \text{BDA} = 2/12 \times .08 \times \$86{,}409.67$$

$$\text{BDA} = \$152.13$$

Hence, the entry on June 30, 19X0, would be:

6/30/X0	Bond Interest Expense	$1,152.13	
	Discount on 6% Bonds Payable		$ 152.13
	Accrued Bond Interest Payable		1,000.00

To record the accrual of bond interest and amortization of bond discount on ten-year, six percent bonds payable at 6/30.

This entry would be followed by a reversing entry on July 1, 19X0, and the regular journal entry to record the payment of bond interest on October 31, 19X0:

7/1/X0	Discount on 6% Bonds Payable	$ 152.13	
	Accrued Bond Interest Payable	1,000.00	
	Bond Interest Expense		$1,152.13

To reverse the 6/30/X0 accrual of bond interest on ten-year, six percent bonds payable sold at a discount of $13,590.33.

10/31/X0	Bond Interest Expense	$3,456.39	
	Discount on 6% Bonds Payable		$ 456.39
	Cash		3,000.00

To record the payment of interest and amortization of discount on ten-year, six percent bonds payable sold at a discount of $13,590.33.

The reversing entry is necessary in this case because continuously computing the amortization of the bond discount using a 1.33 percent (1/6 × .08) market interest rate is inconsistent with the original computation of the bond discount in which a semiannual four percent (1/2 × .08) market interest rate was used. The effect of compounding 1.33 percent every two months is not the same as the effect of compounding four percent semiannually. Hence, the bond discount amortization for each semiannual payment period must be computed using the four percent semiannual market interest rate.

Bond Retirement

The final economic event in the life of the bond is retirement. Bond retirement occurs when the face value of the bonds is paid to the bondholders. This event usually occurs at the end of the term of the bond. However, a decline in the market rate of interest may make early retirement economically desirable. Furthermore, if the institution fails to comply with any of the restrictions included in the bond indenture, the bonds will be in default and must be retired immediately. Hence, there are two basic types of bond retirement: retirement at maturity and early bond retirement.

Retirement at Maturity

At the end of the term of the bond, or when the bonds mature, the face value is paid to the bondholders. This transaction almost always occurs in conjunction with the payment of interest. Hence, the total cash disbursement to the Memorial Hospital bondholders on the bond retirement date would be $103,000. If the bonds are sold at face value, the following journal entry should be made on the bond retirement date:

6% Bonds Payable	$100,000.00	
Bond Interest Expense	3,000.00	
Cash		$103,000.00

To record the final interest payment and retirement of ten-year, six percent bonds sold at face value.

If the bonds are sold when the market rate of interest is eight percent, the journal entry on the bond retirement date should be:

6% Bonds Payable	$100,000.00	
Bond Interest Expense	3,961.54	
Discount on 6% Bonds Payable		$ 961.54
Cash		103,000.00

To record the final interest payment, final amortization of bond discount and retirement of ten-year, six percent bonds sold at a discount of $13,590.33.

Similarly, the following entry should be made to record the final payment on the Memorial Hospital bonds if the bonds are sold when the market rate of interest is four percent:

6% Bonds Payable	$100,000.00	
Bond Interest Expense	2,019.61	
Premium on 6% Bonds Payable	980.39	
Cash		$103,000.00

To record the final interest payment, final amortization of bond premium and retirement of ten-year, six percent bonds sold at a premium of $16,351.43.

Sinking Fund

If Memorial Hospital is subject to a sinking fund restriction that requires equal payments to the sinking fund on every interest payment date during the second half of the term of the bond, or if the hospital elects to participate in such a sinking fund arrangement, the journal entries to retire the bonds at maturity will be slightly different. If the restricted earnings account to which the sinking fund payments are made earns eight percent interest annually, then the hospital will have to make payments of $8,329.09[8] to the sinking fund on each interest payment date beginning with the first interest payment date in the second half of the term of the bond (see Problem 5-5). Hence, the following entry must be made in Memorial Hospital's accounting records on each interest payment date in the second half of the term of the bond:

Sinking Fund	$8,329.09	
Cash		$8,329.09

To record cash payments to the sinking fund for ten-year, six percent bonds payable.

As interest payments are made to the sinking fund, the hospital should debit the Sinking Fund account and credit an Interest Revenue account. Then, on the last bond interest date, the following entries should be made, assuming the bonds have been sold at face value:

Sinking Fund	$8,329.09	
Cash		$8,329.09

To record cash payments to the sinking fund for ten-year, six percent bonds payable.

6% Bonds Payable	$100,000.00	
Bond Interest Expense	3,000.00	
Sinking Fund		$100,000.00
Cash		3,000.00

To record the final interest payment and retirement of ten-year, six percent bonds sold at face value.

Hence, the journal entries required to retire bonds at maturity, given a sinking fund arrangement, are not substantially different from the entires to retire bonds at maturity when no sinking fund arrangement is in effect.

Early Bond Retirement

An early bond retirement occurs when the face value of the bonds is paid to the bondholders before the bonds mature. Early bond retirement may be elective, as in the case where a call provision is exercised, or compulsory, as in the case of default. These two types of early retirement are similar, and are distinguished from bond retirement at maturity, in that the retirement date is not always coincident with an interest payment date and in that any discount or premium on the bonds is not completely amortized on the retirement date. Hence, early bond retirement often gives rise to accrued interest payments and to gains or losses from the early retirement of premiums or discounts.

For example, assume that the Memorial Hospital bonds sold at face value on May 1, 19X0 are in default and are payable on May 31, 19X4, due to an inability to comply with the financial ratio restrictions of the bond indenture. The total payment to the bondholders will include the interest for the month of May, 19X4, in addition to the face value of the bonds. When this payment is made, the following journal entry will be recorded in Memorial Hospital's accounting records:

5/31/X4	6% Bonds Payable	$100,000.00	
	Bond Interest Expense	500.00	
	Cash		$100,500.00

To record the payment of accrued interest and early retirement of ten-year, six percent bonds sold at face value.

If the defaulted bonds have been sold at a discount of $13,590.33 and the effective interest rate method is used to amortize the discount, on the date of default Memorial Hospital's accounting records will show:

6% Bonds Payable	
	$100,000

Discount on 6% Bonds Payable	
$9,385.09	

Before the bonds can be retired, the accrued interest and the amortization of the discount must be computed for the month of May, 19X4. The accrued interest payable is $500 (1/12 × .06 × $100,000) and the amortization of the discount is computed as:

$$\text{CIP} + \text{BDA} = \text{MIR} + \text{NBP}$$

$$\$500 + \text{BDA} = (1/12 \times .08) \times \$90{,}614.91$$

$$\text{BDA} = \$104.10$$

Hence, two entries must be made to record the retirement of the defaulted bonds.

5/31/X4	Bond Interest Expense	$604.10	
	Discount on 6% Bonds Payable		$104.10
	Accrued Bond Interest Payable		500.00

To record the accrued interest and amortization of discount at 5/31/X4.

6% Bonds Payable	$100,000.00	
Accrued Bond Interest Payable	500.00	
Loss on Defaulted Bonds	9,280.99	
Discount on 6% Bonds Payable		$ 9,280.99
Cash		100,500.00

To record the payment of interest, early retirement, and loss on ten-year, six percent bonds sold at a discount of $13,590.33.

The journal entries to record the elective early retirement of the Memorial Hospital bonds are identical to the entries to record the retirement of the defaulted bonds except that the Loss on Defaulted Bonds account would be replaced by a Loss on Bond Retirement account. However, before the hospital elects to exercise the call provision and retire the bonds early, a detailed analysis must be made of the economics of early retirement because the bond indenture often specifies that a call premium, which is some percentage of the face value of the bonds or some percentage of the future interest payments or both, be paid to the bondholders when the call provision is exercised. The early retirement analysis evaluates the net cash outflows of retirement against the net cash inflows of reissuance at the lower interest rate. This type of analysis is illustrated below using the Memorial Hospital bonds.

Assume that on May 1, 19X0, Memorial Hospital issues the six percent bonds when the market interest rate is eight percent. Further assume that the bonds have a call provision that specifies that the bonds must be retired at 110[9] if called before May 1, 19X4, and that the bonds must be retired at 105 if called after May 1, 19X4. During May 19X4, the market rate of interest falls to four percent. Since the current market rate of interest is substantially below the market rate when the bonds were issued, the management wishes to determine the economic feasibility of calling the bonds on May 31, 19X4, and reissuing the same bonds on July 1, 19X4 (see Problem 5-4).

The first part of the early retirement analysis involves calculating the total cash outflow to call and retire the bonds. The hospital must pay the bondholders $105,000 (105 percent × $100,000) plus any accrued interest, which is $500 (1/12 × .06 × $100,000) in this case. The total cash outflow will include any general and administrative costs of calling, retiring, and reissuing the bond. In this case, these costs are assumed to be negligible. Hence, on the date of retirement, the following entries must be made in Memorial Hospital's accounting system.

5/31/X4	Bond Interest Expense	$ 604.10	
	Discount on 6% Bonds Payable		$104.10
	Accrued Bond Interest Expense		500.00

To record the accrued interest and amortization of discount at 5/31/X4.

6% Bonds Payable	$100,000.00	
Accrued Bond Interest Payable	500.00	
Loss on Bond Retirement	14,280.99	
Discount on 6% Bonds Payable		$ 9,280.99
Cash		105,500.00

To record the payment of interest, early retirement, and loss on ten-year, six percent bonds sold at a discount of $13,590.33.

The second portion of the analysis involves calculating the cash inflows from reissuing the bonds on July 1, 19X4. On that date, the hospital will receive cash equal to the present value of the future cash flows in the remaining 11 5/6 periods in the term of the bond, or $110,445.01[10] in this case, plus any accrued interest on the date of sale, or $1,000 (2/12 × .06 × $100,000). Hence, on the date of reissuance, the following journal entry would be made in Memorial Hospital's accounting system.

7/1/X4	Cash	$111,445.01	
	Bond Interest Expense		$ 1,000.00
	Premium on 6% Bonds Payable		10,445.01
	6% Bonds Payable		100,000.00

To record the reissuance of ten-year, six percent bonds with a remaining life of 71 months at a premium of $10,445.01.

In this case, Memorial Hospital should recall the bonds because the cash inflows of reissuance exceed the cash outflows of retirement. However, if the market rate of interest had fallen to six percent, the hospital would have received only $100,000 for the bond plus the accrued interest amounting to $1,000. In this second case, calling the bonds would not be economically advantageous because the cash outflows exceed the cash inflows.[11]

Sale of Bonds after the Authorized Issue Date

The full term of the bond is defined in the bond indenture as the length of time between a specific authorized issue date and a specific retirement date. The authorized issue date is the first date on which the bonds may be sold, while the retirement date is the last date on which the bonds may be retired. The length of time between the authorized issue date and the retirement date usually can be expressed in a number of years.

Of course, the actual term of the bond is not necessarily identical to the full term. As discussed in the previous section, the term of the bond may be shortened through early retirement. Similarly, it may be shortened through sale of the bond after the authorized issue date. However, in no case may the term be lengthened without the bond being in default.

Pricing Bonds Sold after the Authorized Issue Date

Although the previous sections on bond pricing were based on the assumption that the bonds were sold on the authorized issue date, the calculations required to price bonds sold after this date do not differ significantly from the bond pricing calculations of the previous sections. The important differences are that (1) there will be fewer periods than in the full term of the bond, and (2) since interest begins to accrue on the authorized issue date, purchasers will be willing to pay for the interest that has accrued between the authorized issue date and the date of sale. Hence, the price of bonds sold after the authorized issue date would be calculated as follows:[12]

$$\text{Price} = \text{Present value (on the sale date) of the Future Cash Flows} + \text{Accrued Interest}$$

For example, suppose that the ten-year, six percent Memorial Hospital bonds are authorized to be issued on May 1, 19X0, but are not actually issued until July 1, 19X0 (see Problem 5-3). Given that the market rate of interest is six percent and that interest payments are made semiannually on October 31 and on April 30, the price of the bonds on the date of sale would be:

$$\begin{aligned}\text{Price} &= \text{Present Value of Future Cash Flows} + \text{Accrued Interest}\\ &= (\$3{,}000 \times 14.694731 + \$100{,}000 \times .55915807) + \$3{,}000 \times 2/6\\ &= \$100{,}000 + \$1{,}000\\ &= \$101{,}000\end{aligned}$$

where: 14.694731 is the present value of an annuity of $1 invested at three percent for 19⅔ periods (the time remaining in the term of the bond); and
.55915807 is the present value of $1 invested at three percent for 19⅔ periods.

In this case, the purchaser would be willing to pay an amount equal to the face value of the bond plus the accrued interest on the sale date.

Of course, if the bonds are sold two months after the authorized issue date and if the market rate of interest is eight percent on the sale date, the bonds must sell at a discount. Just as interest accrues over time, discounts diminish over time, and accordingly, the amount of the discount on the bonds sold on July 1, 19X0, should be less than the discount on the bonds sold on May 1, 19X0. This intuitive analysis provides a means of checking the formal calculation.

$$
\begin{aligned}
\text{Price} &= \text{Present Value of Future Cash Flows} + \text{Accrued Interest} \\
&= (\$3{,}000 \times 13.440181 + \$100{,}000 \times .46239274) + \$3{,}000 \times 2/6 \\
&= \$86{,}559.82 + \$1{,}000 \\
&= \$87{,}559.82
\end{aligned}
$$

where: 13.440181 is the present value of an annuity of $1 invested at four percent for 19⅔ periods; and
.46239274 is the present value of $1 invested at four percent for 19⅔ periods.

As expected, the discount of $13,440.18 ($100,000 − 86,559.82) in this case is less than the $13,590.33 discount on the bonds sold on the issue date when the market rate of interest was eight percent. In this case, however, the purchasers are willing to pay an extra $1,000 for the accrued interest.

Similarly, bond premiums diminish over time. Hence, the premium on the six percent Memorial Hospital bonds sold on July 1, 19X0, when the market rate of interest is four percent should be less than the premium on the same bonds sold on the issue date when the market rate of interest is four percent. The price of the bond on July 1, 19X0 can be calculated as follows:

$$
\begin{aligned}
\text{Price} &= \text{Present Value of Future Cash Flows} + \text{Accrued Interest} \\
&= (\$3{,}000 \times 16.128588 + \$100{,}000 \times .67742825) + \$3{,}000 \times 2/6 \\
&= \$116{,}128.59 + \$1{,}000 \\
&= \$117{,}128.59
\end{aligned}
$$

where: 16.128588 is the present value of an annuity of $1 invested at two percent for 19⅔ periods; and
.67742825 is the present value of $1 invested at two percent for 19⅔ periods.

Note that the discount of $16,128.59 ($116,128.59 − $100,000.00) is indeed less than the $16,351.43 discount for the bonds sold on the authorized issue date. However, the purchasers again are willing to pay $1,000 for the interest that has accrued on the bond between the authorized issue date and the sale date.

The journal entries to record the July 1, 19X0, sale of the bonds in all three cases are given below.

7/1/X0	Cash	$101,000.00	
	Bond Interest Expense		$ 1,000.00
	6% Bonds Payable		100,000.00

To record the sale of ten-year, six percent bonds at face value two months after the issue date and to record the receipt of accrued interest on the sale date.

7/1/X0	Cash	$ 87,559.82	
	Discount on 6% Bonds Payable	13,440.18	
	Bond Interest Expense		$ 1,000.00
	6% Bonds Payable		100,000.00

To record the sale of ten-year, six percent bonds at a discount of $13,440.18 two months after the issue date and to record the receipt of accrued bond interest on the sale date.

7/1/X0	Cash	$117,128.59	
	Bond Interest Expense		$ 1,000.00
	Premium of 6% Bonds Payable		16,128.59
	6% Bonds Payable		100,000.00

To record the sale of ten-year, six percent bonds at a premium of $16,128.59 two months after the issue date and to record the receipt of accrued interest on the sale date.

Note that the $1,000 received for accrued interest is credited to bond interest expense in each case. This credit reduces the amount in the Bond Interest Expense account in the year of sale because the hospital does not incur any interest expense before the bond is sold. Also note that the amount recorded in six percent Bonds Payable account is still $100,000 because this amount must be paid to the bondholders on the retirement date.

Payment of Interest on Bonds Sold after the Authorized Issue Date

The cash interest payment to the Memorial Hospital bondholders will be \$3,000 on every interest payment date, regardless of when the bonds are sold. If the bonds have been sold at face value, the interest expense recorded on each interest payment date will be \$3,000 also. However, if the bonds have been sold at a discount or a premium, this discount or premium must be amortized over the actual term of the bond.

Again, the institution may elect either the straight line or the effective interest rate method of interest amortization. If the straight line method is used, the total discount or premium can be divided into monthly segments. Then, on the first interest payment date, the amortization is calculated as the monthly allocation multiplied by the number of months that the bonds have been outstanding. On subsequent interest payment dates, the amortization is equal to the monthly allocation multiplied by the number of months that have passed since the previous interest payment date. If the fiscal year ends between interest payment dates, the number of months in the interim are used to calculate the amount of the amortization.

If the effective interest rate method of amortization is elected, the calculation of the amortization on the first interest payment date will be unique and all subsequent amortizations will be identical to the amortizations for bonds sold on the issue date. For example, consider the six percent Memorial Hospital bonds that are sold on July 1, 19X0, when the market rate of interest is eight percent. These bonds sell at a discount of \$13,440.18. To calculate the amortization of this discount on the first interest payment date, the discount outstanding on the first interest payment date must be computed. This figure is equal to the face value of the bond less the price of the bond on the first interest payment date excluding the accrued periodic interest. In this case, the discount outstanding on October 31, 19X0, would be computed as follows.

$$\begin{aligned}\text{Discount Outstanding} &= \text{Face Value} - \text{Price on Interest Payment Date Excluding Accrued Interest}\\ &= \$100{,}000.00 - \$86{,}866.06\\ &= \$13{,}133.94\end{aligned}$$

Hence, \$306.24 (\$13,440.18 − \$13,133.94) of the discount must be amortized on October 31, 19X0. This amortization brings the value of the net bonds payable to \$86,866.06 (\$86,559.82 + \$306.24), which is identical to the value of the net bonds payable after the first interest payment when the bonds are sold on the issue date (\$86,409.67 + \$456.39). Therefore, subsequent discount amortizations will be identical to those calculated for bonds sold on the issue date.

A similar calculation is used to compute the bond premium amortization when the bonds are sold after the issue date. The premium amortization on the first interest payment date for the Memorial Hospital bonds sold at a premium of $16,128.59 would be as shown.

Premium Outstanding = Price Excluding Accrued Interest − Face Value
= $115,678.46 − $100,000.00
= $15,678.46

Premium Amortization = Premium on Sale Date − Premium on Interest Payment Date
= $16,128.59 − $15,678.46
= $450.13

This amortization makes net bonds payable equal to $115,678.46 ($116,128.49 − $450.13) after the first interest payment date, which is the same value recorded in the same account on the same date when the bonds are sold on the issue date.

These computations highlight the fact that the accounting for bonds is relatively complex. A good deal of technical information must be developed to record the issuance of bonds, the payment of bond interest, and the retirement of bonds in the institution's accounting system. In addition, to evaluate the bond as a financing alternative, the other provisions and restrictions of the bond indenture must be considered with respect to changing market conditions and alternative means of financing (see Appendix 5-B).

FINANCING ALTERNATIVES

In the past, debt financing was not considered a viable means of obtaining the funds needed to expand the services of health care institutions[13] because banks and other lenders considered these institutions to be highly specialized, high risk investments that would be difficult to salvage in the event of default. Although short-term loans could be obtained through local banks, only a few major insurance companies would make long-term loans to health care institutions in need of funds. In addition, a number of institutional bond houses would underwrite bond offerings marketed to the public by health care institutions; however, in these instances, the provisions of the debt agreements were restrictive and the interest costs high. Most lenders were interested in the value of the institution's real estate as security for loans and seldom lent any health care institutions more than 50 percent of the appraised value of the institution's property, plant, and equipment. As a result, most health care institutions found debt financing to be a difficult and expensive means of raising capital. Therefore, these institutions turned to debt financing only after all other sources of financing had been exhausted.

In today's capital markets, however, many lenders consider health care institutions to be among the safest forms of investment. This change in attitude is due primarily to the implementation of the Medicare and Medicaid programs and, more recently, to federal health planning legislation. By significantly increasing the percentage of patient service revenues flowing to health care institutions directly from the federal government, Medicare and Medicaid have provided health care institutions with a stable and dependable revenue source that forms a basis for loan security. Federal health planning legislation has provided added security for institutional lenders by requiring that states establish Health Systems Agencies (HSAs) that (1) evaluate the current and future needs for health care facilities, (2) develop comprehensive health care plans, and (3) issue Certificate of Need approval to health care institutions before any major capital improvements are undertaken. Many investors view this planning legislation as a federal franchising program which protects the institution from future competition. In summary, federal legislation has made it easier for health care institutions to seek financing in the capital markets by enabling them to obtain highly leveraged[14] loans from a wide variety of lending sources at more favorable interest costs.

The new attitude toward health care debt financing is one of the reasons that long-term debt has become the single dominant source of capital financing in health care institutions today. A variety of debt financing alternatives are available to health care institutions, including tax-exempt revenue bonds, Federal Housing Administration (FHA) insured mortgage loans with a Government National Mortgage Association (GNMA) guarantee, conventional mortgage financing, and public taxable bonds.

Selecting the Appropriate Financing Alternative

Many factors affect the selection of the appropriate financing alternative. These factors can be grouped into the five general categories shown in Table 5-1: (1) financial community factors, (2) requirements of the financing alternative, (3) institutional and management restrictions, (4) other financial considerations, and (5) timing factors.

Financial Community Factors

General conditions and attitudes in the financial community at a particular time may either encourage or prohibit the selection of a particular financing alternative. For example, the financial condition of the nation's cities and municipalities can affect investor acceptance of municipal debt significantly. New York City's financial crisis in 1975 almost eliminated the market for tax-exempt municipal financing in New York State and raised tax-exempt municipal interest rates substantially in other parts of the country. Similarly, governmental health care policies and the financial community's institutional investment policies and attitudes can affect the ability of health care institutions to obtain various types of financing. For example, in an attempt to minimize risk rather than maximize return, certain institutional investors may adopt a policy of only entering into loans which are guaranteed by the federal government. On the other hand, pensions funds, which are tax-exempt, generally will not invest in tax-exempt securities marketed by hospitals because the interest rates on tax-exempt securities are lower than those on taxable securities.

Requirements of the Financing Alternative

The requirements of the financing alternatives also affect the selection of a particular alternative. For example, the refinancing provisions of 2½ percent FHA insured mortgage loans with a GNMA guarantee may make this type of financing more desirable than tax-exempt financing when interest rates are expected to decline because if such a decline occurs, the hospital probably will not be able to refinance the loan economically. Prepayments amounting to 15 percent of the original principal amount of the loan may be made without penalty on FHA insured mortgage loans in any calendar year prior to maturity. Prepayment in excess of this limit also may be made, but at a negotiated penalty (see Table 5-2).

Internal Restrictions

Managerial policies and attitudes also have an impact on the selection or rejection of a specific financing alternative. For example, where institutional policy precludes the intervention of a municipal authority in the institution's decision-making process, tax-exempt financing may not be an acceptable financing alternative. Most tax-exempt financing requires management (1) to meet specified working capital ratios, (2) to provide for funding of depreciation, and (3) to provide for funding of one year's debt service (i.e., the average principal and interest payment required in any year). If these requirements are not satisfied, the institution is in technical default and

Table 5-1 Factors Affecting the Selection of Appropriate Financing Alternative

Financial Community Factors
Governmental health care policies
Financial condition of the nation's cities and municipalities
Institutional investment policies and attitudes
General supply and demand for investment funds

Requirements of the Financing Alternative (See Appendix 5-B)
Term to maturity
Interest rate
Prepayment provisions
Refinancing provisions
Default provisions
Additional debt restrictions
Working capital restrictions
Funding requirements (debt service reserve, depreciation, sinking fund, etc.)

Institutional and Management Restrictions
Board of managers' policies
Management attitudes toward government involvement in construction programs and institutional operations
Future borrowing requirements
Equity requirements

Other Financial Considerations
Institutional management
Financial position of the institution
Results of feasibility study
Results of bond ratings (see Appendix 5-A)
Availability of working capital
Availability of government grants, guarantees, and subsidies
Availability of philanthropic contributions
Size of financing

Timing Factors
Length of time required to obtain funds
Length of construction period

the issuing municipal authority may hire consultants to analyze and evaluate the institution's management at the institution's expense. The authority also may require the institution to implement the suggestions of the consultant, which could include a restructuring of the administration, a curtailment of certain programs, and a reduction of the staff. Concern over this type of government involvement and control in institutional decision making has led many Catholic hospitals to avoid tax-exempt financing and to select other forms of debt financing. Hence, in the event of technical default, tax-exempt financing would not comply with institutional policy.

Other Financial Considerations

A number of other financial factors also must be considered before selecting a particular financing alternative. For example, an institution must obtain an acceptable bond rating (see Appendix 5-A) to issue either tax-exempt or taxable bonds in the public market. Similarly, an institution must be well managed and have a satisfactory financial history to encourage prospective investors. On the other hand, government grants, guarantees, and subsidies can enhance the desirability of a particular financing alternative by reducing the interest rate associated with a specific alternative. Philanthropic contributions also may enhance the desirability of a particular financing alternative; if philanthropic contributions are expected in the near future, financing alternatives that can be prepaid with little or no penalty may be more desirable. Each of these factors should be considered before a financing alternative is selected.

Timing Factors

Timing factors also affect the selection of a particular financing alternative. For example, if financing is needed in a relatively short period of time, mortgage financing or taxable bonds, which usually are the least desirable means of financing, may be attractive alternatives because these forms of financing can be obtained in a relatively short period of time. Similarly, if the construction period is lengthy, mortgage financing may be an attractive alternative because this form of financing usually permits the borrower to accept the loan proceeds over the construction period as funds are needed; whereas tax-exempt bond financing, generally a more desirable financing alternative, usually requires the institution to accept the proceeds of the loan when the loan agreement is formally closed (i.e., when the lender and the borrower sign the loan agreement). Hence, the interest payments under mortgage financing could be substantially less than the interest payments under tax-exempt bond financing when the construction period is lengthy.[15]

Summary

The selection of the most appropriate financing alternative must be based on a detailed understanding of the institution's financial and management priorities and a knowledge of the relationship between these priorities and the available methods of financing. To cope more effectively with this complex decision, the board of managers in many institutions has established a finance committee to select an investment banker who is experienced in health care financing. The investment banker collects information from the institution's management, architect, attorney, feasibility consultant, auditor, and director of financial management before recommending a particular financing alternative.

Capital Financing Alternatives

Selecting the appropriate financing alternative is no simple task. The operational needs of the institution must be considered, as well as the benefits and limitations of the various financing alternatives. Each of the four major sources of debt financing will be discussed in an effort to stimulate general discussion regarding the advantages and disadvantages of the various sources of financing.

Tax-exempt Revenue Bonds

Tax-exempt revenue bonds (see Appendix 5-B) have two basic features: the interest payments to the bondholders are not subject to federal income taxation, and the bonds are secured by the *gross* revenues of the organization being financed. These bonds are issued on behalf of tax-exempt institutions by a state finance authority, a municipal finance authority established by a county or city government, or the institution itself, under Section 63-20 of the Internal Revenue Code.[16] In addition to the basic features, in most states the interest income on the bonds is also exempt from state income taxation if the bondholders live in the state in which the bonds are issued. Furthermore, in many cases, the bondholders are able to maintain a first mortgage on the institution's assets as additional security.

Currently, tax-exempt revenue bonds have become the most popular hospital financing alternative for several reasons. First, investors who realize a tax saving on interest payments usually are willing to accept interest rates on these bonds that are from 1 to 2½ percent lower than the interest rates on taxable bond issues of similar quality. Second, the term to maturity on these bonds can be as long as 30 years, thus allowing ample time to accumulate the funds to retire the debt. Furthermore, a high ratio of financing usually is available with tax-exempt revenue bonds. In fact, many institutions are able to finance 100 percent of total project costs, including reserve requirements, financing expenses and interest during construction. (See Table 5-2 for additional advantages of tax-exempt revenue bond financing.)

Tax-exempt revenue bonds also have undesirable aspects for the borrowing institution. If the bonds are issued through a state or municipal finance

Table 5-2[17] Advantages and Disadvantages of Tax-Exempt Revenue Bonds

Advantages	Disadvantages
1. Interest costs are usually 1–2½ percent lower than other methods of financing.	1. When the bonds are issued under a state or local authority, title to the facility may have to be transferred to the authority during the life of the issue.
2. The term of the loan can be as long as 30 years.	2. If a nonprofit institution issues its own tax-exempt bonds under a state's nonprofit corporation statute, Internal Revenue Service guidelines require that the institution pass title to a municipality at the end of the term of the bonds. (However, operational control would remain with the institution.)
3. Since the loan amount is determined by the ability of the facility to generate revenue, up to 100 percent of total project costs might be financed.	3. A comprehensive feasibility study executed by a recognized consulting firm is required.
4. Bond proceeds are available before construction, thus eliminating the need for interim construction financing.	4. Financing expenses, including the feasibility study, bond counsel, other legal fees, and printing costs generally are higher than in some other methods of financing.
5. Interest payments can be capitalized during construction.	5. A debt-service reserve fund, usually equaling one year's average principal and interest payment may be required. (The reserve fund, however, is used to pay off the last maturing bond principal and earns interest income.)
6. Tax-exempt bond issues are usually structured with open-ended provisions that allow for issuance of additional bonds, provided certain levels of financial performance are maintained.	6. A bond discount, typically between two and three percent, is required.
7. Existing debt usually can be refinanced.	7. Prepayment of the bonds usually cannot be made during the first ten years of the issue; thereafter, the bonds are callable at a premium decreasing from approximately 3 percent to zero in the 11th through 15th years.
8. Tax-exempt bond issues often can be privately placed.	8. A bond rating usually is required. Investors require an "A" rating before accepting tax-exempt revenue bonds (see Appendix 5-A).
9. Principal repayment schedules may be structured so that the principal payments in the early years of the loan are reduced. This results in the loan being tailored to the institution's ability to repay. First repayment is normally scheduled for one or two years after completion of the project.	

authority, title to the institution technically is transferred to the issuing authority, which has the option of exercising the control associated with ownership until the bonds are retired. However, no intervention in the institution's internal affairs generally occurs unless the institution is unable to meet all of the requirements of the loan agreement. Similarly, if the institution issues its own tax-exempt bonds under the provision of Section 63-20 of the Internal Revenue Code, title to the institution must pass to the municipality in which the institution is located when the bonds are retired. Of course, as stated previously, these title transfers usually are of little or no consequence because as long as the institution remains in a financially viable position, the new owner or trustee generally does not assume control over operations. (See Table 5-2 for additional disadvantages of tax-exempt revenue bond financing.)

FHA-insured Mortgage Loans with GNMA Guarantees

FHA-insured mortgage loans with GNMA guarantees are mortgage loans that are insured primarily by the FHA and have a secondary guarantee provided by the GNMA. This double federal insurance lowers the risk inherent in this type of financing and aids in attracting investors who are willing to receive a lower interest rate for their funds. FHA-insured mortgage loans with GNMA guarantees may be obtained by proprietary, as well as nonprofit, institutions.

An institution may select this financing technique for several reasons. For example, in addition to attracting investors at interest rates that are lower than conventional mortgage interest rates, the term of FHA-insured mortgage loans can extend as long as 25 years after the completion of construction. In addition, FHA-insured mortgage loans with GNMA guarantees allow the institution to obtain insured mortgages amounting to 90 percent of the appraised replacement cost of the facility, including equipment. In fact, 100 percent financing actually may be obtained because filing and inspection fees, commitment fees, closing costs, interest during construction, financing charges, and legal and title fees also may be included as costs before applying the 90 percent financing percentage (see Table 5-3 for additional advantages of FHA-insured mortgage loans with a GNMA guarantee).

On the other hand, FHA-insured mortgage loans have disadvantages. For example, the maximum interest rate on these mortgages is established by the FHA. Although this interest rate is adjusted periodically to reflect changes in the market, if the maximum interest rate is below the current market rate, the institution must discount the mortgage in order to attract investors. In addition, the institution must conform to federal building

Table 5-3 Advantages and Disadvantages of FHA-Insured Mortgage Loans with GNMA Guarantee(s)

Advantages	Disadvantages
1. Loan-to-value ratio can be as high as 90 percent.	1. Processing of the FHA application can be time-consuming.
2. The value of the land, existing buildings, and major movable equipment may satisfy the institution's equity requirement.	2. Construction must conform to FHA/HEW standards.
3. Most preparation and application costs can be included in eligible costs.	3. Construction labor costs can be higher than under other methods of financing because of strict government regulations.
4. The full faith and credit guarantee of the U.S. government allows the institution to secure an attractive interest rate.	4. If the FHA interest rate is below current money market rates, the institution must discount the mortgage to bring the yield to the investor up to market levels.
5. The GNMA Construction Loan Certificate enables the institution to obtain both construction and permanent financing in a single package at the same interest rate.	5. The institution must pay an annual mortgage insurance premium of 0.5 percent of the unamortized principal amount.
6. If the institution is undergoing an expansion or modernization program, eligible debt can include refinancing of existing debt.	6. The institution must pay front-end inspection and filing fees totaling 0.8 percent of the principal amount.
7. The term of the loan can be as much as 25 years after completion of construction.	7. Many investment bankers involved with this program lack expertise, or are not capable, in all aspects of the FHA/GNMA program.
8. Prepayment of 15 percent of the original principal amount is permitted in a calendar year without penalty. In addition, the loan can be structured to allow for prepayment in excess of this amount at any time for a negotiated penalty.	

codes, wage scales, and hiring practices when using FHA-insured mortgage loan financing. Furthermore, the time required to obtain the needed funds may be lengthy because (1) the Department of Health, Education and Welfare (DHEW) must conduct a feasibility study before the loan application can be processed, and (2) the experience, attitude, and workload of the local FHA office originating the loan agreement can speed or retard the completion of the agreement. However, if the loan application is prepared with the assistance of an experienced investment banker who is also an authorized GNMA issuer, the time required to process the loan application can be minimized. (See Table 5-3 for additional disadvantages of FHA-insured mortgage loan financing with GNMA guarantees.)

Conventional Mortgage Financing

Under a conventional mortgage, the investor (usually a savings bank) agrees to convey funds to the institution in exchange for the title to the facility (including plant, major equipment, and land) which is pledged as security until the mortgage is repaid. The expertise provided by an investment banker is extremely important in this type of financing because lending policies, interest rates, and attitudes toward health care institutions vary among institutional lenders. Although this financing technique is not designed specifically for health care institutions, the investment banker often can negotiate an agreement that makes conventional mortgages a viable debt financing alternative.

Conventional mortgage financing provides several advantages to the institution. For example, this method of financing permits maximum flexibility by allowing the institution to structure a financing package that is best suited to the institution's financial priorities. In addition, conventional mortgage financing usually can be obtained more quickly than any other means of debt financing. (See Table 5-4 for other advantages of conventional mortgage financing.)

However, conventional mortgage financing also has disadvantages. The primary disadvantage is that lenders often will not issue mortgage loans for amounts greater than 75 percent of the total appraised value of the facility. This loan-to-value ratio is substantially less than the loan-to-value ratios of tax-exempt bond financing and FHA-insured mortgage loans. Hence, under conventional mortgage financing, a greater amount of equity capital may have to be raised to finance project costs. In addition, this financing alternative is generally only available to highly rated, well endowed, and well known institutions. (See Table 5-4 for additional disadvantages of conventional mortgage financing.)

Public Taxable Bonds

Public taxable bond financing has two basic features: (1) bond indentures (see the first part of this chapter) are issued to the public in exchange for cash, and (2) the interest payments on the bonds are subject to federal, state, and local income taxation. This type of financing traditionally was the method most widely used by health care institutions. However, the advent of new financing techniques designed specifically for health care institutions has caused a decline in the use of public taxable bonds as a means of debt financing.

The advantages of public taxable bond financing are not overwhelming. The penalties levied on early debt retirement are relatively lenient and the financing can be arranged in a relatively short period of time. In addition, the institution usually is able to issue additional debt, as needed,

Table 5-4 Advantages and Disadvantages of Conventional Mortgage Financing

Advantages	Disadvantages
1. This method takes the shortest amount of time to implement.	1. The loan-to-value ratio usually is lower than that of other financing techniques. Therefore, the institution must contribute a high percentage of equity or utilize alternative methods of financing.
2. This method of financing allows the institution the greatest amount of flexibility to structure a financing package most suitable to its financial priorities.	2. The loan term may be shorter than the terms of alternative methods of financing.
3. The institution does not have to conform to DHEW/FHA construction standards.	3. The loan covenants usually are more restrictive than the covenants under other methods of financing.
4. Flexible interest rates obviate the need for substantial discounting.	4. The interest rate usually will be higher than the interest rates of alternative methods of financing.
5. Since the interest rate is negotiated well before closing, the institution can predict total costs more accurately and easily.	5. Funds may be difficult to obtain when money markets are tight, or if the hospital is located in an unattractive area.
6. A feasibility study frequently is not required, printing expenses are reduced or avoided, and legal fees usually are less expensive than with other alternatives.	
7. This method does not require many of the reserve funds required in a tax-exempt issue.	

provided that certain financial performance levels are maintained. (See Table 5-5 for other advantages of public taxable bond financing.)

The disadvantages of public taxable bond financing, on the other hand, are substantial. First, the term of the loan is short (15 to 20 years), and refinancing often is necessary. Furthermore, the financing fees associated with public taxable bonds may be high in relation to the financing fees of the other financing alternatives. These high financing fees often offset the savings that result from the lower interest rate available in the public bond market. In many cases, these disadvantages combine to make public taxable bond financing an uneconomical financing alternative. (See Table 5-5 for other disadvantages to public taxable bond financing.)

Summary

Because many factors affect the selection of the appropriate financing alternative, the best method of financing will vary with the financial

Table 5-5 Advantages and Disadvantages of Public Taxable Bonds

Advantages	Disadvantages
1. Traditionally, the prepayment provisions have been more liberal than the prepayment provisions of any other financing alternative.	1. Traditionally, the loan-to-loan value ratio has been less than 60 percent. However, greater reliance on the revenue-generating capacity of the institution is affecting this ratio.
2. Generally, the stated interest rate will be lower than the interest rate associated with a private placement.	2. If high ratio financing is involved, an extensive feasibility study is required.
3. These issues normally are structured with an open-ended provision which allows for the issuance of additional debt, provided that certain financial performance levels are maintained.	3. Usually, the loan term is shorter than the terms for alternative methods of financing.
4. The effect of serialized maturities frequently reduces the net effective cost to the institution.	4. Front-end fees, including the underwriters' spread and legal and printing expenses, are substantial. As a result, the net effective cost to the institution usually is higher than alternative methods of financing.
5. The institution does not have to conform to DHEW/FHA construction standards.	5. The preparation and placement of the issue can be time consuming.
6. Bond proceeds are available before construction, alleviating the need for interim construction financing.	

priorities of the institution and the money market conditions at the time of financing (see Question 5-1). Hence, each institution should develop and delineate the financial priorities of prospective projects to insure an appropriate capital financing program. In addition, an investment banker who is familiar with the financing techniques applicable to health care institutions should be engaged to aid in evaluating the debt financing alternatives in the current market.

NOTES

1. Federal or state hospital authorities may place interest ceilings on tax-exempt revenue bonds.
2. The present value of an annuity of \$1 is calculated as $(1 - (1 + i)^{-n})/i$, where i is the periodic interest rate and n is the number of periods.
3. The present value of \$1 is calculated as $(1 + i)^{-n}$, where i is the periodic interest rate and n is the number of periods.

4. To calculate the amortization of a bond premium, the following formula should be used: Cash Interest Payment (CIP) − Bond Premium Amortization (BPA) = Market Interest Rate (MIR) × Net Bonds Payable (NBP). The interest expense in this case would be equal to the cash payment less the bond premium amortization.
5. In the case of a bond premium, the effective interest rate method of amortization would yield declining interest expense in ensuing periods.
6. The effective interest rate amortization of the bond premium for the first period of the Memorial Hospital bonds would be calculated as:

$$\text{CIP} - \text{BPA} = \text{MIR} \times \text{NBP}$$

$$\$3000 - \text{BPA} = .02 \times \$116{,}351.43$$

$$\text{BPA} = \$672.97$$

   where: BPA represents the bond premium amortization.

7. See Appendix A for a description and analysis of reversing entries.
8. This value is computed using the formula for the future value of an ordinary annuity:

$$\text{FV} = \text{A}\,\frac{(1 + i)^n - 1}{i},$$

   where: FV is the future value ($100,000), A is the annuity ($8,329.09), i is the periodic interest rate (4%), and n is the number of periods (10).
9. Retiring the bonds at 110 means that the bondholders will receive 110 percent of the face value of the bonds upon retirement.
10. See the section on Pricing Bonds Sold after the Authorized Issue Date for the method of calculating this value. This computation assumes that the stated interest rate on the new bond issue remains at six percent. If the interest rate on the new issue is reduced to the market rate of interest, the present value of cash flows inherent in the new issue, including the costs of retiring the old issue, should be compared with the present value of the cash flows inherent in the old issue.
11. If the Memorial Hospital had issued $100,000 in new bonds with a 71-month life and a stated interest rate of four percent, the present value of the difference between the interest payments of the old issue and the interest payments of the new issue would have to be included as a cash inflow in the analysis. However, this amount would not be included in the journal entries of retirement or reissuance.
12. These calculations also pertain to pricing bonds that have been called and are going to be reissued.
13. Note that although any health care institution may seek funds from the various sources to be discussed, hospitals to date have constituted the market for these types of financing. Therefore, the examples in this section will be drawn from hospital experiences.
14. The term "leverage" as used here, refers to the ratio of debt to assets pledged to secure the debt. A high degree of leverage occurs when a small pledge of assets is required to secure a large debt. Therefore, if two hospitals borrow $11 million each, and Hospital A pledges $400,000 worth of assets while Hospital B must pledge $5 million worth of assets, Hospital A has negotiated a more highly leveraged loan than Hospital B.
15. The institution may invest the excess tax-exempt loan proceeds during the period when they are not needed, partially offsetting the higher interest costs during the period of construction.

16. Generally, 63-20 tax-exempt financing is used only in the four states with no tax-exempt enabling legislation: Alaska, California, Hawaii, and Washington.
17. The information contained in the tables represented in this chapter has been contributed by Blyth, Eastman Dillon Health Care Financing, Inc.

Appendix 5-A

The Bond Rating

A bond rating provides investors with a simple means of evaluating the credit worthiness of an institution. A common scale is used to evaluate all bonds in the market, thus allowing interinstitutional comparisons. Institutions with higher bond ratings are able to attract investors at lower interest rates than institutions with lower bond ratings. Hence, an institution's bond rating is important both in attracting investors and in determining the interest rate that the institution will pay for debt financing. Currently, only hospitals have access to tax-exempt bond markets; therefore, this appendix will consider the rating process from a hospital perspective. However, the process would not differ substantially for other types of health care institutions.

The importance of bond ratings in the health care industry has increased in recent years for several reasons. For example, with the advent of tax-exempt revenue bond financing, the importance of the hospital bond rating has increased because investors require the bond rating to compare potential investments. In addition, several of the major bond funds have established policies of not investing in bonds below a specific rating (usually "A" or better). Finally, the concern over hospital bankruptcy and default, accompanied by fears of the possible impact of proposed cost containment legislation, has made bond ratings almost mandatory. These factors have caused hospital bond investors to require bond ratings as criteria for selecting an investment.

The Bond Rating Scale

Three major credit rating services list bond ratings: Moody's Investors' Services, Inc., Standard and Poor's Corp., and Fitch's Investor Service,

Inc. Each of these services rates bonds on a scale consisting of a series of A's and B's with pluses and minuses attached to show further gradations. The most secure investments are given a rating of Aaa by Moody's and AAA by Standard and Poor's, while slightly lower quality issues are rated as Aa and AA by the two agencies, respectively. Upper medium risk bonds are given a rating of A at both services. The scale continues with ratings of Baa and BBB for medium grade bonds, etc. If further gradations are needed, a plus or minus, or a 1 is placed next to the letter rating.

The most common bond rating for a hospital is an A. This rating indicates that most hospital bonds are upper medium risk bonds. With few exceptions, better ratings, which result in lower interest rates, are given only to well established, nationally known, well endowed, financially solvent, multispecialty teaching hospitals.

Planning and Preparing for the Bond Rating

The bond rating is based on a detailed review of a broad range of financially relevant information, including a meeting with the hospital's administration, the hospital's board members, the investment banker, the feasibility study consultant, and key members of the medical staff. Hence, careful planning is needed to prepare for the credit rating process. The information required by the rating service must be accurate and timely. In addition, the hospital's representatives must be prepared to answer a number of probing questions.

The credit rating agency usually will want to gather information regarding the specific financing alternative selected, the proposed project, the hospital's financial status, and the general operation of the hospital. Detailed information about the financing alternative can be obtained from the prospectus, official statement, or loan offering memorandum. In addition, all legal documents, including the trust indenture, bond resolution, and all closing documents, must be given to the credit rating agency. Similarly, the information required to describe the proposed project must include the architect's reports, the Certificate of Need and other approvals, the results of the feasibility study, and a map of the service area that identifies the location of all competing organizations and describes the construction plans of these competing organizations. In addition to this information, the details describing the financial status and the general operation of the hospital must be provided.

A substantial amount of financial information is required by the credit rating agency to determine the financial status of the hospital. The hospital must have certified audit reports for the preceding five years, including letters of explanation from the hospital's counsel regarding past or present litigation and the expected outcome of any current litigation. In addition, the hospital must have the most recent interim financial statements with comparable statements for the prior year, as well as operating and capital budgets for the forthcoming year, copies of monthly budget reports distributed to departmental heads, a description of the performance variance reporting system, and a description of the means employed to rectify unfavorable variances. The hospital also must give the credit rating agency a copy of all lease agreements and a list of all banks with which the hospital has established lines of credit. Furthermore, the hospital must make cash flow projections which include an analysis of accounts receivable. This analysis of accounts receivable should include a calculation of the average number of days that accounts are outstanding, a description of any pending rate appeals or disputes with third party payers, and a list of all cost ceilings, reimbursement rates, per diem costs, and routine costs. All of this information should be gathered and consolidated prior to the rating.

The information required to describe the general operations of the institution is almost as difficult to collect as the financial information. First, the hospital must compile a list of all approvals, licenses, and accreditations. Second, historical patient statistics, including admissions, average length of stay, patient days, occupancy, average daily census, outpatient and emergency visits, and ancillary service procedures, must be compiled. Furthermore, the hospital must prepare a profile of its medical staff which specifies the age of the staff, the distribution of admissions, the location of the physicians' offices relative to the location of the hospital, the staff usage of competing facilities, and the staffing of the emergency room. Finally, the hospital must compile a list of the occupations and employers of all board members and must obtain resumes from members of the administration and key members of the medical staff. All of this information should be distributed to the rating agency several weeks before the rating is desired.

During the meeting between representatives of the credit rating agency and the hospital administration, the hospital board members, the investment banker, the feasibility study consultant and key members of the hospital staff are asked to discuss various aspects of the project, the hospital's financial status, and the general operation of the organization. Generally, the credit rating agency is interested particularly in comments regarding the hospital's long range plans, as well as expected changes in the service area and the hospital's plans to cope with these changes.

The community support for the project and the assumptions underlying the feasibility study are scrutinized in this meeting also. The hospital's representatives may be asked to discuss the history, philosophy, goals, and objectives of the hospital, as well as its organizational structure. In addition, the hospital's representatives may have to discuss the methodology used to project demands, the hospital's budgeting process and analysis of performance, the expected impact of existing or proposed cost controls and rate regulations, the hospital's policy toward risk management, and any recent experience that the hospital has had with malpractice litigation.

The Bond Rating Process

The two steps required by the bond rating process have been discussed above: (1) the hospital must compile a considerable amount of financially relevant information for the credit rating agency, and (2) after this information has been reviewed and analyzed by the credit rating agency, hospital representatives must meet with the rating committee to discuss the institution's current and future financial outlook. Once the hospital has compiled the necessary information regarding the specific financing alternative to be used, the proposed project, the hospital's financial status, and the general operation of the hospital, this information must be submitted to the credit rating agency for analysis and review. The rating analysts abstract the information submitted by the hospital so that comparisons can be made between this hospital and comparable institutions. In many cases, the subjective nature of the information requires that the hospital be compared to an abstract of the "ideal" institution as perceived by the analyst. The analysis is complete when the rating analyst presents the rating committee with a report of the analysis and a list of recommendations.

The rating process begins with a review of the analyst's report and a review of the analyst's recommendations by the rating committee. This committee then meets with the hospital's representatives to ask a series of probing questions that further clarify the analyst's report. In addition, the rating committee reviews the various loan covenants that are designed to provide extra security for the bondholders. Any other measures which may have an impact on the hospital's ability to make interest payments or on the hospital's ability to retire this debt also are reviewed. The final duty of the rating committee is to evaluate the hospital, assign a rating, and prepare a short report for the hospital's management to explain the rating assigned.

Conclusion

The impression that the hospital's representatives make on the rating committee can have a significant effect on the eventual bond rating and, indirectly, on the interest rate that the hospital will be required to pay. One means of improving the rating committee's impression of the hospital is to have the investment banker coordinate the rating meeting. The investment banker often can direct the course of events in this meeting to highlight the hospital's strong points. The rating meeting should be conducted at the hospital so that the rating committee can tour the premises, perceive the impact of any proposed construction, and meet the administrators, board members, and medical staff in their environment. Furthermore, the hospital's representatives must be prepared for the rating meeting so that the rating committee leaves with a favorable impression. Hence, it behooves the hospital's management to plan and prepare for all aspects of the bond rating.

Appendix 5-B

Selected Sections of a Preliminary Official Statement Detailing Various Aspects of the Tax-Exempt Revenue Bonds of the Good Samaritan Hospital and Medical Center, Portland, Oregon

PRELIMINARY OFFICIAL STATEMENT DATED JULY 22, 1977

NEW ISSUE **†Rating: Standard & Poor's: A+ (prov.)**

Interest on the Series 1977 Bonds is exempt in the opinion of Bond Counsel, under existing statutes and court decisions, from Federal income taxes, and under Oregon Law, from all personal income tax in the State of Oregon.

$36,300,000*

The Hospital Facilities Authority of the City of Portland, Oregon

Hospital Revenue Bonds, Series 1977

(Good Samaritan Hospital and Medical Center Project)

Dated: August 1, 1977 **Due: July 1, as shown below:**

Principal and interest (payable January 1, 1978 and semi-annually each July 1 and January 1 thereafter) are payable at the principal corporate trust office of First National Bank of Oregon, Portland, Oregon or at Bankers Trust Company, New York, New York. The Series 1977 Bonds are subject to redemption prior to maturity as described herein. The Series 1977 Bonds are being issued to provide funds which will be used to pay the Project Costs as defined herein.

The Series 1977 Bonds are not an obligation of or a charge upon the tax revenues of the City of Portland but are solely the obligation of the Authority, which has no taxing power. The Series 1977 Bonds will be secured under the provisions of the Indenture, the Lease, the Sublease and the Guaranty as each is referred to herein, and will be equally and ratably payable from rental revenues of the Authority pursuant to its Sublease with, and additionally secured by the Guaranty of

Good Samaritan Hospital & Medical Center

$10,060,000 Serial Bonds*

Amount*	Maturity*	Interest Rate	Amount*	Maturity*	Interest Rate
$415	1980	%	$ 690	1988	%
440	1981		735	1989	
470	1982		780	1990	
500	1983		835	1991	
535	1984		885	1992	
570	1985		945	1993	
605	1986		1,010	1994	
645	1987				

$21,240,000* Term Bonds Due July 1, 2007.

$5,000,000* Term Bonds Due July 1, 2009.

The Hospital covenants to provide funds to the Authority which will be sufficient to redeem at par all the $5,000,000 principal amount of Series 1977 Bonds due July 1, 1987 (which Series 1977 Bonds are not subject to redemption by the Authority) at the bondholders' option on July 1, 1987 and on each July 1 thereafter upon prior written notice (see page 3 herein).

All Prices 100%

(Plus accrued interest on all Series 1977 Bonds from August 1, 1977)

The Series 1977 Bonds are offered subject to prior sale, when, as and if issued by the Authority and accepted by the Underwriters, subject to the approval of legality by Rankin, McMurry, Osburn & Gallagher, Portland, Oregon, Bond Counsel. Certain legal matters will be passed upon by Souther, Spaulding, Kinsey, Williamson & Schwabe, Portland, Oregon, Counsel for the Hospital and Brown, Wood, Ivey, Mitchell & Petty, New York, New York, Counsel to the Underwriters. It is expected that the Series 1977 Bonds in definitive form will be available for delivery in New York, New York on or about August 25, 1977.

Kidder, Peabody & Co.
Incorporated

Blyth Eastman Dillon & Co.
Incorporated

Dean Witter & Co.
Incorporated

† For an explanation of the Rating, see "Rating" herein.

* Estimates, subject to change.

The Date of this Official Statement is August , 1977.

IN CONNECTION WITH THIS OFFERING, THE UNDERWRITERS MAY OVER-ALLOT OR EFFECT TRANSACTIONS WHICH STABILIZE OR MAINTAIN THE MARKET PRICE OF THE SERIES 1977 BONDS AT A LEVEL ABOVE THAT WHICH MIGHT OTHERWISE PREVAIL IN THE OPEN MARKET. SUCH STABILIZING, IF COMMENCED, MAY BE DISCONTINUED AT ANY TIME.

No dealer, broker, salesman or other person has been authorized by The Hospital Facilities Authority of the City of Portland, Oregon, or the Underwriters or Good Samaritan Hospital and Medical Center to give any information or to make any representations, other than those contained in this Official Statement, and if given or made, such other information or representations must not be relied upon as having been authorized by any of the foregoing. This Official Statement does not constitute an offer to sell or the solicitation of an offer to buy, nor shall there be any sale of the Series 1977 Bonds by any person in any State in which it is unlawful for such person to make such offer, solicitation or sale. The information set forth herein has been obtained from The Hospital Facilities Authority of the City of Portland, Oregon, Good Samaritan Hospital and Medical Center and other sources which are believed to be reliable but is not guaranteed as to accuracy or completeness by, and is not to be construed as a representation by, the Underwriters or, as to information from other sources, by the Authority. The information and expressions of opinion herein are subject to change without notice and neither the delivery of this Official Statement nor any sale made hereunder, shall under any circumstances, create any implication that there has been no change in the affairs of The Hospital Facilities Authority of the City of Portland, Oregon or Good Samaritan Hospital and Medical Center since the date hereof.

TABLE OF CONTENTS

PRELIMINARY OFFICIAL STATEMENT

$36,300,000*

The Hospital Facilities Authority of the City of Portland, Oregon

Hospital Revenue Bonds, Series 1977

(Good Samaritan Hospital and Medical Center Project)

INTRODUCTORY STATEMENT

Purpose of this Official Statement. The purpose of this Official Statement, including the cover page and the appendices hereto, is to set forth information in connection with the offering of $36,300,000* Hospital Revenue Bonds, Series 1977 (Good Samaritan Hospital and Medical Center Project) (the "Series 1977 Bonds") of The Hospital Facilities Authority of the City of Portland, Oregon (the "Authority") to be issued under and secured by a Trust Indenture, to be dated as of August 1, 1977 (the "Indenture") by and between the Authority and First National Bank of Oregon, Portland, Oregon, as trustee (the "Trustee"). The proceeds of the Series 1977 Bonds and other funds available for the purpose will be used to provide funds which will be used to pay the Project Costs as herein defined.

The Hospital Facilities Authority of the City of Portland, Oregon. The Authority is the issuer of the Series 1977 Bonds. The Authority was created pursuant to Oregon Revised Statutes 441.525 to 441.595, inclusive, for the purpose of issuing revenue bonds to provide hospital facilities for lease and sale to private nonprofit hospital corporations.

Good Samaritan Hospital and Medical Center. The Hospital, an Oregon nonprofit corporation, was founded in 1875 to provide health care to the residents of Portland. It is licensed for 539 beds, of which 450 are currently in operation. Appendix A contains information on the history, organization, operations, and financial performance of the Hospital.

Purpose of the Series 1977 Bonds. The proceeds from the sale of the Bonds, together with certain funds to be made available by the Hospital, will be used to pay the cost of the replacement and modernization of the existing Hospital facilities, including the refinancing of bank indebtedness incurred to commence the initial phase of the Project. See the caption "The Project" herein for a more detailed description of the Project.

Security. A Hospital Facilities Lease will be entered into between the Authority and the Hospital whereby the Hospital will lease the Hospital Facilities to the Authority. At the same time, a Sublease will be entered into between the Authority and the Hospital whereby the Authority will sublease the Hospital Facilities to the Hospital. The Sublease will be a general obligation of the Hospital and the Hospital will pledge its credit to the payments thereunder, which payments will be in amounts sufficient to pay the principal of and the interest on the Series 1977 Bonds as the same become due. In addition, the Hospital will execute and deliver to the Trustee a Guaranty Agreement, dated as of August 1, 1977 (the "Guaranty"), in which the Hospital will guarantee to the Trustee the full and prompt payment of principal, premium, if any, and interest on the Series 1977 Bonds. See the caption "The Series 1977 Bonds" and the summaries of the Lease, the Sublease, the Indenture and the Guaranty in Appendix C for a more detailed description of the security for the Series 1977 Bonds.

Rate Covenant. The Hospital covenants that commencing with the delivery of the Series 1977 Bonds, it will fix, charge and collect and revise from time to time, subject to applicable requirements or restrictions imposed by law, rates, fees and charges for the use of and for the services furnished or to be furnished by the Hospital so that the Net Revenues in each Fiscal Year will be in an amount not less than 110% of the Annual Debt Service for such Fiscal Year. See the subcaption "Rates, Fees and Charges" under the caption "The Sublease" in Appendix C for the complete text of the Hospital's covenants as to rates.

Bonds in Addition to the Series 1977 Bonds. The Authority, upon compliance with the terms and conditions and for the purposes described under the subcaption "Bonds in Addition to the Series 1977 Bonds" under the caption "The Indenture" in Appendix C, may issue additional revenue bonds on a parity as to security and payment with the Series 1977 Bonds.

---

* Estimates, subject to change.

THE AUTHORITY

General

The Authority was created by Resolution No. 31894, adopted by the Portland City Council on June 22, 1977 pursuant to Oregon Revised Statutes 441.525 to 441.595, inclusive, for the purpose of assisting in providing hospital facilities to serve the residents of the City of Portland and the State of Oregon.

The Authority is empowered to acquire, own, lease and dispose of hospital facilities and to issue revenue bonds to achieve its purposes. However, revenue bonds or other obligations issued by the Authority are not an obligation of the City of Portland or a charge upon its revenues. The Authority has no taxing power.

Directors of the Authority

The Board of Directors of the Authority consists of seven members appointed by the Portland City Council to serve a term of three years.

The present directors of the Authority are as follows:

Name	Office	Position
Mildred Schwab	Chairman	Commissioner of Public Affairs of the City of Portland
A. Leighton Platt, C.P.A.	Vice-Chairman	Partner, Peat, Marwick, Mitchell & Co.
Herbert L. Amerson	Secretary/Treasurer	Commercial Accounts Manager, Pacific Northwest Bell
Arnold Biskar, C.P.A.	Director	Partner, Laventhol & Horwath
William Branson	Director	President, Blue Cross of Oregon
Dennis Keenan	Director	Executive Director, Cascade Health Care
Steven A. Lowenstein, Esq.	Director	Manager, Oregon Legal Services, Corp.

BONDHOLDERS' RISKS

General

The Series 1977 Bonds are limited obligations of the Authority, payable from and secured by moneys to be received by the Authority from the Hospital under the Sublease. *No representation or assurance can be made or given that revenues and receipts will be realized by the Hospital in amounts necessary to make payments under the Sublease or to make other payments in amounts sufficient to pay principal of, whether at maturity or upon redemption or prepayment, and interest on the Series 1977 Bonds.* Future economic and other conditions which are unpredictable, may adversely affect revenues and receipts and, consequently, payment of principal of and interest on the Series 1977 Bonds.

Factors That Could Affect The Future Financial Condition Of The Hospital

The future financial condition of the Hospital could be affected adversely by, among other things, legislation and regulatory actions and by increased competition from other health care providers.

A. *Hospital Cost Containment Act of 1977*

On April 25, 1977 a bill (the "Hospital Cost Containment Act of 1977") was introduced into Congress with the support of the President of the United States of America. The bill would act to limit the annual increase of inpatient revenues for an acute care hospital although exceptions are anticipated to be granted to hospitals involved in capital additions. The Feasibility Report prepared by Booz, Allen & Hamilton, Inc. attached hereto as Appendix B did not assume the bill would be enacted in its present form. If it were enacted in its present form, the Feasibility Report would be changed. It is not possible at this time to predict if the bill were enacted what its effect would be on the Hospital.

B. *Regulatory Actions That Could Affect The Hospital*

The Hospital is subject to regulatory actions by those governmental and private agencies that administer Medicare and the State Welfare Programs, Blue Cross of Oregon ("Blue Cross"), the National Labor Relations Board, the Professional Standards Review Organization (PSRO), the Joint Commission on the Accreditation of

Hospitals, the various federal, state, and local agencies created by the National Health Planning Resources Development Act of 1974 (the "National Health Planning Act"), and other federal, state and local governmental agencies. The impact that certain of these organizations could have on the potential reimbursement of the Hospital is explained in more detail below. No mention is made of the possible impact of a national health insurance program, as there is now no reasonable method of determining the effect any such program would have.

The following general factors could adversely affect the level of reimbursement planned for the Hospital:

(1) *Increased Costs Without a Comparable Increase In Revenue*

Cost increases could result from among other factors: increases in the salaries, wages, and fringe benefits of hospital employees, increases in costs associated with advances in medical technology, and increases in the costs of operating the physical plant of the Hospital.

Third Party Reimbursement—If certain costs attributable to patients are viewed by third party payors as unnecessary for patient service and are not reimbursed by them, the Hospital may lose the associated income. In addition, the result of future contract negotiations with Blue Cross could adversely affect levels of reimbursement. Third party payors include Medicare, the State Welfare Program, and Blue Cross.

Other Private Third Party Payors—Other private third party payors may adversely alter the amounts payable under their reimbursement contracts with their members, without notice to or recourse by the Hospital.

Certificate of Need Approval—The National Health Planning Act requires each state to initiate "Certificate of Need" legislation in order to insure that certain future medical expenditures (for a hospital, generally those in excess of $150,000) will be reviewed by a local "Health Systems Agency" (HSA). Approval by the HSA will be necessary in order for the expenditure to be eligible for reimbursement by Medicare and Medicaid.

(2) *Future Limits or Reductions on the Level of Support for Medicare and the State Welfare Program*

Future actions by the federal government for Medicare and by the State government for its welfare program, limiting or reducing the total amount of funds available for either or both of these programs, could lower the amount of reimbursement available to the Hospital.

(3) *Disallowance of Presently Reimbursable Costs*

If third party cost reimbursement regulations are adversely changed in the future, the income of the Hospital would be reduced. If such changes in the regulations reduce or eliminate the reimbursements related to interest or depreciation expense without other provision being made therefor, there could be a significant adverse effect on the Hospital. In addition, a number of third party payors are currently evaluating the initiation of prospective reimbursement programs that could limit reimbursement for costs not planned for at the beginning of the budget period.

(4) *Actions to Limit the Service or Financial Support of a Particular Diagnosis or Class of Patients*

Recent PSRO legislation is directed in part at regulating the amount of reimbursement of costs based upon certain criteria applicable to different types of diagnoses and treatments for particular medical problems.

C. *Factors That Could Result in Increased Competition*

The following factors, among others could result in increased competition:

(1) *Alternative Sources of Health Care and Alternative Hospitals*

The Hospital could face competition in the future from other hospitals and from other forms of health care delivery that could offer comparable health care services to the population which the Hospital presently serves. This could include the construction of new or the renovation of existing hospitals, health maintenance organizations, ambulatory surgical centers, and private laboratories and radiological services.

In addition, competition could come from forms of health care delivery that could offer lower priced services to the same population. These services could be used to substitute for some of the revenue generating services presently offered by the Hospital. The services that could be used to substitute for hospital treatment include: skilled and specialized nursing facilities, home care, intermediate nursing home care, preventive care, and drug and alcohol abuse programs. One of the stated goals of the National Health Planning Act is to develop alternative forms of health care delivery to replace acute inpatient care. The text of the law cites several methods the HSA's are encouraged to promote as a matter of policy to reduce acute inpatient care within their service area.

(2) *Social and Economic Factors Affecting the Service Area Population*

The Hospital could also face increased competition for patients if the population residing in the area it serves is less than the projections used in the Feasibility Report, attached hereto as Appendix B, or there is an increase in the proportion of patients who are unable to pay the full cost of their care.

Other Risk Factors—In the future, the following factors, among others, may adversely affect the operations of health care facilities, including the Hospital, to an extent that cannot be determined at this time:

(1) Adoption in the State of Oregon of legislation which would establish a rate-setting agency with statutory control over hospitals in the State of Oregon.

(2) Employee strikes and other adverse labor actions which could result in a substantial reduction in revenues without corresponding decreases in costs.

(3) The reduced need for hospitalization or other services arising from future medical and scientific advances.

(4) Efforts by insurers and governmental agencies to limit the cost of hospital services, and to reduce utilization of hospital facilities by such means as preventive medicine, improved occupational health and safety, and outpatient care.

(5) Cost and availability of medical malpractice insurance in the State of Oregon. See "Medical Malpractice Considerations" herein.

(6) Utility costs could increase materially in the future due to an energy shortage, and to the extent that they are not reimbursed, could have an adverse impact on the finances of the Hospital.

MEDICAL MALPRACTICE CONSIDERATIONS

Medical Malpractice Insurance Coverage

The Hospital currently carries the following malpractice professional liability insurance:

(1) *Primary:* $1,000,000 on an occurrence basis with no annual aggregate for a term beginning August 22, 1975 until cancelled. This policy is cancellable by the insurer on 60 days' notice. This policy obligates the insurer to pay on behalf of the insured (defined to include the Hospital, Medical Building Land Company, Good Samaritan Medical Building (a partnership) and Good Samaritan Foundation) all sums which the insured shall become legally obligated to pay as damages because of (a) injury, sickness or disease, including death, sustained by any person, (b) injury to or destruction of property, (c) malpractice, error or mistake in performing autopsies and (d) damages sustained by present, prospective or former employees caused by any negligent act, error or omission of the insured. Since the risks covered by the policy include risks other than those related to malpractice, the coverage available at any time for malpractice is subject to diminution.

(2) *First Excess Liability:* $4,000,000 in excess of $1,000,000 on an occurrence basis with no annual aggregate for a term beginning August 22, 1976 and ending August 22, 1977.

(3) *Second Excess Liability:* $5,000,000 in excess of $5,000,000 on an occurrence basis with no annual aggregate for a term beginning August 22, 1976 and ending August 22, 1977.

(4) *Third Excess Liability:* $10,000,000 in excess of $10,000,000 on an occurrence basis with no annual aggregate for a term beginning October 29, 1976 and ending October 29, 1977.

The excess policies numbered (2), (3) and (4) above cover the same risks as the primary policy. Each excess policy refers to and assumes the existence of the underlying insurance coverages as a condition to its obligation. Each policy contains certain exclusions for damages sustained by reason of war, government confiscation and nuclear incident. There can be no assurance given that the above-mentioned insurance policies, or any of them, can be renewed, or that the primary policy may not be cancelled by the insurer or that medical malpractice insurance will at any time be available at reasonable cost or at any cost. While the policies mentioned above are currently in force, the Hospital has not agreed to maintain such policies or like coverages. See the subcaption "Insurance" under the caption "The Sublease" in Appendix C of this Official Statement.

Malpractice Litigation Affecting the Hospital

The Hospital advises that as of June 17, 1977 there were nine pending civil actions seeking damages against the Hospital for alleged medical malpractice. The Hospital further advises that medical malpractice insurance contracts will cover the amount sought in each such civil action. The highest recovery sought in any such action is $288,000.

PENDING LITIGATION

The Hospital advises that in addition to the litigation mentioned above under the subcaption "Malpractice Litigation Affecting the Hospital", there are six unresolved charges pending based upon discrimination as to race, sex or physical handicap. One pending lawsuit seeks recovery for damages in excess of $1 million, alleging race discrimination. The Federal District Court has dismissed the class action aspect of this lawsuit and Hospital management believes that the plaintiff's chance of success is minimal. In the opinion of Hospital management there is little financial exposure to the Hospital from the balance of the charges based on discrimination.

SERIES 1977 BONDS NOT A DEBT

The Series 1977 Bonds will not constitute or create any debt or debts, liability or liabilities on behalf of the State of Oregon or any political subdivision thereof, or of the City of Portland or any public corporation other than the Authority, or a loan of the credit of the State of Oregon or a pledge of or a charge upon the tax revenues of the State of Oregon or of any such political subdivision, or of the City of Portland or any public corporation but will be payable solely from funds paid by the Hospital under the Sublease.

ABSENCE OF MATERIAL LITIGATION

There is no controversy or litigation of any nature now pending or threatened restraining or enjoining the issuance, sale, execution or delivery of the Series 1977 Bonds, or in any way contesting or affecting the validity of the Series 1977 Bonds or any proceedings of the Authority taken with respect to the issuance or sale thereof, or the pledge or application of any moneys or security provided for the payment of the Series 1977 Bonds or existence or powers of the Authority.

APPROVAL OF LEGALITY

Legal matters incident to the authorization, issuance and sale of the Series 1977 Bonds by the Authority are subject to the unqualified approving opinion of Rankin, McMurry, Osburn & Gallagher, Portland, Oregon, Bond Counsel. Certain legal matters will be passed upon for the Hospital by its counsel, Souther, Spaulding, Kinsey, Williamson & Schwabe, Portland, Oregon and for the Underwriters by their counsel, Brown, Wood, Ivey, Mitchell & Petty, New York, New York.

TAX EXEMPTION

In the opinion of Bond Counsel, under existing statutes and court decisions, interest on the Series 1977 Bonds is exempt from Federal income taxes, and under Oregon law, such interest is exempt from all personal income tax in the State of Oregon.

UNDERWRITING

The Series 1977 Bonds are being purchased by the Underwriters, for whom Kidder, Peabody & Co. Incorporated is acting as Representative. The Underwriters have jointly and severally agreed to purchase the Series 1977 Bonds at an aggregate discount of $726,000 from the initial offering price set forth on the cover page. The Contract of Purchase provides that the Underwriters will purchase all the Series 1977 Bonds, if any are purchased, and requires the Hospital to deliver to the Underwriters on the date the Series 1977 Bonds are sold its Letter of Representation constituting the agreement of the Hospital in accordance with its terms to indemnify the Underwriters and the Authority against losses, claims, damages and liabilities arising out of any incorrect statements or information contained in the Preliminary Official Statement and the Official Statement pertaining to the Hospital and other matters. The initial public offering prices set forth on the cover page may be changed by the several Underwriters, and the Underwriters may offer and sell the Series 1977 Bonds to certain dealers (including dealers depositing Series 1977 Bonds into investment trusts) and others at prices lower than the offering prices set forth on the cover page.

RATING

As noted on the cover page hereof, Standard & Poor's Corporation has given the Series 1977 Bonds a rating of A+ (prov.). Any explanation of the significance of this rating may only be obtained from the rating agency. The Hospital and the Authority furnished to such rating agency certain information and materials respecting the Series 1977 Bonds and themselves. Generally, a rating agency bases its rating on such information and materials and investigations, studies and assumptions by the rating agency. There is no assurance that such rating will obtain for any given period of time or that it may not be lowered or withdrawn entirely by the rating agency, if in its judgment circumstances so warrant. Any such downward change in or withdrawal of such rating may have an adverse effect on the market price of the Series 1977 Bonds.

EXPERTS

The Financial Feasibility Study included in Appendix B hereto has been prepared by Booz, Allen & Hamilton, Inc. and has been included in reliance upon the expertise of such firm as management consultants knowledgeable in projecting the future operations of health care institutions. Such study is based on estimates, assumptions, forecasts and other information as stated in Appendix B.

OTHER MATTERS

The Hospital has furnished all information herein relating to the Hospital. Any statements herein involving matters of opinion, whether or not expressly so stated, are intended as such and not as representations of fact.

The foregoing summaries or descriptions of provisions of the Series 1977 Bonds, the Lease, the Sublease, the Indenture and the Guaranty and all references to other materials not purporting to be quoted in full, are only brief outlines of some of the provisions thereof and do not purport to summarize or describe all of the provisions thereof.

The Official Statement will be issued by the Authority and approved by the Hospital.

THE HOSPITAL FACILITIES AUTHORITY OF THE CITY OF PORTLAND, OREGON

By

Chairman

APPROVED:

GOOD SAMARITAN HOSPITAL AND MEDICAL CENTER

By

President

Questions and Problems

Question 5-1. You are asked by the medical director of a large medical group, organized as a profit-making organization, to prepare a report detailing the economic differences between a bond issue and an ownership method of securing investment capital. The medical director indicates that $500,000 of investment capital is required. The medical group currently has $1 million of owners' equity. The tax rate for the group is 48 percent. The interest rate for the proposed bond issue is 8.5 percent. The required percentage return on owners' equity is equal to the bond interest rate. For tax purposes, the returns to owners are considered dividends and, hence, do not qualify as expenses.

Required:
Assume the before-tax and before-interest expense income is $208,000. Prepare a report detailing the economic impact of the bond financing alternative and the equity financing alternative. What is the economic impact of bond financing versus equity financing if only $200,000 of investment capital is required?

Question 5-2.

a. Construct a diagram where institutional risk is plotted on the horizonal axis, and face value, market rate of interest, stated rate of interest, number of restrictive covenants, dollar value of assets pledged, and first date when sinking fund payments must be made (recall that for most organizations sinking fund payments begin in the second half of the term of the bonds) are *individually* plotted on the vertical axis. (Note: six diagrams are required.)
b. Define institutional risk.
c. What do you infer from the term "risk management"?

Question 5-3. You are the administrator of a large teaching hospital. Your investment banker suggests that tax-exempt revenue bonds will be the best method of financing for the institution. The board of managers requests that you submit a plan outlining the steps required to obtain a favorable bond rating. Prepare such a report.

Problem 5-1.

a. The Reynolds Prepaid Medical Plan is planning to issue a bond which has a face value of $75,000. The stated rate of interest is 8.5 percent payable semiannually and the term is 15 years. The probability that the market rate of interest will be 8.5 percent is .4.

The probability that the market rate of interest will be six percent is .4; and the probability that it will be 11 percent is .2. Assuming these estimates are accurate, how much cash is likely to be generated by the sale of the bond?
Note that expected value may be computed as follows:

$$EV = \sum_{i=1}^{n} P_i X_i$$

where: P_i represents the probability that the ith event occurs;
X_i represents the dollar valuation of the ith event; and
n represents the number of events.

b. Assume the least likely event occurs, record the sale of the bonds and the first interest payment (assume straight line amortization). Assume the bond interest is payable on January 1 and July 1, and the bonds are sold on January 1.

Problem 5-2. The Bellevue Memorial Hospital is issuing a taxable bond. They wish to secure exactly $91,750.00. The market rate of interest is 8.75 percent. Prepare four proposals which would yield $91,750.00 for various face values, stated interest rates, and terms. For example, one of the four proposals may be:

Cash Received	Face Value	Stated Interest Rate	Term
$91,750	$91,750	8.75%	variable

Problem 5-3. On April 1, 19X1, the Stratford Prepaid Group sold a $100,000 bond with interest payable February 1 and August 1. The stated interest rate was 9 percent. The market rate of interest on April 1 was 9.25 percent. The term of the bond was ten years.

a. Record the sale of the bonds.
b. Make the appropriate journal entries on April 1, 19X1, August 1, 19X1, December 31, 19X1, January 1, 19X2, and February 1, 19X2 (assume straight line amortization).
c. If the compound amortization method were used, how would the total debits to the interest expense account in part (b) above change? Would there by any difference over the total life of the bond?

Problem 5-4. The administrator of the Americas HMO has called you in for a consultation. On January 1, 19X1, a bond was sold with the following terms:

Face value	$250,000
Stated interest rate	12.5 percent
Term	20 years
Interest payable	semiannually

It is now January 1, 19X8, and the market interest rate is 8.3 percent. The administrator has noticed that the bonds have an early retirement penalty provision which indicates that a three percent payment penalty must be paid on the face value of the bonds if they are retired before the 20-year term expires. Assume the cost of reissuing the bonds (for a term of at least 13 years) is one percent of the face value of the bonds to be issued.

a. Should the Americas HMO retire the bonds and reissue another bond at the market rate of interest?
b. What payment penalty would make the administrator indifferent between refinancing and not refinancing?

Problem 5-5. Given the information in Problem 5-3, record the first and second sinking fund payments, assuming a sinking fund is to be established in 19X5. The sinking fund payments are to be made on February 1 and should provide for $100,000 at the end of the term of the bond. The sinking fund earns 8.5 percent annually.

Chapter 6

The Statement of Changes in Financial Position

You gave me the work
I finally heard.
I'm doing the best that I can.
I've got to admit it's getting better;
It's getting better all the time.

J. Lennon and P. McCartney

Traditionally, two questions have been relevant in evaluating the financial performance of an organization:

1. What is the financial position, or net worth, of the organization at a particular point in time?
2. How well has the organization managed its resources as measured by the results of operations during the current period?

A balance sheet (a statement of financial position) and an income statement (a statement of operations) provide the information needed to answer these questions. However, in today's dynamic economic environment, a third question has become relevant.

3. How well has the organization managed its current assets (cash and assets which are readily convertible into cash) and its current liabilities (liabilities which require cash for payment during the period)?

A statement detailing the organization's financing and investing activities provides the information needed to answer this question. Therefore, since September 30, 1971, the Accounting Principles Board (APB) Opinion #19 has required that a statement detailing the changes in financial position be included along with the balance sheet and statement of operations in an organization's annual report. The Opinion notes that this statement should (1) be entitled a *Statement of Changes in Financial Position*, (2) be based on a broad concept embracing all changes in financial position, and (3) disclose all important aspects of the organization's financing and investing activities, regardless of whether cash or other elements of working capital are affected directly. The Opinion further stipulates that the form, content, and terminology of the statement should be flexible so that the information relevant in differing circumstances can be provided. In this chapter, two bases for reporting the changes in financial position, working capital and cash, are examined.

WORKING CAPITAL

Working capital (WC), which is defined as the difference between current assets (CA) and current liabilities (CL) (see Appendix A), can be computed from information contained in the balance sheet. Although the *amount* of working capital at any particular time is of little importance, the *change* in working capital from one period to another indicates how well the organization's current assets and current liabilities are being managed.

The change in working capital for the period between time t_{n-1} and time t_n may be computed as follows.

Working Capital at Time t_n	Working Capital at Time t_{n-1}	Change During Period t_{n-1} to t_n
CA_n	CA_{n-1}	$CA_n - CA_{n-1} = \Delta CA$
(CL_n)	(CL_{n-1})	$(Cl_n) - (CL_{n-1}) = \Delta(CL)$
WC_n	WC_{n-1}	$WC_n - WC_{n-1} = \Delta WC$

For example, assume that Memorial Hospital's current assets and current liabilities are shown in Exhibit 6-1. In this case, working capital is $185,000 and $153,000 on December 31, 19X2, and December 31, 19X1, respectively. During the period, working capital has increased by $32,000.

This $32,000 change in working capital may be detailed in accordance with APB Opinion #19 as shown in Exhibit 6-2. However, ascertaining whether this increase of $32,000 reflects favorably or unfavorably on the management of the hospital is difficult without knowing how the increase has been generated. For example, a $32,000 increase in working capital could result from either of the following situations:

Situation A: The hospital experiences an operating loss of $192,000 during the period and obtains an 18-month note for $224,000 at 11 ¾ percent interest.

Exhibit 6-1 Partial Comparative Balance Sheets for Memorial Hospital

MEMORIAL HOSPITAL
Partial Comparative Balance Sheets
December 31, 19X2 and 19X1

	December 31, 19X2			December 31, 19X1		
Current Assets:						
Cash		$41,000			$19,000	
Accounts Receivable	$160,000			$193,000		
Less: Allowance for Bad Debts	10,000	150,000		12,000	181,000	
Inventory		53,000			63,000	
Total Current Assets			$244,000			$263,000
Current Liabilities:						
Notes Payable		$34,000			$64,000	
Accounts Payable		14,000			38,000	
Accrued Interest Payable		11,000			8,000	
Total Current Liabilities			$59,000			$110,000

Situation B: The hospital experiences an operating surplus of $96,400 and retires debit of $64,400 during the period.

Although the management implications are very different in these two situations, both situations result in an increase in working capital of $32,000! Therefore, the causes of a change in working capital must be known to interpret the change in working capital.

Working Capital Transactions

The causes of a change in working capital can be isolated by analyzing the transactions that affect working capital during the period. However, before defining, isolating, and analyzing working capital transactions, the definition, isolation and analysis of income transactions will be considered. An income transaction is any transaction which affects both a revenue or expense account (income accounts) *and* some asset, liability, or owners' equity account (nonincome accounts). For example, if a patient is billed $25 for an emergency medical service (EMS) visit, an income transaction occurs. The journal entry to record this transaction is:

Patient Accounts Receivable (·)	$25	
EMS Revenue		$25

Exhibit 6-2 Memorial Hospital: Change in Working Capital Accounts

MEMORIAL HOSPITAL
Partial Statement of Changes in Financial Position:
Working Capital Basis
for the Year Ending December 31, 19X2

Working Capital Accounts	Balances December 31 19X2	Balances December 31 19X1	Working Capital Increase ⟨Decrease⟩
Current Assets:			
Cash	$41,000	$19,000	$22,000
Accounts Receivable	160,000	193,000	(33,000)
Allowance for Bad Debts	(10,000)	(12,000)	2,000
Inventory	53,000	63,000	(10,000)
Total Current Assets	244,000	263,000	
Current Liabilities:			
Notes Payable	34,000	64,000	30,000
Accounts Payable	14,000	38,000	24,000
Accrued Interest Payable	11,000	8,000	(3,000)
Total Current Liabilities	59,000	110,000	
Working Capital	$185,000	$153,000	$32,000

This is an income transaction because both an income account (EMS Revenue) and a nonincome account (Patient Accounts Receivable) have been affected. However, if brain scanning equipment is purchased for $10,000, an income transaction does not occur. The entry to record this transaction is:

Equipment (Brain Scanning Equipment)	$10,000	
Accounts Payable		$10,000

In this case, assets and liabilities (both nonincome accounts) are increased, but revenues and expenses (income accounts) are unaffected. These two examples illustrate that a change in income occurs only when an economic transaction affects both an income and nonincome account.

Similarly, a change in working capital results only when a transaction affects a working capital *and* a nonworking capital account (see Problem 6-2). Since working capital is defined as the difference between current assets and current liabilities, these accounts are the working capital accounts. All other accounts are nonworking capital accounts. Therefore, a working capital transaction is any transaction that affects a current asset (CA) or a current liability (CL) account *and* affects a noncurrent asset (NCA), a noncurrent liability (NCL), a revenue (R), an expense (E), or an owners' equity (OE) account.

Consider the schematic shown in Figure 6-1. The only working capital transaction in the schematic is T_5. The transaction represented by T_5 is the only one that affects both a working capital account, CA, and a nonworking capital account, R. An example of T_5 is:

Cash (CA)	$55	
Patient Revenue (R)		$55

To record the delivery of service for $55 cash.

Examples of the other transactions are:

T_1: Accounts Payable (CL)	$1064	
Cash (CA)		$1064

Figure 6-1 Schematic Showing Various Types of Economic Transactions

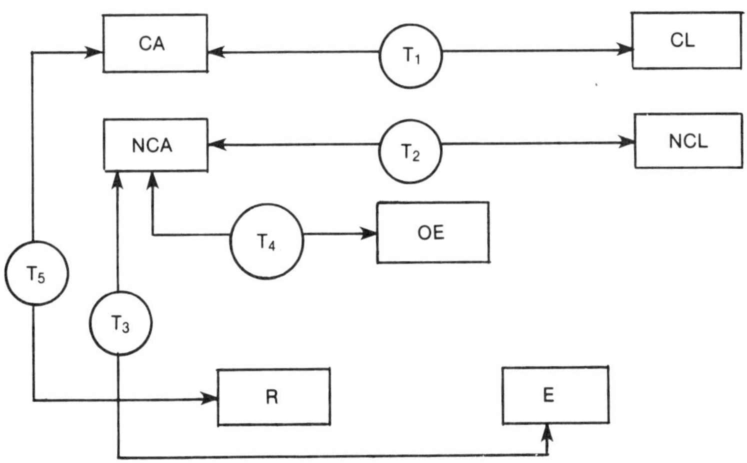

Where: T_i are economic transactions affecting particular account categories CA, CL, NCA, NCL, OE, R or E.

To record the payment of $1,064 of accounts payable.

T_2:	Land (NCA)	$10,000	
	Long-Term Bonds Payable (NCA)		$10,000

To record the purchase of land in exchange for long-term bonds with a market value of $10,000.

T_3:	Depreciation Expense (E)	$7,800	
	Accumulated Depreciation (NCA)		$7,800

To record the annual depreciation of fixed assets.

T_4:	Equipment (NCA)	$6,000	
	Contribution (OE)		$6,000

To record the contribution of an asset with a market value of $6,000.

Note that none of these transactions affect both a working capital and a nonworking capital account.

Stating Changes in Working Capital in Terms of the Nonworking Capital Accounts

The change in working capital can be stated in terms of the nonworking capital accounts, as well as in terms of the working capital accounts, because (1) all working capital transactions affect both a working capital and a nonworking capital account, and (2) the debits always equal the credits in the double entry accounting system (see Appendix A). For example, the accounting equation[1] at time t_{n-1}

$$(A = L + OE + R - E)_{n-1}$$

can be reformulated as:

(6-1) $$CA_{n-1} + NCA_{n-1} = CL_{n-1} + NCL_{n-1} + OE_{n-1} + R_{n-1} - E_{n-1}.$$

Similarly, the accounting equation at time t_n can be stated as:

(6-2) $$CA_n + NCA_n = CL_n + NCL_n + OE_n + R_n - E_n.$$

To compute the amount of working capital in each period, $WC_i = CA_i -$

CL_i, where $i = n - 1, n$, equations (6-2) and (6-1) can be rearranged, respectively, as follows.

(6-3) $CA_n - CL_n = -NCA_n + NCL_n + OE_n + R_n - E_n$

(6-4) $CA_{n-1} - CL_{n-1} = -NCA_{n-1} + NCL_{n-1} + OE_{n-1} + R_{n-1} - E_{n-1}$

Then, if equation (6-4) is subtracted from equation (6-3), the change in working capital from time t_{n-1} to time t_n, $\Delta WC_{n-(n-1)} = (CA_n - CL_n) - (CA_{n-1} - CL_{n-1})$ can be computed as:

(6-5) $\Delta WC_{n-(n-1)} = -(NCA_n - NCA_{n-1}) + (NCL_n - NCL_{n-1}) + (OE_n - OE_{n-1}) + (R_n - R_{n-1}) - (E_n - E_{n-1})$.

Equation (6-5) demonstrates that the causes for a change in working capital can be stated in terms of changes in the nonworking capital accounts. In fact, since changes occur in the nonworking capital accounts as a result of financing activities from which working capital is derived (sources of working capital) and investing activities to which working capital is applied (applications of working capital), the nonworking capital accounts are useful in describing the changes in working capital in the statement of changes in financial position. By delineating the causes for changes in working capital, the statement of changes in financial position produces information that is useful in evaluating the management of the organization's current assets, current liabilities, and the management of the organization's financing and investing activities.

PREPARING A STATEMENT OF CHANGES IN FINANCIAL POSITION: WORKING CAPITAL BASIS

A statement of changes in financial position prepared on a working capital basis provides information regarding the causes for any change in working capital during a particular period. The sources and applications of working capital are delineated in the statement. The difference between the total sources and total applications equals the change in working capital computed from the comparative balance sheets at the beginning and end of the period.

Preparing the statement of changes in financial position can be a very complex task. Fortunately, however, a systematic methodology has been developed to gather the information required. However, before discussing this methodology, some special conceptual problems concerning adjustments needed to convert an institution's net income to working capital generated from operations will be considered.

Working Capital Generated from Operations

The last two expressions of equation (6-5), $(R_n - R_{n-1}) - (E_n - E_{n-1})$, can be restated as $(R_n - E_n) - (R_{n-1} - E_{n-1})$, which indicates that a change in working capital will occur if the net income of period n is different from the net income of period $n - 1$ (see Question 6-1). However, when the accounting records are closed at the end of period $n - 1$, the net income for that period is incorporated in the owners' equity account. Hence, when the information required to compute the change in the owners' equity account between time t_{n-1} and time t_n is extracted from the accounting records, the owners' equity account at time t_{n-1} will reflect some amount, OE_{n-1}^*, which is equal to $OE_{n-1} + (R_{n-1} - E_{n-1})$. Since $(R_{n-1} - E_{n-1})$ is incorporated in OE_{n-1}^*, equation (6-5) can be restated as:

$$(6\text{-}6)\quad \Delta WC_{n-(n-1)} = -(NCA_n - NCA_{n-1}) + (NCL_n - NCL_{n-1}) + (OE_n - OE_{n-1}^*) + (R_n - E_n).$$

This equation indicates that the change in working capital for any particular period is a function of that period's net income, as well as a function of the changes that occur in the noncurrent asset accounts, the noncurrent liability accounts, and the owners' equity accounts[2] during that period.

Since net income measures the results of operations for any particular period and most net income transactions are working capital transactions, the amount of working capital generated by operations is approximated well by net income (see Question 6-5). However, working capital from operations is strictly defined as the amount of working capital generated as a result of pursuing the normal operations of the institution (i.e., rendering health care services). Therefore, net income transactions that do not affect working capital must not be included in working capital from operations. Similarly, net income transactions that affect working capital, but do not arise from pursuing the normal operations of the institution, must be excluded from working capital from operations. In other words, if net income is used as the first approximation of working capital from operations, adjustments must be made to eliminate the effects of net income transactions (1) that are not working capital transactions and (2) that do not arise through the normal operations of the institution. Some of the usual adjustments needed to convert net income to working capital from operations are given in Figure 6-2.

Depreciation

Assume that the accounts of a nursing agency have the following balances on January 1, 19X1.

Cash		Equipment		Accounts Payable		Equity	
$10,000		$10,000			$5,000		$15,000

During 19X1 the following transactions take place.

1. $10,000 of skilled nursing services are performed.

Entry: Patient Accounts Receivable (·)	$10,000	
Service Revenue (D)		$10,000

2. Nursing wages paid during the year amount to $5,000.

Entry: Nursing Wage Expense	$5,000	
Cash		$5,000

3. An EKG machine, purchased at the end of 19X0 for $10,000 and expected to have a two-year life, is depreciated on a straight line basis.

Entry: Depreciation Expense	$5,000	
Accumulated Depreciation		$5,000

Figure 6-2 Adjustments Required to Convert Net Income to Working Capital from Operations

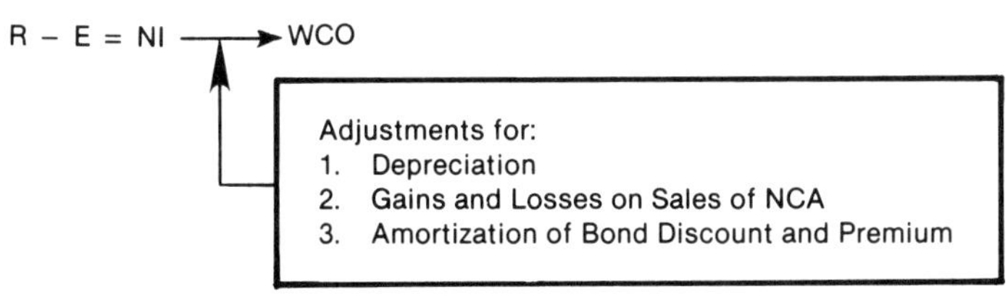

Where: NI represents net income; and
WCO represents working capital from operations

In this example, the change in working capital can be calculated from the working capital accounts as follows.

Change in Working Capital Accounts:	Working Capital Increase (Decrease)
Cash	($5,000)
Patient Accounts Receivable	10,000
Current Liabilities	– 0 –
Working Capital	$5,000

Therefore, an analysis of the nonworking capital accounts should show a $5,000 increase in working capital for 19X1.

The only source of working capital for this year is generated from operations. However, net income (contribution to equity), as measured by generally accepted accounting principles, is:

Nursing Revenue		$10,000
Less: Nursing Wages	$5,000	
Depreciation	5,000	10,000
Net Income		$ - 0 -

Thus, the analysis of the nonworking capital accounts *seems* to show no change in working capital. To resolve this apparent discrepancy, the working capital implications of the three transactions that occurred during 19X1 must be examined.

The transaction to record the performance of $10,000 of skilled nursing services is a working capital transaction because it affects a working capital account (Patient Accounts Receivable) and a nonworking capital account (Service Revenue). Both net income and working capital from operations are increased by $10,000 as a result of this transaction.

Similarly, the transaction to record the payment of $5,000 of nursing wages is a working capital transaction because it affects a working capital account (Cash) and a nonworking capital account (Nursing Wage Expense). Net income, as well as working capital, is reduced by $5,000 as a result of this transaction.

However, the transaction to record the annual depreciation of the EKG machine is not a working capital transaction because it affects two nonworking capital accounts (Depreciation Expense and Accumulated Depreciation). Although this transaction reduces net income by the $5,000 depreciation expense, no corresponding reduction in working capital from

operations has occurred. Therefore, to adjust net income to working capital from operations, depreciation must be *added* to net income.
to net income.

In the nursing agency example, the statement of changes in financial position should show the following.

Sources of Working Capital

From operations:		
Net Income	$ - 0 -	
Add: Adjustments for income transactions not affecting working capital:		
Depreciation	$5,000	
Working capital from operations		$5,000
Total sources of working capital		$5,000

Since none of the transactions affecting the nursing agency were applications of working capital, the statement of changes in financial position for the nursing agency would show an increase in working capital of $5,000. This increase agrees with the $5,000 increase calculated from the working capital accounts.

Gains on Sales of Noncurrent Assets

Assume that an HMO sells an asset for $8,000 cash. If the asset had an original value of $10,000 and has accumulated depreciation to date of $6,000, the entry to record the sale is as shown.

Cash	$8,000	
Accumulated Depreciation	6,000	
Equipment		$10,000
Gain on Sale of Equipment		4,000

This transaction is a working capital transaction because it affects a working capital account (Cash) and three nonworking capital accounts (Equipment, Accumulated Depreciation, and Gain on Sale of Equipment). Working capital is increased by $8,000 as a result of this sale. Net income is increased by the $4,000 gain on the sale (a revenue account).

Assume that the HMO's net income during the period is $10,000, including the $4,000 gain on the sale of equipment. The sources of working capital section of the statement of changes in financial position would include the following.

Sources of Working Capital		
From Operations:		
Net Income	$10,000	
Total working capital from operations		$.....
From other sources:		
Sale of equipment	8,000	
	.....	
	.....	
	.....	
Total working capital from other sources		.....
Total sources of working capital		$.....

Since the $4,000 gain included in net income has not been generated from operations (i.e., it has not been generated as a result of rendering health care services), it must be subtracted from net income to compute working capital from operations. Furthermore, the $8,000 cash received from the sale of the asset can be separated into two parts, the conversion of the book value[3] of the asset to cash, $4,000, and the gain of $4,000 representing the cash received in excess of the book value. Therefore, subtracting the gain from net income avoids a double counting of the gain, in addition to stating the amount of working capital generated from operations properly.

In this case, if no other adjustments are needed to adjust net income to working capital from operations, the sources of working capital section of the statement of changes in financial position would be as shown.

Sources of Working Capital		
From Operations:		
Net Income	$10,000	
Add (deduct) adjustments for net income transactions not affecting working capital:		
Gain on sale of equipment	(4,000)	
Total working capital from operations		$6,000

From other sources:		
Sale of equipment	$8,000	
	.....	
	.....	
	.....	
Total working capital from other sources		.....
Total sources of working capital		$.....

Any other sources of working capital would be listed under the sale of equipment. Thus, the total sources of working capital could be computed. The applications of working capital would be listed in the section of the statement following the sources of working capital.

Losses on Sales of Noncurrent Assets

The entry to record the sale of the asset in the previous example, if the asset were sold for $2,000, would be:

Cash	$2,000	
Accumulated Depreciation	6,000	
Loss on Sale of Equipment	2,000	
Equipment		$10,000

This transaction is a working capital transaction because it affects a working capital account (Cash) and three nonworking capital accounts (Equipment, Accumulated Depreciation, and Loss on Sale of Equipment). Working capital is increased by $2,000 as a result of the sale and net income is reduced by the $2,000 loss on the sale.

The $2,000 decrease in net income has not been generated from operations and must be added back to net income to state working capital from operations properly. Again, the $2,000 cash received in exchange for the asset consists of two parts: the conversion of the book value of the asset to cash, $4,000, and a loss on the disposition of the asset, $2,000. Therefore, the $2,000 loss has affected working capital by reducing the amount of cash received. Adding the loss back to net income properly states working capital from operations and avoids double counting the loss.

Bond Discount Amortization

Recall from Chapter 5 that when bonds are issued at a price less than their face value, the bonds are said to be issued at a discount equal to the difference between their face value and their selling price. This discount is recorded in an account called Discount on Bonds Payable, a contra-account to Bonds Payable, which must be amortized (written off) over the term of the bonds so that the total amount due to the bondholders (the face value of the bond) is reflected in the accounts at the end of the term of the bond. The effect of bond discount amortization is to increase bond interest expense and thus reduce net income. An examination of the working capital implications of bond discounts follows.

Assume that an institution wants to issue ten-year bonds with a face value of $100,000 and a stated interest rate of six percent (interest payable annually), but can only market the bonds at a discount of $2,000. The entry to record the issuance of these bonds is:

Cash	$98,000	
Discount on 6% Bonds Payable	2,000	
6% Bonds Payable		$100,000

To record the sale of ten-year, six percent bonds, face value of $100,000, for $98,000.

Hence, a $2,000 discount must be amortized over a ten-year period. If the bond discount is amortized on a straight line basis, $200 of the discount will be amortized each year.

The entry to record the annual payment of interest and the amortization of the bond discount is:

Bond Interest Expense	$6,200	
Discount on 6% Bonds Payable		$ 200
Cash		6,000

To record the payment of interest and the amortization of bond discount on a ten-year, six percent bonds sold at a discount of $2,000.

This transaction is a working capital transaction because it affects a working capital account (Cash) and two nonworking capital accounts (Bond Interest Expense and Discount on 6% Bonds Payable). Working capital is decreased by $6,000 as a result of the cash expenditure to pay the bond interest. However, the Bond Interest Expense account, which decreases net income, includes the $200 discount amortization as well as the $6,000 cash outflow. Since the bond discount amortization portion of this entry affects two nonworking capital accounts (Bond Interest Expense and Discount on 6% Bonds Payable), the amortization of the discount does not affect working capital. Therefore, to state working capital from operations properly, the $200 bond discount amortization must be added back to net income.

Bond Premium Amortization

When bonds are issued at a price greater than their face value, the bonds are said to be issued at a premium equal to the difference between the selling price and the face value of the bonds. This premium is recorded in an account called Premium on Bonds Payable which, like the Discount on Bonds Payable account, must be amortized over the term of the bond. The effect of amortizing the bond premium is to decrease bond interest expense, thereby increasing net income. The working capital implications of bond premium amortization will be analyzed in the following example.

Assume that the institution in the previous example issues ten-year, six percent bonds (interest payable annually) with a face value of $100,000. If the market is willing to pay a premium of $2,000 for these bonds, the entry to record the issuance of the bonds is:

Cash	$102,000	
Premium on 6% Bonds Payable		$ 2,000
6% Bonds Payable		100,000

To record the sale of ten-year, six percent bonds, face value $100,000, for $102,000.

If the premium is amortized on a straight line basis, $200 of the premium must be amortized each year.

The entry to record the annual payment of interest and the amortization of the bond premium is:

Bond Interest Expense	$5,800	
Premium on 6% Bonds Payable	200	
Cash		$6,000

To record the payment of interest and the amortization of bond premium on ten-year, six percent bonds sold at a premium of $2,000.

This transaction is a working capital transaction because it affects a working capital account (Cash) and two nonworking capital accounts (Bond Interest Expense and Premium on 6% Bonds Payable). Working capital is reduced by $6,000 as a result of this transaction, but net income is reduced by only $5,800. Therefore, to state working capital from operations properly, the $200 bond premium amortization must be subtracted from net income.

A Methodology for Preparing a Statement of Changes in Financial Position

The methodology for preparing a statement of changes in financial position on a working capital basis was introduced by William J. Vatter. Vatter's methodology uses the basic working capital relationship (i.e., working capital is affected only when a transaction affects both a working capital account *and* a nonworking capital account). The steps in the methodology for preparing the statement of changes in financial position on a working capital basis are as follows.

STEP 1—Set up a T account for (a) each nonworking capital account, (b) a Net Income Conversion account,[4] and (c) a Working Capital account. Record the beginning balances (noted with a (✓)) in the nonworking capital T accounts.

STEP 2—Isolate the journal entries that have affected the nonworking capital accounts during the period (from the time the opening balances are recorded to the end of the accounting period) and reformulate these entries so that the balancing debit or credit in each journal entry[5] is made (a) to the Net Income Conversion account, if working capital from operations is affected, or (b) to the Working Capital account, if working capital other than that from operations is affected. Economic transactions that affect only nonworking capital accounts also must be entered in the Working Capital account so that all of the institution's financing and investing activities during the period will be recorded in the Working Capital account or in the Net Income Conversion account. The debit entries to the Working Capital account as a result of these "nonworking capital" transactions must equal the credit entries to the Working Capital account as a result of these transactions.

STEP 3—Post all of the journal entries from step 2 in the T accounts set up in step 1. When the balances in the nonworking capital accounts equal their year-end balances, the Net Income Conversion account should be closed to the Working Capital account.

STEP 4—The statement of changes in financial position can be prepared directly from the Working Capital account. The *debit* entries in this account are the *sources* of working capital and the *credit* entries are the *applications* of working capital. The details for the Working Capital from Operations section of the statement of changes in financial position can be obtained from the debits and credits in the Net Income Conversion account.

The following example illustrates the application of these steps.

Consider the comparative balance sheets shown in Exhibit 6-3 for the Memorial Hospital.

Exhibit 6-3 Comparative Balance Sheets for Memorial Hospital

MEMORIAL HOSPITAL
Comparative Balance Sheets
December 31, 19X2 and 19X1

	December 31, 19X2			December 31, 19X1		
ASSETS						
Current Assets:						
Cash		$ 41,000			$ 19,000	
Accounts Receivable	$160,000			$193,000		
Less: Allowance for Bad Debts	10,000	150,000		12,000	181,000	
Inventory		53,000			63,000	
Total Current Assets			$ 244,000			$ 263,000
Fixed Assets:						
Hospital Building and Equipment	423,000			373,000		
Less: Accumulated Depreciation	200,000	223,000		89,000	284,000	
Land		596,000			500,000	
Construction in Process		337,000			180,000	
Total Fixed Assets			1,156,000			964,000
Total Assets			$1,400,000			$1,227,000
LIABILITIES						
Current Liabilities:						
Notes Payable		34,000			64,000	
Accounts Payable		14,000			38,000	
Accrued Interest Payable		11,000			8,000	
Total Current Liabilities			59,000			110,000
Long-Term Liabilities						
6% Bonds Payable		469,000			419,000	
Discount on 6% Bonds Payable		43,900			41,000	
Total Long-Term Liabilities			425,100			378,000
Total Liabilities			484,100			488,000
OWNERS' EQUITY						
Contributed Capital		500,000			400,000	
Earnings Retained from Previous Periods		415,900			339,000	
Total Owners' Equity			915,900			739,000
Total Liabilities and Owners' Equity			$1,400,000			$1,227,000

STEP 1—Set up T accounts

Given the comparative balance sheets for 19X2 and 19X1, the following T accounts, with the associated beginning balances, should be created:

Hospital Equipment	
(✓) $373,000	

Accumulated Depreciation	
	(✓) $89,000

Land	
(✓) $500,000	

Construction in Process	
(✓) $180,000	

6% Bonds Payable	
	(✓) $419,000

Discount on 6% Bonds Payable	
(✓) $41,000	

Contributed Capital	
	(✓) $400,000

Retained Earnings	
	(✓) $339,000

Income Conversion	

Working Capital	

STEP 2—Isolate working capital transactions and reformulate journal entries.

A perusal of the journal entries made during the period yields the following additional information regarding the changes in the nonworking capital accounts:

A. D. Gannon, philanthropist, contributed land valued at $96,000.
B. During 19X2, $157,000 of construction was completed on the hospital's new wing.
C. On June 15, 19X2, four EKG machines were purchased for $20,000 each.
D. On August 8, 19X2, three EKG machines with historical costs of $10,000 each (book value $4,000 each) were sold for $5,000 each.
E. Six percent, ten-year bonds, face value $50,000, were sold for $46,000, excluding interest.
F. A grateful patient contributed $4,000 to the hospital's cardiac research fund.
G. The revenues for the year were $281,200 and the expenses were $207,300.

Given this additional information and the comparative balance sheets, the entries to record the changes in the nonworking capital accounts can be reformulated as follows.

A. (i) Land	$96,000	
Working Capital		$96,000

To record the contribution of land valued at $96,000 as an application of working capital.

(ii) Working Capital	$96,000	
Contributed Capital		$96,000

To record the contribution of land valued at $96,000 as a source of working capital.

B. Construction in Process	$157,000	
Working Capital		$157,000

To record construction completed on the hospital's new wing as an application of working capital.

C. Hospital Building and Equipment	$80,000	
Working Capital		$80,000

To record the purchase of four EKG machines, valued at $20,000 each, as an application of working capital.

D. Working Capital	$15,000	
Accumulated Depreciation	18,000	
Net Income Conversion		$ 3,000
Hospital Building and Equipment		30,000

To record the sale of three EKG machines, book value $4,000 each, for $5,000 each, as a source of working capital and to adjust the Net Income Conversion account for the $3,000 gain on the sale of the EKG machines, which increased net income but is not working capital from operations.

E. Working Capital	$46,000	
Discount on 6% Bonds Payable	4,000	
6% Bonds Payable		$50,000

To record the sale of ten-year, six percent bonds, face value $50,000, for $46,000 as a source of working capital.

F. Working Capital	$4,000	
Contributed Capital		$4,000

To record the contribution of $4,000 to the cardiology department as a source of working capital.

G. Net Income Conversion	76,900	
Retained Earnings		76,900

To record the contribution of net income to retained earnings as working capital from operations. (See Question 6-8.)

H. Net Income Conversion	129,000	
Accumulated Depreciation		129,000

To adjust the Net Income Conversion account for the depreciation on the hospital's depreciable assets that reduced net income but does not reduce working capital.

I. Net Income Conversion	1,100	
Bond Discount		1,100

To adjust the Net Income Conversion account for the amortization of the bond discount that reduced net income but does not reduce working capital.

STEP 3—Post journal entries to the appropriate T accounts.

The journal entries from step 2 must be posted to the T accounts set up in step 1. Once all of these journal entries have been posted, the balances in the nonworking capital accounts should equal their year-end balances. Then, the Net Income Conversion account should be closed to the working capital account as follows.

J. Working Capital	204,000	
Income Conversion		204,000

To close the Net Income Conversion account to the Working Capital account and record working capital from operations as a source of working capital.

The resultant balances in the T accounts are:

Hospital Building and Equipment	
$373,000	$30,000 (D)
80,000	
$423,000	

Accumulated Depreciation	
(D) $18,000	$ 89,000
	129,000 (H)
	$200,000

Land	
(✓) $500,000	
(Ai) 96,000	
$596,000	

Construction in Process

Debit	Credit
(✓) $180,000	
(B) 157,000	
$337,000	

6% Bonds Payable

Debit	Credit
	(✓) $419,000
	50,000(E)
	$469,000

Discounts on 6% Bonds Payable

Debit	Credit
(✓) $41,000	$1,100 (I)
(E) 4,000	
$43,900	

Contributed Capital

Debit	Credit
	(✓) $400,000
	96,000 (Aii)
	4,000 (F)
	$500,000

Retained Earnings

Debit	Credit
	(✓) $339,000
	76,900 (G)
	$415,000

Net Income Conversion

Debit	Credit
(G) $ 76,900	$ 3,000 (D)
(H) 129,000	
(I) 1,100	
$204,000	$204,000 (J)

Working Capital

Debit	Credit
(Aii) $ 96,000	$ 96,000 (Ai)
(D) 15,000	157,000 (B)
(E) 46,000	80,000 (C)
(F) 4,000	
(J) 204,000	
269,000	237,000
	32,000 Increase in working capital
$269,000	$269,000

The sources of working capital are represented by the five debits in the working capital account, and the applications of working capital are represented by the three credits in the working capital account.

STEP 4—Preparing the statement of changes in financial position.

Using the information recorded in the Working Capital and the Net Income Conversion T accounts in step 3, the following statement of changes in financial position can be prepared for the Memorial Hospital.

MEMORIAL HOSPITAL

Statement of Changes in Financial Position: Working Capital Basis for the Year Ended December 31, 19X2

Sources of Working Capital	
From operations:	
Net income	$76,900
Add (deduct) adjustments for income transactions not affecting working capital:	
Depreciation	129,000
Amortization of bond discount	1,100
Gain on sale of equipment	(3,000)
Total working capital from operations	$204,000

Statement of Changes in Financial Position: Working Capital Basis for the Year Ended December 31, 19X2 Continued

From other sources:		
Sale of equipment	15,000	
Sale of bonds	46,000	
Philanthropic contributions (Note 1)	100,000	
Total working capital from other sources		161,000
Total sources of working capital		365,000
Applications of Working Capital		
Land (Note 1)	96,000	
Construction	157,000	
Purchase of equipment	80,000	
Total applications of working capital		333,000
Increase in working capital		$32,000

NOTE 1—Philanthropic contributions included:
Land: $96,000 (market value)
Cash contribution to cardiac research fund: $4,000

Working Capital Accounts	Balances December 31 19X2	Balances December 31 19X1	Working Capital Increase (Decrease)
Current Assets:			
Cash	$ 41,000	$ 19,000	$22,000
Accounts Receivable	160,000	193,000	(33,000)
Allowance for Bad Debts	(10,000)	(12,000)	2,000
Inventory	53,000	63,000	(10,000)
Total Current Assets	$244,000	$263,000	
Current Liabilities:			
Notes Payable	34,000	64,000	30,000
Accounts Payable	14,000	38,000	24,000
Accrued Interest Payable	11,000	8,000	(3,000)
Total Current Liabilities	59,000	110,000	
Working Capital	$185,000	$153,000	$32,000

Analyzing the statement of changes in financial position prepared on a working capital basis aids in evaluating the financial management of the institution. In this case, the hospital appears to be in a strong financial position because working capital generated from operations financed 61 percent of the applications of working capital. However, working capital is not the only basis for evaluating the financial management of an institution. The change in cash is another useful basis for evaluation.

PREPARING A STATEMENT OF CHANGES IN FINANCIAL POSITION: CASH BASIS

Recall that APB Opinion #19 stipulates that the form and content of the statement of changes in financial position may differ, given varying institutional situations. For some health care institutions, the sources and applications of cash provide a more meaningful basis of evaluation than the sources and applications of working capital. If this is the case, these institutions should prepare a statement of changes in financial position on a cash basis.

The preparation of the statement of changes in financial position on a cash basis and a working capital basis are similar. However, the primary focus of the statement prepared on a cash basis is to delineate the sources of cash (inflows of cash) and applications of cash (outflows of cash). The typical form of the statement of changes in financial position prepared on a cash basis is shown in Exhibit 6-4.

Note that the types of adjustments to revenues and expenses in the statement prepared on a cash basis are similar to the net income adjustments required to convert periodic net income to the working capital generated from operations in the statement prepared on a working capital basis. The adjustments to revenue should convert the revenue developed under the accrual basis of accounting to cash generated from operations for the period. For example, consider the following revenue and accounts receivable transactions for the Memorial Hospital during 19X2.

Patient Accounts Receivable (·)	$218,250	
Revenue		$218,250

To record the creation of accounts receivable during the year.

Cash	$62,950	
Revenue		$62,950

To record the collection of cash from patients for services provided.

Exhibit 6-4 Form of Statement of Changes in Financial Position: Cash Basis

MEMORIAL HOSPITAL
Statement of Changes in Financial Position: Cash Basis
for the Year Ended December 31, 19X2

Sources of Cash		
From operations:		
Revenues	$XXXX	
Add (deduct) adjustments to convert revenues to a cash basis:		
Specific adjustments	XXX	
	(XX)	
Cash generated from revenues		$XXX
Expenses	XXXX	
Add (deduct) adjustments to convert expenses to a cash basis:		
Specific adjustments	XXX	
	(XX)	
Cash disbursed for expenses		XXX
Total cash from operations		XXX
From other sources:		
Specific other sources	XXX	
	XXX	
Total cash from other sources		XXX
Total sources of cash		XXX
Applications of Cash		
Specific applications	XXX	
	XXX	
	XXX	
Total applications of cash		XXX
Increase (decrease) in cash		$ XX

Cash	$251,250	
Patient Accounts Receivable (·)		$251,250

To record the collection of certain patient accounts.

In this case, the total cash generated from revenues is the sum of the two debit entries in the cash account:

Cash	
$ 62,950	
251,250	
$314,200	

However, the total cash generated from revenues also may be measured as:

Cash Generated from Operations = Revenues $-$ Δ Accounts Receivable

where: Δ Accounts Receivable represents the change in the accounts receivable during the period.

This relationship exists because the cash collected during the period for services rendered is equal to the revenues recorded for services rendered during the period, less the accounts receivable created during the period that are still outstanding at the end of the period, plus the accounts receivable outstanding at the end of the prior period that are collected during the current period.

In the case of the Memorial Hospital, revenues have amounted to \$281,200 (\$218,250 + \$62,950) and accounts receivable have decreased by \$33,000 (\$218,250 − \$251,250)[6] during the year. Therefore, cash generated from operations is as shown.

Cash Generated from Operations = Revenue $-$ Δ Accounts Receivable

$$\$314{,}200 = \$281{,}200 - (-\$33{,}000)$$

The adjustments required to convert expenses to cash disbursed for expenses during the period are similar to the revenue adjustments already described. All noncash expenses and the changes in working capital accounts which affect cash expended during the year must be isolated to adjust the recorded expenses to cash disbursed for expenses during the year. For example, the depreciation expense recorded for the year increases the recorded expenses but does not affect cash disbursed for expenses. On the other hand, a decrease in the Accounts Payable account requires a cash disbursement but does not affect the expenses recorded during the period. Therefore, in the statement of changes in financial position prepared on a cash basis, the depreciation expense should be deducted from the recorded expenses and the net decrease in the Accounts Payable account should be added to the recorded expenses to compute the amount of cash disbursed for expenses during the year. A methodology similar to the methodology discussed for preparing a statement of changes in financial position on a working capital basis may be used (see Problem 6-8). On the other hand, each adjustment may be analyzed individually, as demonstrated for the Memorial Hospital revenue adjustment above (see Problem 6-7). The completed statement of changes in financial position on a cash basis for the Memorial Hospital is shown in Exhibit 6-5.

Exhibit 6-5 Memorial Hospital's Statement of Changes in Financial Position: Cash Basis

MEMORIAL HOSPITAL
Statement of Changes in Financial Position: Cash Basis
for the Year Ended December 31, 19X2

Sources of Cash		
From Operations:		
Revenues	$281,200	
Add (deduct) adjustments to convert revenues to a cash basis:		
Accounts receivable decrease	33,000	
Cash generated from revenues		$314,200
Expenses	207,300	
Add (deduct) adjustments to convert expenses to a cash basis:		
Depreciation expense	(129,000)	
Allowances for bad debts decrease	2,000	
Inventory decrease	(10,000)	
Notes payable decrease	30,000	
Accounts payable decrease	24,000	
Accrued interest payable increase	(3,000)	
Amortization of bond discount	(1,100)	
Cash disbursed for expenses		$120,200
Total cash from operations		194,000
From other sources:		
Sale of equipment	15,000	
Sale of bonds	46,000	
Philanthropic contributions (Note 1)	100,000	
Total cash from other sources		161,000
Total sources of cash		355,000
Applications of Cash:		
Land (Note 1)	96,000	
Construction	157,000	
Purchase of equipment	80,000	
Total applications of cash		333,000
Increase in cash during the period		$22,000

NOTE 1—Philanthropic contributions included:
Land: $96,000 (market value)
Cash contribution to cardiac research fund: $4,000.

The statement of changes in financial position prepared on a cash basis provides valuable information which may be used to ascertain how the institution derives and uses its cash. In addition, this statement can provide management with valuable planning information regarding the operational management of the institution (see Questions 6-2 and 6-3). For example, consistent with the information provided in the analysis of working capital, the analysis of cash indicates an effectively managed institution. Note that 58 percent of the applications of cash are provided by cash generated from operations.

NOTES

1. See Appendix A for a discussion concerning the fundamental accounting equation, A = L + OE.
2. Note that $(R_{n-1} - E_{n-1})$ is included in OE_n also, since the beginning balances in the owners' equity accounts for period n is equal to the ending balances in the owners' equity accounts for period $n - 1$. Therefore, $(OE_n - OE^*_{n-1})$ indicates all changes in the owners' equity accounts other than those arising through the generation of income.
3. The book value of an asset is the recorded value of the asset, less the amount of depreciation taken to date on the asset.
4. The Net Income Conversion account is used to convert the net income measured by conventional accounting principles to working capital generated from operations.
5. These journal entries are not journalized in the institution's accounting system, nor are they posted to the institution's ledgers. They are only used to prepare the statement of changes in financial position.
6. The decrease in accounts receivable also can be computed from the comparative balance sheets for the Memorial Hospital at December 31, 19X1 and 19X2 (p. 207). The Memorial Hospital's accounts receivable on December 31, 19X1 and 19X2 are $193,000 and $160,000, respectively. Therefore, accounts receivable have decreased by $33,000 ($160,000 − $193,000) during 19X2.

Questions and Problems

Question 6-1. The change in working capital is defined as:

$$(6\text{-}5)\ \Delta WC_{n-(n-1)} = -(NCA_n - NCA_{n-1}) + (NCL_n - NCL_{n-1}) + (OE_n - OE_{n-1}) + (R_n - R_{n-1}) - (E_n - E_{n-1}).$$

Discuss the form of this equation for a nonprofit institution. How does the working capital analysis change for a non-profit institution?

Question 6-2. The administrator of a prepaid group practice is confused about the value of the information contained in the Statement of

Changes in Financial Position: Cash Basis. The administrator argues that this same information is available by analyzing the cash receipts and cash disbursements books. Discuss this assertion and relate it to the information represented in the Statement of Changes in Financial Position: Cash Basis.

Question 6-3. Consider the Statement of Changes in Financial Position: Cash Basis, p. 216 and respond to the following: The Statement of Changes in Financial Position: Cash Basis can be misleading if one believes that all the adjustments result in changes in cash. For example, during the year the institution may satisfy an account payable with inventory. This transaction does not affect cash, yet the changes in these two accounts (inventory and accounts payable) will be used to adjust reported expenses to reflect cash disbursed for expenses during the period.

Question 6-4. Recast the Statement of Changes in Financial Position: Cash Basis so that the change in working capital is adjusted to reflect the change in cash (also see Problem 6-9). Discuss this form of presentation.

Question 6-5. Discuss the following statement: Since the purpose of nonprofit institutions is to break even, operations will never be a *net* source of working capital.

Question 6-6. After carefully reading the Statement of Changes in Financial Position: Working Capital Basis for the year, the chief of medicine writes the following memo to the controller:

> I have a fair understanding of the many relationships represented in our Statement of Changes in Financial Position, but I must confess I cannot conceptualize how depreciation can be a "source of working capital." After all, depreciation is an expense. How are expenses sources of working capital?

Required: Respond to this memo.

Question 6-7. As indicated in the chapter, when the working capital basis is selected to delineate the changes in financial position, APB Opinion #19 requires the statement of changes in financial position to have two parts:

1. The analysis of the changes in the nonworking capital accounts, and
2. The analysis of the changes in the working capital accounts.

Discuss the relationship between these two parts of the statement. Why does APB Opinion #19 require both to be included whenever an income statement is published?

Question 6-8. On page 208 the reported revenues for the Memorial Hospital were $281,200 and the reported expenses, $207,300. However, the net income reported for Memorial Hospital on page 210 was $76,900. Explain this apparent discrepancy.

Question 6-9. How can the Statement of Changes in Financial Position: Working Capital Basis and the Statement of Changes in Financial Position: Cash Basis be used to provide information relevant in preparing the cash budget?

Question 6-10. The Projected Cash Flow Statement presented below for the City General Hospital has been included in a preliminary bond offering prospectus. The purpose of the bond issue is to modernize the existing structure and provide funds for new facility construction.

CITY GENERAL HOSPITAL
PROJECTED CASH FLOW, 19X1 to 19X6
(Dollars in Thousands)

	19X1	19X2	19X3	19X4	19X5	19X6
Beginning Cash Balance	$ 94	$ 1,512	$2,026	$2,210	$1,490	$1,835
Add: Net Income Before Interest and Depreciation	827	883	949	1,276	3,532	3,582
Proceeds of Federal Grant	—	200	200	100	—	—
Proceeds of Bond Issue	—	10,839	8,591	4,295	—	—
Interest Earnings	—	766	766	383	—	—
Cash on Hand	1,100	—	—	—	—	—
Less: Increase in Working Capital Requirements	$ 334	$ 194	$ 216	$ 445	$ 975	$ 301
Construction Payments (Net)	—	7,553	7,553	3,776	—	—
Replacement of Equipment	175	125	50	50	50	50
Interest Payments	—	2,037	2,037	2,036	—	—
Bond Discount	—	698	—	—	—	—
Payments to Debt Service Reserve Fund	—	1,567	466	467	—	—
Cash Available for Debt Service	$1,512	$ 2,026	$2,210	$1,490	$3,997	$5,066
Estimated Debt Service	—	—	—	—	2,162	2,497
Ending Cash Balance	$1,512	$ 2,026	$2,210	$1,490	$1,835	$2,569

Required: Consider the category "Increase in Working Capital Requirement." List four working capital accounts which probably account for a significant proportion of the anticipated increased demands for working capital. Rationalize why each account you listed will result in an increased demand in working capital.

Problem 6-1. Prepare a Statement of Changes in Financial Position: Working Capital Basis and a Statement of the Changes in Financial Position: Cash Basis given the following information for the Visiting Nurses Society.

VISITING NURSES SOCIETY
Comparative Balance Sheets
June 30, 19X2 and 19X1

	June 30	
Assets	19X2	19X1
Cash	$ 1,100	$ 3,400
Accounts Receivable	7,000	2,000
Allowance for Uncollectables	(2,000)	(300)
Inventory	2,600	1,200
Service Equipment	20,000	25,000
Accumulated Depreciation	(15,000)	(15,000)
Land	18,000	26,000
Construction in Process	19,900	—
Total Assets	$51,600	$42,300
Liabilities and Equity		
Liabilities		
Notes Payable	$ 6,000	$ 5,000
Accounts Payable	7,000	6,000
Accrued Interest Payable	3,400	3,000
Bonds Payable	15,000	10,000
Discount on Bonds Payable	(2,200)	(2,400)
Total Liabilities	$29,200	$21,600
Equity		
Contributed Capital	$13,400	$12,000
Earnings Retained	9,000	8,700
Total Equity	22,400	20,700
Total Liabilities and Equity	$51,600	$42,300

Additional information:

A. Construction on the Maternal and Infant Care Clinic during fiscal 19X1–X2 amounted to $19,900.
B. The Ladies Aid Society contributed $1,400 on January 24, 19X2.
C. Land was sold for book value, $8,000, on August 21, 19X1.
D. Equipment initially worth $5,000, with a book value of $2,000, was sold for $3,000 on December 24, 19X1.
E. On July 1, 19X1, five-year, eight percent bonds with a face value of $5,000 were sold for $4,700.

F. The agency's revenue was $90,100 and the expenses were $90,800 during fiscal 19X1–X2.

Problem 6-2. What effect does each of the following transactions have on working capital?

a. Cash	$12,500	
Land		$12,500

To record the sale of land for $12,500.

b. Cash	$ 11,000	
Building	193,000	
7% Bonds Payable		$204,000

To record the acquisition of a building and renovation capital in exchange for seven percent bonds with a face value of $204,000.

c. Accounts Payable	$5,397.12	
Discounts Lost	102.88	
Cash		$5,500

To record the payment of an account payable after the discount period has expired.

d. Accrued Interest Receivable	$93.47	
Interest Income		$93.47

To record the accrual of interest on a short-term note receivable.

e. Accrued Interest Payable	$ 60	
Interest Expense	30	
Notes Payable	6,000	
Cash		$6,090

To record the retirement of a $6,000, 90-day, six percent note payable.

f. Interest Expense	$5,450	
Discount		$ 450
Cash		5,000

To record the payment of periodic interest and the amortization of the bond discount on $100,000, five percent bonds sold at a discount of $4,500.

Problem 6-3.

K. T. MATERNITY HOSPITAL

Comparative Balance Sheets
December 31, 19X2 and 19X1

ASSETS	19X2	19X1
Cash	$ 37,000	$ 46,000
Accounts Receivable (net)	70,000	92,000
Inventory	55,000	53,000
Building (net)	486,700	493,000
Equipment (net)	284,000	211,000
Land	160,000	120,000
Total Assets	$1,092,700	$1,015,000
LIABILITIES		
Accounts Payable	$ 27,000	$ 36,000
Short-Term Notes Payable	30,000	20,000
Serial Bonds Payable	20,000	40,000
Mortgage Payable	153,000	197,000
Total Liabilities	$230,000	$293,000
OWNERS' EQUITY		
Contribution from owners	$ 520,000	$ 480,000
Profits retained from previous years	242,000	201,000
Current net income after taxes	100,700	41,000
Total Equity	862,700	722,000
Total Liabilities and Equity	$1,092,700	$1,015,000

Additional Information

A. The hospital sold a portion of its building to a private group practice on January 1, 19X2, for $120,000.
B. Additions to the building during 19X2 were completed on July 1, 19X2. The capitalized value of these additions was $140,000.
C. Depreciation is recorded at the rate of ten percent of historical cost per year. The depreciation during 19X2 was recorded properly. The depreciation on the addition was recorded only from July 1, 19X2, until December 31, 19X2.
D. New equipment was purchased on December 31, 19X2.
E. The depreciation on the equipment during the year was $24,500.
F. Land with a market price of $40,000 was acquired in exchange

for serial bonds with a face value and a market value of $20,000 on January 2, 19X2.

G. The private group practice in item A assumed a portion of the hospital's mortgage payable equal to half of the price paid by the group for the building. Mortgage principle payments amounting to $18,500 were made during the year. A new mortgage which is included in the Mortgage Payable account was obtained to finance a portion of a new addition to the hospital in 19X3.

H. Land valued at $20,000 was donated by a physician on December 31, 19X2.

Required:

a. Compute the change in working capital using the current asset and current liability accounts.

b. Prepare a Statement of Changes in Financial Position: Working Capital Basis.

Problem 6-4. Analyze the following transactions and indicate the effect of each transaction on working capital (i.e., increase, decrease, or unchanged). Also state the magnitude of any change in working capital resulting from each transaction.

a. A ten-year, 8.5 percent bond with a face value of $130,000 is sold on January 2, 19X1, in a market where the interest rate is 9.3 percent. Bond interest is payable on January 1 and July 1. A sinking fund provision states that a sum of money must be deposited on each interest payment date so that 80 percent of the face value of the bond is available on the date the bonds are to be retired. The rate of interest that is earned on the sinking fund is seven percent.

b. The accrual of bond interest payable is recorded on December 31, 19X1.

c. Interest is paid to the bondholders and a deposit is made to the sinking fund on January 1, 19X2.

d. The bond is retired at maturity.

Problem 6-5. The following events occurred for the United Nursing Service Agency during 19X1:

a. The agency earned gross revenues of $153,400. Ten percent of these revenues were collected in cash at the time services were rendered.

b. Total expenses for the year amounted to $90,700. Depreciation expense, the only nonworking capital expense, amounted to $35,000.

c. Accounts receivable of $98,700 were collected.
d. Cash disbursed for operational expenses amounted to $51,800 during the year.
e. Equipment was purchased for $6,000 cash and the trade-in on used equipment with a book value of $2,000. The new equipment had a list price of $9,100.
f. Ten-year six percent bonds with a face value of $9,000 and interest payable semiannually were issued in exchange for land on June 30. The market rate of interest at the time of the issuance was eight percent.
g. A building with a book value of $68,000 was sold for $75,000.
h. A 180-day 12 percent note with a face value of $12,000 was received in exchange for equipment with a book value of $15,000.

Required:
What is the effect (direction and magnitude) of each of these eight events on:

1. Cash,
2. Working capital, and
3. Net income?

Problem 6-6. Given the information for the Memorial Hospital, the following statement has been prepared by the hospital's accountant. Discuss the form and content of this statement.

MEMORIAL HOSPITAL

Statement of Changes in Cash
for the Year Ended December 31, 19X1

Sources of Cash		
From operations:		
Net income	$ 76,900	
Add (deduct) adjustments for income transactions not affecting cash:		
Depreciation	129,000	
Amortization of bond discount	1,100	
Gain on sale of equipment	(3,000)	
Patient accounts receivable decrease	31,000	
Inventory decrease	10,000	
Accounts payable decrease	(24,000)	
Accrued interest payable increase	3,000	
Total cash from operations		$224,000
From other sources:		
Sale of equipment	15,000	
Sale of bonds	46,000	
Philanthropic contributions	4,000	
Total cash from other sources		65,000
		289,000
Applications of Cash		
Construction	157,000	
Purchase of equipment	80,000	
Payment on notes payable, short-term (nontrade)	30,000	
		267,000
Increase in cash		$ 22,000

Problem 6-7. In the Statement of Changes in Financial Position: Cash Basis on page 216 there were six adjustments to the reported hospital expenses of $207,300. Evaluate these adjustments and explain how each converts reported hospital expense to cash disbursed for operations.

Problem 6-8. The Vatter methodology was demonstrated for preparing the statement of changes in financial position: working capital basis.

Required:

a. Modify the Vatter methodology in order to generate information useful in preparing the statement of changes in financial position on a cash basis.

b. Demonstrate your methodology by applying it to the Memorial Hospital example in the text.

Problem 6-9. Consider the following comparative balance sheets.

HELPFUL WAY NURSING AGENCY
Comparative Balance Sheets
Years Ended December 31, 19X2 and 19X1

Assets	19X2	19X1
Cash	$ 12,000	$ 8,000
Accounts Receivable	10,000	3,000
Fixed Assets	100,000	90,000
Accumulated Depreciation	(20,000)	(12,000)
Total Assets	$102,000	$89,000
Liabilities and Equity		
Accounts Payable	4,000	6,000
Bonds Payable (19X6)	15,000	10,000
Contributed Capital	83,000	73,000
Revenues	97,000	76,000
Expenses	(97,000)	(76,000)
Total Liabilities and Equity	$102,000	$89,000

Additional information:
No fixed assets have been sold during 19X2.

Required:
Prepare a statement which reconciles the change in working capital with the change in cash (also see Question 6-4).

Problem 6-10. Consider the following Statement of Changes in Financial Position. Discuss the activity and financial condition of the Good Samaritan Hospital and Medical Center for the years reported.

GOOD SAMARITAN HOSPITAL & MEDICAL CENTER*
Statement of Changes in Financial Position—General Fund
For The Years Ended June 30, 1973, June 29, 1974, June 28, 1975 and June 26, 1976

	Years Ended June 30, 1973	June 29, 1974	June 28, 1975	June 26, 1976
	Thousands of Dollars			
Funds Provided:				
Operations:				
Excess of revenue over expenses				
Excess of revenue over expenses from operations............	$ 553	$ 614	$ 397	$ 881
Add—depreciation	1,180	1,228	1,396	1,656
Funds derived from operations	1,733	1,842	1,793	2,537
Nonoperating revenue...........	190	172	141	189
Cumulative effect of vacation pay accrual				(312)
Funds derived from operations and nonoperating revenue ..	1,923	2,014	1,934	2,414
Additions to long-term debt.......		600	1,422	3,457
Donations for the acquisition of plant assets..................	16	170	289	628
Total funds provided.........	1,939	2,784	3,645	6,499
Funds Used:				
Additions to Hospital plant	708	2,722	2,749	2,993
Increase (decrease) in cash and investments designated for plant expansion	469	(306)	1	1,144
Payments on long-term debt	381	103	749	548
Real estate purchased for future use	92	132	140	55
Transfer to (from) other funds.....	26	(97)	(32)	14
Other decreases (increases)	7	(6)	(2)	6
Total funds used	1,683	2,548	3,605	4,760
Increase in Working Capital	$ 256	$ 236	$ 40	$1,739
Increase (Decrease) in Elements of Working Capital:				
Cash and short-term investments ..	$ 333	$ (165)	$ 616	$ 425
Accounts receivable.............	463	392	652	550
Inventory and prepaid expenses ...	(17)	163	(82)	(32)
Notes payable to banks..........			(400)	400
Current portion of long-term debt..	(15)	(125)	(203)	618
Accounts payable and other liabilities....................	(83)	(307)	(1,106)	8
Medicare and welfare settlements..	(330)	331	559	(437)
Due from (to) restricted funds.....	(95)	(53)	4	207
Increase in Working Capital	$ 256	$ 236	$ 40	$1,739

*Abstracted from the Preliminary Official Statement of the Good Samaritan Hospital and Medical Center Project, July 22, 1977. See Appendix 5-B.

Chapter 7

Break-Even Analysis and Responsibility Accounting

The Almighty dollar, that great object of universal devotion throughout our land, seems to have no genuine devotees in these peculiar villages.

W. Irving

While the concept and philosophy of breaking even have been readily embraced by managers of nonprofit institutions, various forms of profitability analysis traditionally have been rejected. However, break-even analysis is, in fact, a special case of cost/benefit profitability analysis, where the benefits are revenues. In addition, break-even analysis is used to evaluate performance in nonprofit institutions for the same reason that profitability analysis is used to evaluate performance in profit-oriented institutions: it provides management with an indication of economic performance. Hence, the difference between break-even analysis and profitability analysis is largely semantic.

This chapter examines break-even analysis for both linear and nonlinear cost and revenue functions. Then, the fundamental premises of responsibility accounting are discussed. Lastly, a case study is presented to illustrate the concepts of responsibility accounting and break-even analysis for a general medical clinic.

BREAK-EVEN ANALYSIS

The concept of breaking even is rather elementary. To break even, the institution must operate at a volume where total revenue equals total cost. This volume is called the break-even point and may be noted as $\hat{X}$ only if:

$$R(\hat{X}) = F(\hat{X}) + V(\hat{X})$$

where: $\hat{X}$ represents the patient or process volume for which there is no profit or loss;
$R(\hat{X})$ represents the revenue generated by volume $\hat{X}$;
$F(\hat{X})$ represents the fixed costs for volume $\hat{X}$; and
$V(\hat{X})$ represents the variable costs generated by volume $\hat{X}$.

These revenue and cost equations are seldom known precisely and often must be estimated. Consequently, the usefulness of break-even analysis often depends upon the reasonability of the estimates of the revenue function, the level of fixed costs, and the variable cost function. Regression analysis (linear or nonlinear) may be used to develop the appropriate function estimates. The reasonability of the regression estimates may be ascertained with measures of the statistical significance of the regression functions (see Appendix B). If the revenue and cost function estimates are statistically insignificant, the information generated by the break-even analysis will be meaningless (see Problem 7-3).

Linear Break-Even Analysis

For a linear break-even analysis, the revenue function ($R(X)$), the fixed cost function ($F(X)$), and the variable cost function ($V(X)$) all have the following general algebraic form:

$$f(X) = bX + c$$

where: $f(X)$ is the revenue or cost function;
b and c are constants; and
X is the volume variable.

Hence, the break-even equation, $R(\hat{X}) = F(\hat{X}) + V(\hat{X})$, may be represented as:

$$b_R\hat{X} + c_R = (b_F\hat{X} + c_F) + (b_V\hat{X} + c_V).$$

Usually, no revenue can be generated when there is no volume. Hence, $c_R = 0$. Similarly, no variable costs are incurred if there is no volume, leaving $c_V = 0$. Furthermore, fixed costs usually do not vary with volume, so $b_F = 0$ (see Problems 7-1 and 7-2). Therefore, for most situations, the break-even equation may be restated as:

(7-1) $$b_R\hat{X} = b_V\hat{X} + c_F.$$

Solving equation (7-1) for $\hat{X}$ yields the break-even point:

$$\hat{X} = \frac{c_F}{b_R - b_V}. \tag{7-2}$$

This equation indicates that the marginal contribution to profit of $\hat{X}$ units, $(b_R - b_V) \times \hat{X}$, must equal fixed costs, c_F, at the break-even volume. Hence, the algebraic solution to linear break-even problems is relatively simple.

The solution to break-even problems may be illustrated graphically by plotting the revenue and the total cost functions in the same axis space. The intersection of these two functions is the break-even point. The graphical representation of the solution for the general case, equation (7-1), is shown in Figure 7-1. Note that the total costs are obtained by adding $V(X)$ to $F(X)$. At the point where the revenue function ($R(X)$) intersects the total cost function ($F(X) + V(X)$) the marginal contribution to profit of $\hat{X}$ units, $(b_R - b_V) \times \hat{X}$, is equal to the fixed cost, c_F. The algebraic solution of break-even problems is further illustrated in the following example.

Department of Radiology: Break-Even Analysis

Assume that the administrator of the radiology department wants to know the break-even volume for certain services performed by the radi-

Figure 7-1 Graphic Presentation of the Break-Even Equations

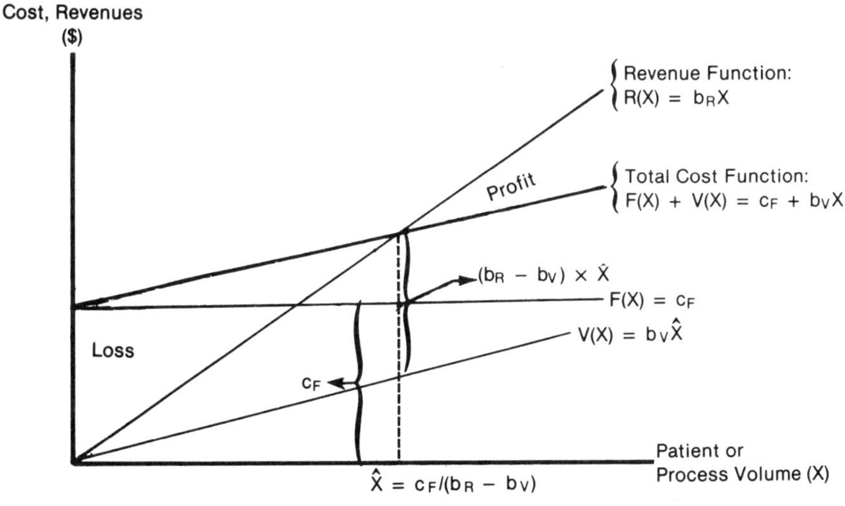

ology department. The administrator estimates that the fixed costs pertaining to these services are approximately $4,500 per month. In addition, the information contained in Table 7-1 is available regarding the radiology department's monthly total cost and monthly volume. Similar information (see Table 7-2) is available regarding monthly service revenue and volume in the radiology department.

If a linear regression analysis is performed for the cost statistics represented in Table 7-1, the monthly total cost function estimate would be:

$$\text{Total Cost Function: } F(X) + V(X) = b_V X + c_F$$
$$= \$20.06X + \$4{,}295.19.$$

The statistics generated for this regression analysis (see Appendix B) are:

$$R = .99,\ R^2 = .99$$
$$t_{13} = 35.7$$
$$S_e = 184.$$

The t statistic is significant at a confidence level of $\alpha < .001$. In addition, the estimate of $4,295.19 for c_F is approximately equal to the $4,500 fixed cost estimate made by the administrator. Hence, the total cost function is capable of providing a meaningful input to the break-even analysis.

Table 7-1 Cost Statistics for Selected Services of the Department of Radiology

Period (Monthly)	Patient Volume (X)	Total Costs	Period (Monthly)	Patient Volume (X)	Total Costs	Period (Monthly)	Patient Volume (X)	Total Costs
1	1,621	$36,991	6	1,043	$25,311	11	1,896	$42,250
2	1,195	27,750	7	1,299	30,644	12	1,572	35,842
3	925	22,991	8	1,501	34,350	13	1,143	27,251
4	1,262	29,654	9	1,662	37,811	14	1,249	29,162
5	1,729	38,856	10	1,194	28,262	15	1,996	44,354

Table 7-2 Monthly Revenue Statistics[a] for the Department of Radiology

Period (Monthly)	Patient Volume (X)	Revenue	Period (Monthly)	Patient Volume (X)	Revenue	Period (Monthly)	Patient Volume (X)	Revenue
1	1,093	$27,327	6	1,251	$31,300	11	1,043	$26,020
2	1,462	26,552	7	1,899	47,471	12	1,763	44,071
3	899	22,477	8	1,096	27,402	13	1,221	30,271
4	1,140	28,500	9	1,521	38,031	14	1,931	48,277
5	1,920	48,060	10	1,664	41,604	15	911	22,780

[a] This cost and revenue information was abstracted from an actual case. The hospital's accounting system recorded patient-related revenue on a basis other than patient volume, as recorded by the department.

A linear regression analysis also may be performed for the revenue statistics reported in Table 7-2. In this case, the monthly revenue regression equation and the related statistics are:

$$\text{Total Revenue Function:} \quad R(X) = b_R X + c_R$$
$$= \$24.66X - \$210.24$$
$$R = .96,\ R^2 = .93$$
$$t_{13} = 13.1$$
$$S_e = 2488.$$

The t statistic for the revenue equation also is significant at a confidence level of $\alpha < .001$, indicating that the revenue function is capable of providing a meaningful input to the break-even analysis. However, as previously discussed, c_R should equal zero for most economic analyses. In this case, since the value assigned to c_R ($-\$210.24$) is relatively close to zero and since a negative fixed element in the revenue function has no economic rationale, c_R will be set equal to zero in the break-even analysis (see Question 7-12).

Once the cost and revenue equations have been developed, the radiology department's break-even point may be determined algebraically as follows.

$$R(\hat{X}) = F(\hat{X}) + V(\hat{X})$$
$$\$24.66\hat{X} = \$4{,}295.19 + \$20.06\hat{X}$$
$$\hat{X} = \frac{\$4{,}295.19}{\$24.66 + \$20.06}$$
$$= 934 \text{ patients}$$

The graphic representation of this solution is shown in Figure 7-2.

In this example, the cost and revenue functions are both linear. However, in cases where they are not linear, management must analyze the functions before selecting the type of break-even analysis.

For example, assume that a laboratory's actual total cost function is F(X) + V(X) as shown in Figure 7-3. This total cost equation may be estimated by a linear regression using data points in the range [0−50,000 units]. The administrator may use this linear regression estimate of the total cost function to aid in setting prices or developing control information for the ensuing period (see Question 7-10). If the laboratory volume in the ensuing period is expected to be 60,000 units, the extrapolation of the

Figure 7-2 Graphic Solution: Radiology Department Break-Even Problem

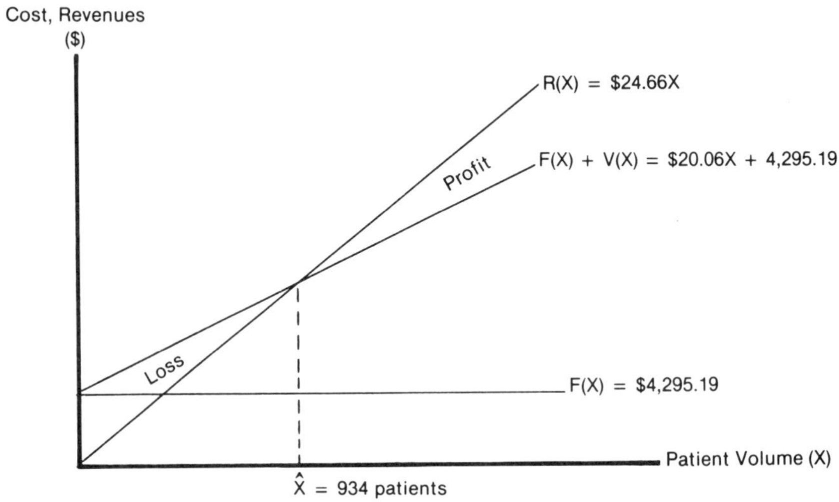

linear regression estimate yields total costs of $367,000. However, the actual total costs at a volume of 60,000 units will be $478,000 (see Question 7-8). Consequently, if the linear regression estimate of total costs at a volume of 60,000 units is used to set prices, these prices will not generate sufficient revenue to cover actual costs. Therefore, where the assumption of linearity is questionable, a nonlinear break-even analysis performed by using nonlinear regression equations should be used to ascertain the break-even point.

Nonlinear Break-Even Analysis: The Quadratic Case

Quadratic break-even analysis is a special case of nonlinear break-even analysis (see Question 7-3). In quadratic break-even analysis, the revenue function ($R(X)$), the fixed cost function ($F(X)$), and the variable cost function ($V(X)$) have the general algebraic form:

$$f(X) = aX^2 + bX + c$$

where: $f(X)$ is the revenue or cost function
a, b and c are constants; and
X is the volume variable.

Figure 7-3 Laboratory Total Costs Represented Graphically

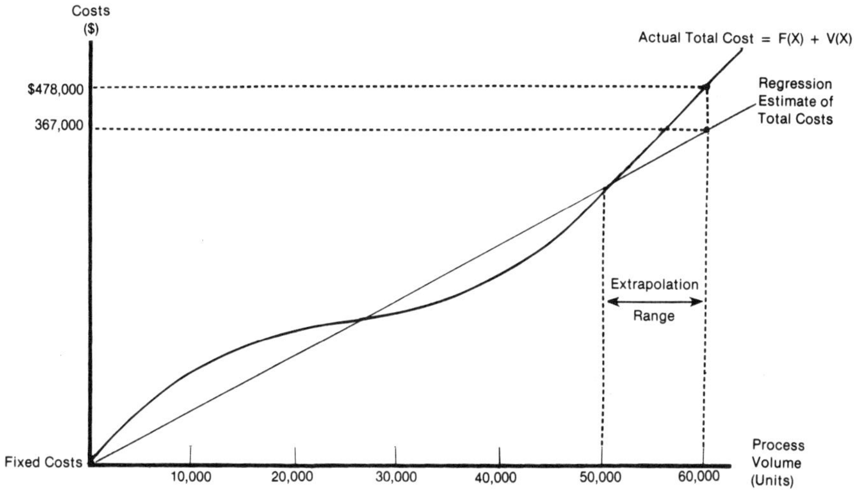

Hence, the break-even equation, $R(X) = F(X) + V(X)$, may be represented as:

(7-3) $$\underbrace{a_R\hat{X}^2 + b_R\hat{X} + c_R}_{\text{Revenue}} = \underbrace{(a_F\hat{X}^2 + b_F\hat{X} + c_F)}_{\text{Fixed Costs}} + \underbrace{(a_V\hat{X}^2 + b_V\hat{X} + c_V)}_{\text{Variable Costs}}.$$

However, c_R, b_F, a_F and c_V usually will equal zero. When this is the case, equation (7-3) can be restated as:

(7-4) $$a_R\hat{X}^2 + b_R\hat{X} = a_V\hat{X}^2 + b_V\hat{X} + c_F$$

Solving equation (7-4) for $\hat{X}$ yields two break-even points.[1]

$$\hat{X}_1 = \frac{-(b_R - b_V) + \sqrt{(b_R - b_V)^2 - 4(a_R - a_V)(-c_F)}}{2(a_R - a_V)}$$

and

$$\hat{X}_2 = \frac{-(b_R - b_V) - \sqrt{(b_R - b_V)^2 - 4(a_R - a_V)(-c_F)}}{2(a_R - a_V)}$$

Hence, the solution to the quadratic break-even analysis is slightly more complex than the solution to the linear break-even analysis. However, it is important to note that the marginal contribution of $\hat{X}$ units at either break-even point, defined as $[(a_R - a_V)\hat{X} + (b_R - b_V)] \times \hat{X}$ in the quadratic break-even solution, again is equal to the fixed costs, c_F.

Just as in the linear case, the solution to quadratic break-even problems may be illustrated graphically. The graphic illustration to the solution of the general case represented by equation (7-4) is shown in Figure 7-4. Note that profit would be maximized at some volume between the two break-even points. This point of profit maximization will be discussed in the following example which illustrates the solution to quadratic break-even problems.

Laboratory Example

Assume that the information in Table 7-3 is available regarding a laboratory department's volume, revenue, and total cost. Further assume that this data is used to develop the following quadratic total revenue and total cost regression equations:[2]

Total Revenue Function: $\text{R(X)} = a_R X^2 + b_R X + c_R$

$$= -\$.0049X^2 + \$9.44X - \$34.$$

Total Cost Function: $\text{F(X)} + \text{V(X)} = a_V X^2 + b_V X + c_F$

$$= \$.0005X^2 + \$3.15X + \$1203.$$

Figure 7-4 Graphic Presentation of Quadratic Break-Even Equations

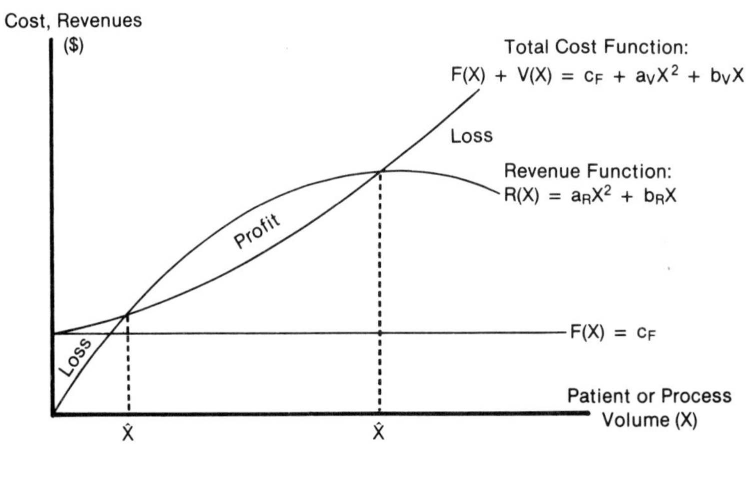

Table 7-3 Laboratory Revenue and Costs

Units Processed	Total Revenue	Total Cost	Profit (Loss)
0	\$ 0	\$1,000	\$(1000)
100	900	1,600	(700)
200	1,600	2,000	(400)
300	2,300	2,300	-0-
400	2,900	2,600	300
500	3,500	2,900	600
600	3,900	3,200	700
700	4,200	3,500	700
800	4,500	3,900	600
900	4,400	4,400	-0-
1,000	4,500	5,000	(500)

Given these regression equations, the break-even analysis may be solved algebraically by substituting the regression equations for $R(\hat{X})$, $F(\hat{X})$, and $V(\hat{X})$ in the break-even equation as follows.

$$R(\hat{X}) = F(\hat{X}) + V(\hat{X})$$

$$-\$.0049\hat{X}^2 + \$9.44\hat{X} - \$34 = \$.0005\hat{X}^2 + \$3.15\hat{X} + \$1203$$

This equation may be simplified as:

$$-\$.0054\hat{X}^2 + \$6.29\hat{X} - 1237 = 0.$$

Then, solving for $\hat{X}$ yields the following break-even points.

$$\hat{X}_1 = \frac{-6.29 + \sqrt{6.29^2 - [4(-.0054)(-1237)]}}{2(-.0054)}$$

$$= 251 \text{ units}$$

$$\hat{X}_2 = \frac{-6.29 - \sqrt{6.29^2 - [4(-.0054)(-1237)]}}{2(-.0054)}$$

$$= 914 \text{ units}$$

Hence, the laboratory breaks even at a processing volume of 251 units and at a volume of 914 units (see Figure 7-5).

Figure 7-5 Graphic Solution: Quadratic Break Even

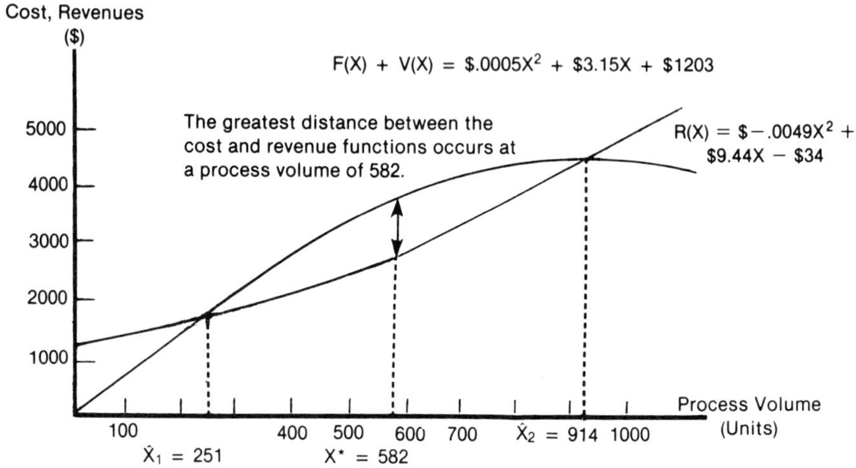

Relationships Between Break-Even and Profitability Analysis

A quick perusal of Figure 7-5 shows that break-even analysis is indeed a form of profitability analysis (see Question 7-11). Note that the excess of revenues over costs in Figure 7-5 is greatest at a volume of 582 units. This is the volume at which profit is maximized.

A close inspection of the break-even equation illustrates the relationship between break-even analysis and profitability analysis. The break-even equation in the laboratory case is:

$$R(\hat{X}) = F(\hat{X}) + V(\hat{X})$$

$$-\$.0049\hat{X}^2 + \$9.44\hat{X} - \$34 = \$.0005\hat{X}^2 + \$3.15\hat{X} + \$1203.$$

This equation may be rewritten as:

$$(-\$.0049\hat{X}^2 + \$9.44\hat{X} - \$34) - (\$.0005\hat{X}^2 + \$3.15\hat{X} + \$1203) = 0.$$

The left-hand portion of this equation is the laboratory profit function

$$\pi = R(X) - [F(X) + V(X)]$$

where: π represents profit.

In break-even analysis, the profit is set equal to zero. However, to find the volume of profit maximization, the equation $d\pi/dX = 0$ must be solved. In this case, the profit function:

$$\pi = (-\$.0049X^2 + \$9.44X - \$34) - (\$.0005X^2 + \$3.15X + \$1203)$$

reduces to:

$$= -\$.0054X^2 + \$6.29X - \$1237. \tag{7-5}$$

Differentiating equation (7-5) gives:

$$\frac{d\pi}{dX} = -\$.0108X + \$6.29 \tag{7-6}$$

Setting equation (7-6) equal to zero yields:

$$-\$.0108X + \$6.29 = 0$$

$$-\$.0108X = -\$6.29$$

$$X^* = 582 \text{ units.}$$

As shown in Figure 7-5, X^* represents the volume at which profit is maximized.

This point of profit maximization could have been found by performing a second order regression analysis on the profit and loss information in Table 7-3. In this case, the resultant quadratic regression equation would have been:

$$\pi = -\$.0054X^2 + \$6.29X - 1238. \tag{7-7}$$

Note that equation (7-7) is almost identical to equation (7-5), the profit equation derived by subtracting the total cost equation from the total revenue equation. Since equations (7-5) and (7-7) differ only in their constant term, they have the same point of profit maximization, $X^* = 582$ units. However, the graphic representation of equation (7-7) differs substantially from the graphic representation of the total cost and revenue function shown in Figure 7-5. Figure 7-6 shows the solution for the point of profit maximization, given the regression equation (7-7), and also contrasts actual profits and losses at various volumes (Table 7-3) with the profits and losses calculated at those volumes from the regression equation (7-7). Figure 7-6 shows that profit is maximized at a volume of 582 units, as expected. Also, note that the profit function crosses the volume axis at the break-even points because profit must equal zero at these points.

Figure 7-6 Graphic Representation of Equation 7-7

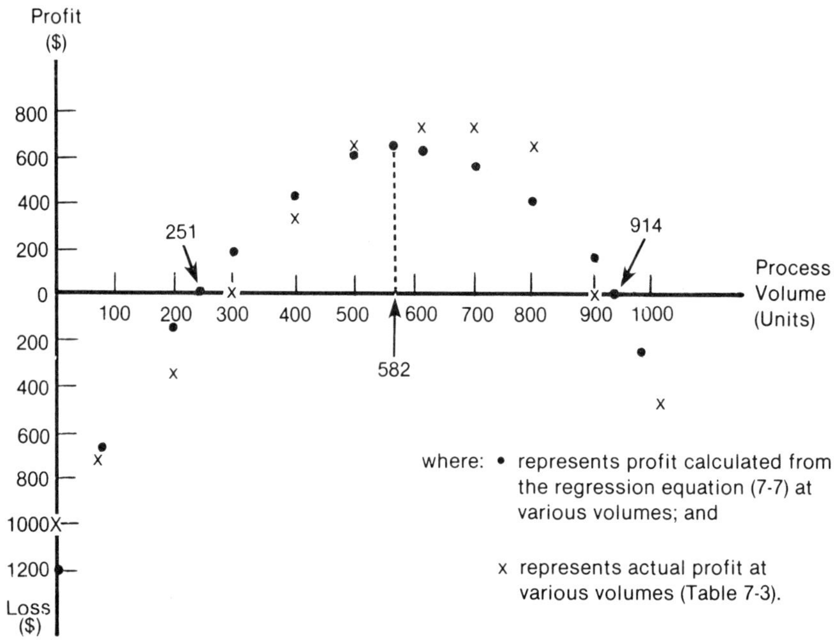

Summary

As indicated previously, the usefulness of break-even analysis and profitability analysis depends upon the accuracy of the revenue function, the fixed cost function, and the variable cost function estimates. Management's control over the processes which generate these functions is another important aspect of break-even and profitability analysis. The effects of managerial intervention on the actual revenue and cost functions, as well as the effects of erroneous classifications between fixed and variable costs, will be discussed in the following section.

WHAT-IF ANALYSIS: A DECISION-MAKING PERSPECTIVE

One means of enriching break-even and profitability analysis is called "what-if" analysis. In what-if analysis, the parameters of a problem are varied systematically and the problem is resolved so that the effects of changes in the parameters can be ascertained. This type of analysis allows management to deal with two important aspects of cost/benefit analysis:

1. What if, through managerial intervention, various parameters may be altered, and
2. What if, through measurement errors and erroneous assumptions, the fixed and variable costs are stated improperly?

Changes in the Break-Even Point Resulting from Managerial Alteration of Costs or Revenue

Managerial intervention may be focused on any of the three parameters: fixed cost, variable cost, or revenue. Alterations in any one of these parameters cause a change in the break-even point. To facilitate the presentation of what-if analysis, the effects of alterations in each of the parameters will be considered separately.

Fixed Cost Alteration

As shown previously, the marginal contribution to profit of $\hat{X}$ units must equal fixed costs at the break-even volume.

$$[(a_R - a_V)\hat{X} + (b_R - b_V)] \times \hat{X} = c_F$$

In linear break-even analysis, $a_R = a_V = 0$ so that the relationship between fixed costs and the marginal contribution to profit at the break-even volume becomes:

$$(b_R - b_V)\hat{X} = c_F$$

which may be stated as:

(7-2) $$\hat{X} = \frac{c_F}{b_R - b_V}.$$

If through management intervention, fixed costs can be reduced by some amount, Δc_F, while no changes occur in the revenue and variable cost functions, then the break-even point will change by some amount, $\Delta\hat{X}$. The direction and relative magnitude of $\Delta\hat{X}$ may be derived as follows.[3]

(7-8) $$\hat{X} - \Delta\hat{X} = \frac{c_F - \Delta c_F}{b_R - b_V}$$

Dividing both sides of equation (7-8) by $\hat{X}$ yields:

$$1 - \frac{\Delta\hat{X}}{\hat{X}} = \frac{c_F - \Delta c_F}{b_R - b_V} \div \hat{X}.$$

However, $\hat{X} = c_F/(b_R - b_V)$. Hence, by substitution:

$$1 - \frac{\Delta\hat{X}}{\hat{X}} = \frac{c_F - \Delta c_F}{b_R - b_V} \div \frac{c_F}{b_R - b_V},$$

and

$$1 - \frac{\Delta\hat{X}}{\hat{X}} = 1 - \frac{\Delta c_F}{c_F},$$

or

(7-9)
$$\frac{\Delta\hat{X}}{\hat{X}} = \frac{\Delta c_F}{c_F}.$$

Therefore, in linear break-even analysis, if fixed costs can be altered, then the percentage alteration in fixed costs ($\Delta c_F/c_F$) will cause a direct and identical percentage alteration in the break-even point ($\Delta\hat{X}/\hat{X}$).

For example, in the linear break-even analysis presented above for the radiology department, $\hat{X}$ = 934 patients, b_R = \$24.66, b_V = \$20.06 and c_F = \$4,295.19. However, suppose through managerial intervention fixed costs can be reduced by \$644.28 to \$3,650.91, a 15 percent reduction. The new break-even point would be:

$$\hat{X} = \frac{\$3{,}650.91}{\$24.66 - \$20.06}$$

$$= 794 \text{ patients.}$$

This is a total reduction of 140 patients, or a 15 percent reduction in the break-even point.

The relationships between fixed cost alterations and changes in the break-even point in nonlinear break-even analysis are quite complex, for reasons most easily seen graphically (see Figure 7-7). This figure shows that whenever the total cost function, the revenue function, or both are quadratic, the direction and magnitude of changes in the break-even point arising through fixed cost alterations cannot be determined solely from the percentage change in fixed costs. However, note that in any linear or quadratic case, regardless of the magnitude or direction of change in the break-even point from reducing fixed costs, the profit potential is increased.

Figure 7-7 The Effects of Fixed Cost Alterations on the Break-Even Point

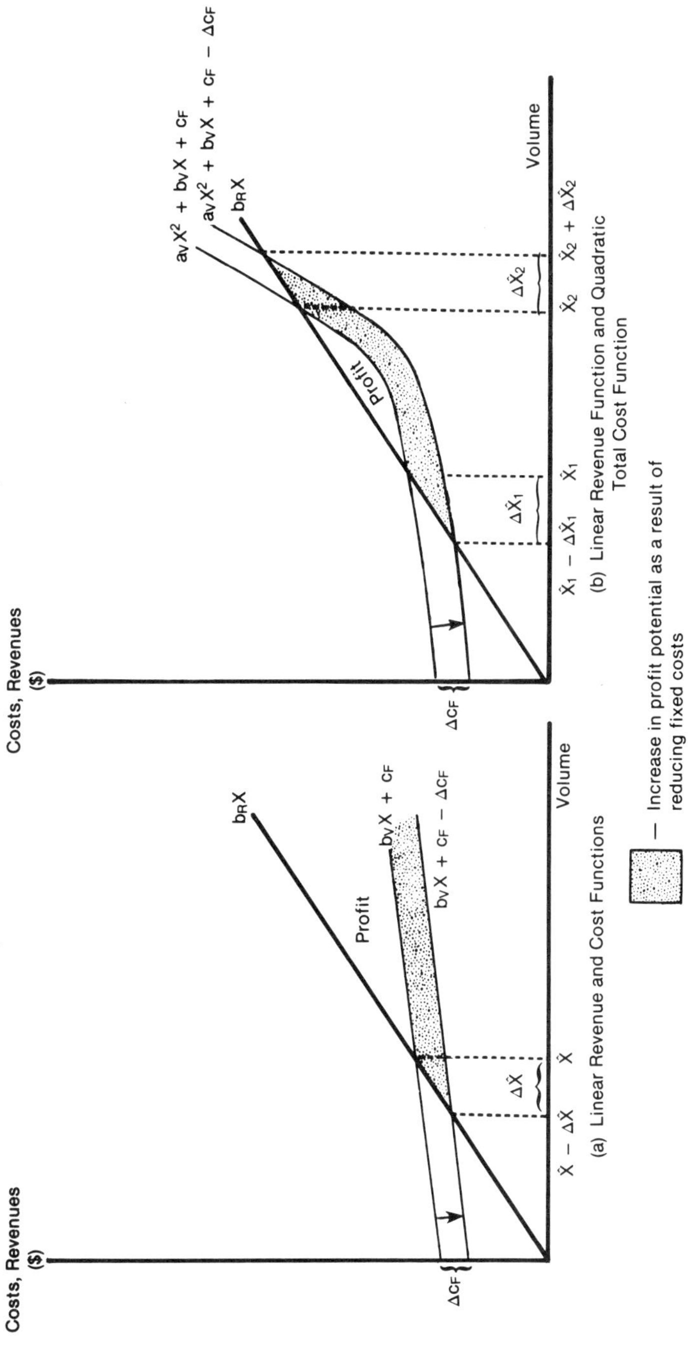

Figure 7-7 Continued

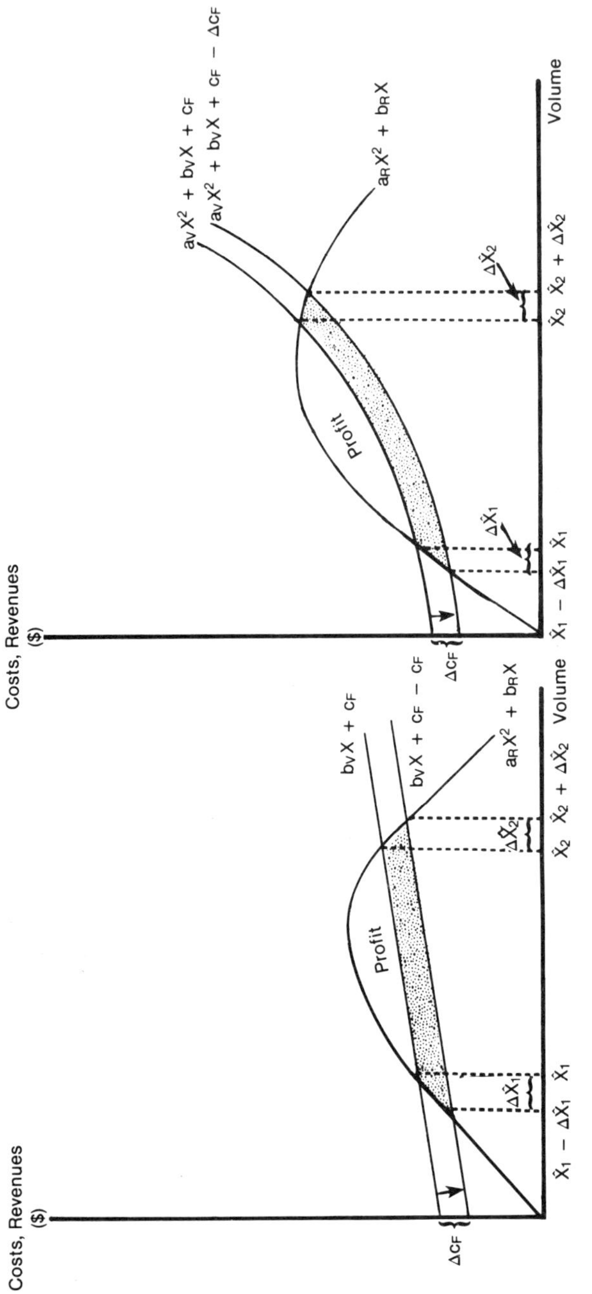

(c) Quadratic Revenue Function and Linear Total Cost Function

(d) Quadratic Revenue and Cost Functions

Variable Cost Alterations and Revenue Alterations

Like fixed costs, if variable costs can be reduced by some amount, Δb_V, through management intervention while no changes occur in the revenue and fixed cost functions, then the break-even point will change by some amount, $\Delta\hat{X}$. To derive the direction and magnitude of this $\Delta\hat{X}$, given linear total cost and revenue functions, again consider the basic relationship between fixed costs and the marginal contribution at the break-even volume.

(7-2) $$\hat{X} = \frac{c_F}{b_R - b_V}$$

Assuming a reduction in variable costs of Δb_V, equation (7-2) may be stated as shown.[4]

(7-10) $$\hat{X} - \Delta\hat{X} = \frac{c_F}{b_R - (b_V - \Delta b_V)}$$

Dividing both sides of equation (7-10) by $\hat{X}$ yields:

$$\frac{\hat{X} - \Delta\hat{X}}{\hat{X}} = \frac{c_F}{b_R - b_V + \Delta b_V} \div \hat{X}.$$

Since $\hat{X} = c_F/(b_R - b_V)$, by substitution:

$$\frac{\hat{X} - \Delta\hat{X}}{\hat{X}} = \frac{c_F}{b_R - b_V + \Delta b_V} \div \frac{c_F}{b_R - b_V}.$$

Hence,

$$\frac{\hat{X} - \Delta\hat{X}}{\hat{X}} = \frac{b_R - b_V}{b_R - b_V + \Delta b_V},$$

or

(7-11) $$(\hat{X} - \Delta\hat{X})(b_R - b_V + \Delta b_V) = (b_R - b_V)\hat{X}.$$

Rearranging the terms in equation (7-11) yields:

(7-12) $$(b_R - b_V)\hat{X} + \Delta b_V\hat{X} - (b_R - b_V + \Delta b_V)\Delta\hat{X} = (b_R - b_V)\hat{X}.$$

Then, $(b_R - b_V)X$ can be subtracted from both sides of equation (7-12), yielding:

$$\Delta b_V \hat{X} - (b_R - b_V + \Delta b_V)\Delta \hat{X} = 0,$$

or

$$\Delta b_V \hat{X} = (b_R - b_V + \Delta b_V)\Delta \hat{X}.$$

Hence,

$$\frac{\Delta b_V}{b_R - b_V + \Delta b_V} = \frac{\Delta \hat{X}}{\hat{X}}.$$

Since $\Delta b_V > 0$,

$$\frac{\Delta b_V}{b_R - b_V} > \frac{\Delta b_V}{b_R - b_V + \Delta b_V},$$

and therefore,

$$\frac{\Delta b_V}{b_R - b_V} > \frac{\Delta \hat{X}}{\hat{X}}. \tag{7-13}$$

Therefore, in linear break-even analysis, if variable costs can be altered through management intervention, then the percentage alteration in the marginal contribution to profit ($\Delta b_V/(b_R - b_V)$) will cause a direct but smaller percentage alteration in the break-even point ($\Delta \hat{X}/\hat{X}$).

A similar analysis can be conducted assuming that revenues can be increased by some amount, Δb_R, for a linear revenue function. In this case, the relationship between fixed costs and the marginal contribution to profit at the break-even volume would be:

$$\hat{X} + \Delta \hat{X} = \frac{c_F}{(b_R + \Delta b_R)^{-}b_V}. \tag{7-14}$$

Following the same derivation given above for Δb_V,

$$\frac{\Delta b_R}{b_R - b_V + \Delta b_R} = \frac{-\Delta \hat{X}}{\hat{X}}$$

and

$$\left|\frac{\Delta b_R}{b_R - b_V}\right| > \left|\frac{-\Delta \hat{X}}{\hat{X}}\right| \tag{7-15}$$

Therefore, in linear break-even analysis, if revenues can be altered through management intervention, the percentage alteration in the marginal contribution to profit $(\Delta b_R/(b_R - b_V))$ will cause an inverse but smaller percentage alteration in the break-even point $(\Delta \hat{X}/\hat{X})$.

The effects of alterations in variable costs or revenues in nonlinear break-even analysis are most simply described graphically. Figure 7-8 indicates the complexity of the relationships which exist between alterations in the break-even point and alterations in the variable cost function or the revenue function. Note that the direction and magnitude of alterations in the break-even point are not easily predictable when alterations are made in variable cost or revenue functions which are quadratic. However, in either the linear or the quadratic case, when variable costs are reduced or revenues are increased, the profit potential is increased. Also note that given any particular set of revenue and cost functions and changes in one or more of the functions, the direction and magnitude of the change in the break-even points can be computed from equations (7-2) or (7-4).

Ascertaining the Desirability of Managerial Actions

Management may take various actions which alter the break-even point and ultimately increase the range over which profit may be generated. The effects of various managerial actions are summarized in Table 7-4. As indicated previously, the absolute effect on the break-even point can be computed, given the estimates of the fixed cost, variable cost, and revenue functions and the specific effect of the managerial action on the functions. However, generally, a cost is associated with managerial actions. Hence, the economic benefits derived from taking a particular action must be greater than the costs of taking that action, if the action is to improve overall economic performance.

For example, assume that the radiology department in the example on page 232 is operating at the break-even point (i.e. $\hat{X} = 934$ patients). Assume further that the administrator is reasonably certain that fixed costs can be reduced by 12 percent at an annual cost of \$493.27, or, alternatively, variable costs can be reduced by \$.53 per patient[5] at an annual cost of \$427.55. The total profit derived at an expected operating volume of 934 patients, given the reduced fixed cost of \$3,779.78, will be:

$$\begin{aligned}\pi &= (\$24.66 - \$20.06) \times 934 - \$3{,}779.78 \\ &= \$516.62\end{aligned}$$

Hence, the net economic benefit of altering fixed costs will be:

$$\begin{aligned}\text{Net economic benefit} &= \$516.62 - \$493.27 \\ &= \$23.35.\ \text{per year}\end{aligned}$$

Figure 7-8 The Effects of Variable Cost Alterations and Revenue Alterations on the Break-Even Point

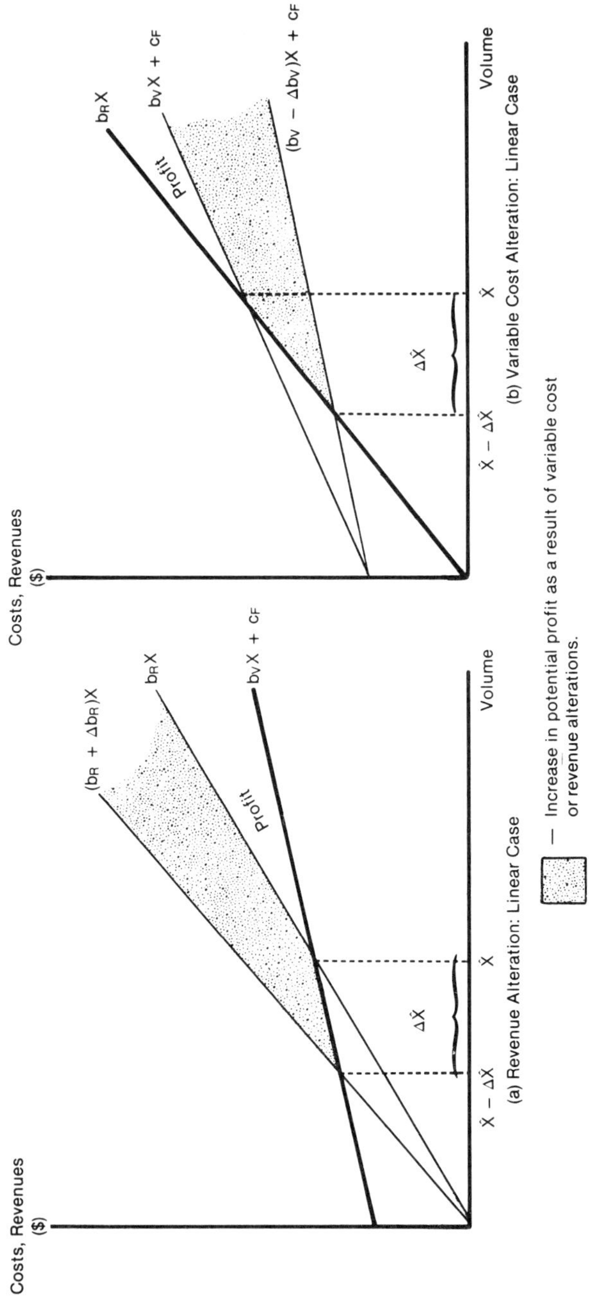

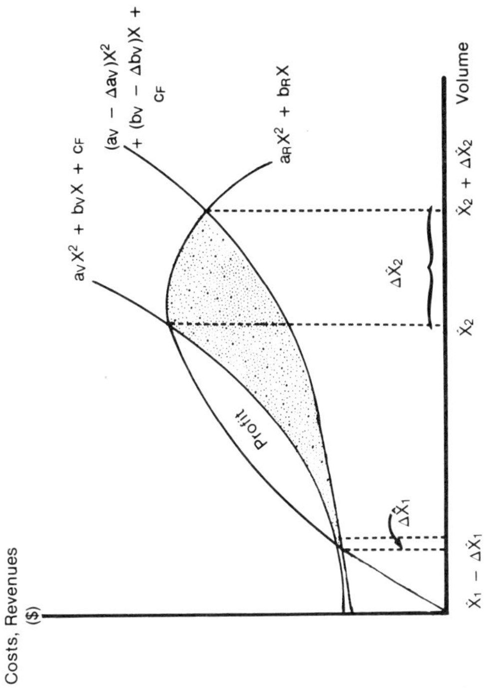

(d) Variable Cost Alteration: Quadratic Case

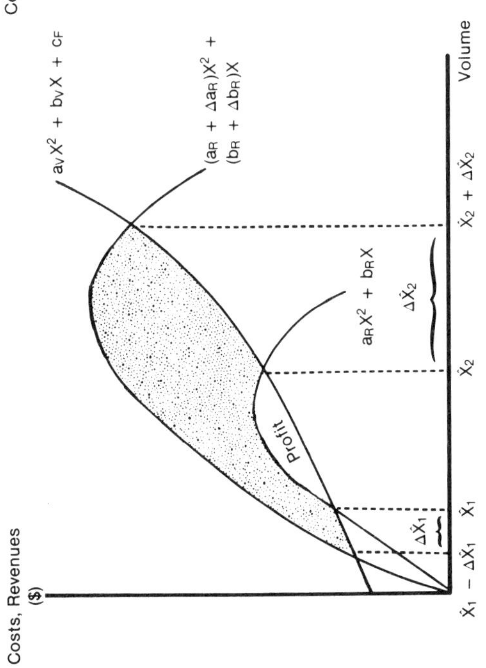

(c) Revenue Alteration: Quadratic Case

Table 7-4 The Effects of Managerial Intervention on the Break-Even Point

Action	Effect of Action on Break-Even Point		
		Quadratic Case[a]	
	Linear Case	Lower Break-Even Point	Upper Break-Even Point
Reduce fixed costs			
Effect, Magnitude	Direct, 1:1	Direct, Uncertain	Inverse, Uncertain
Reduce variable costs			
Effect, Magnitude	Direct, Fraction of $\Delta V(X)/(R(X) - V(X))$	Direct, Uncertain	Inverse, Uncertain
Increase revenues			
Effect, Magnitude	Inverse, Fraction of $\Delta R(X)/(R(X) - V(X))$	Inverse, Uncertain	Direct, Uncertain

[a] The magnitude of changes in the break-even point arising through managerial intervention is dependent on the specific quadratic cost and revenue functions.

Alternatively, if variable costs are reduced, the total profit derived at the expected operating volume of 934 patients will be:

$$\pi = (\$24.66 - \$19.53) \times 934 - \$4{,}295.19$$
$$= \$496.23.$$

In this case, the net economic benefit of altering variable costs will be:

$$\text{Net economic benefit} = \$496.23 - \$427.55$$
$$= \$68.68. \text{ per year}$$

Since the net economic benefit of altering the variable costs in this case is greater than the net economic benefit of altering the fixed costs (and since the larger net economic benefit is greater than zero), the administrator should reduce the variable costs in the radiology department. (See Question 7-13.) Note that this decision is dependent upon the expected volume of patients, in this case assumed to be 934 patients (see Problem 7-6).

Changes in the Break-Even Point as a Result of Reclassifying Fixed and Variable Costs

When the fixed and variable costs are improperly classified, one cost category is understated while the other one is overstated. Properly classifying the costs causes a change in both the fixed costs and the variable costs of equations (7-2) and (7-4). Therefore, reclassifying fixed and variable costs often alters the break-even point determined using the improperly classified costs.

To ascertain the effect of a cost reclassification on the break-even point, the magnitudes of changes in the fixed and variable costs must be computed. Then the revised fixed and variable costs must be included in equation (7-2) or equation (7-4) so that the proper break-even point can be computed. For example, assume that the total recorded costs in an EMS unit with linear total cost and revenue functions are \$262,641.39. If fixed costs are measured as \$163,043.00 and the EMS unit's patient volume is 19,653 patients, the variable costs per patient are:

$$V(X) = \frac{\$262{,}641.39 - \$163{,}043.00}{19{,}653}$$
$$= \$5.07 \text{ per patient.}$$

If the average revenue per patient is \$19.87, the break-even point is:

$$\hat{X} = \frac{\$163{,}043.00}{\$19.87 - \$5.07}$$

$$= 11{,}016 \text{ patients.}$$

However, if the fixed costs erroneously include \$89,623.81 in physicians' salaries, fixed costs should be \$73,419.19 (\$163,043.00 − \$89,623.81) and variable costs per patient should be:

$$V(X) = \frac{\$262{,}641.39 - \$73{,}419.19}{19{,}653}$$

$$= \$9.63 \text{ per patient.}$$

These revised costs should be included in equation (7-2) so that the proper break-even point can be computed as follows:

$$\hat{X} = \frac{\$73{,}419.19}{\$19.87 - \$9.63}$$

$$= 7{,}170 \text{ patients.}$$

Hence, by reclassifying the physicians' salaries from fixed to variable costs, the break-even point is reduced. Of course, managers should not attempt to alter cost classifications for the sole purpose of altering the break-even point. However, the fact that a questionable cost classification may cause the break-even point to change from 11,016 patients to 7,170 patients is managerially relevant information (see Question 7-10).

Extension to a Broader Control Perspective

Break-even analysis, as a special case of profitability analysis, is only one element in the organizational evaluation process. To attain the break-even volume and actually break-even, departmental managers must monitor departmental resources carefully. The manager's ability to control resources provides a basis for evaluating managerial performance. This concept of making managers responsible for the utilization of specific resources is the basic principle underlying responsibility accounting systems.

RESPONSIBILITY ACCOUNTING

Numerous technical definitions exist regarding responsibility accounting systems. Unfortunately, most of them are overly complex, attempting to incorporate all of the important aspects of systems control and authority to embellish the following basic concept: *to effect resource control, one or more individuals must be held responsible for each controllable aspect of performance.* If the individual has complete control over the resources in a particular performance area, that individual should be solely responsible for performance deviations arising from the use of those resources. If two or more individuals have joint control over particular resources, those individuals should be held jointly responsible for performance deviations arising from the use of those resources. Finally, an individual should not be held responsible for performance deviations in areas over which he has no control.

Practical Issues Regarding Resource Control

These delineations clarify the basic control concept underlying responsibility accounting systems. However, three important practical issues regarding resource control in a responsibility accounting system must be considered before such a system can be implemented. First, the evaluation of individuals must be coordinated with the degree of control that those individuals exert over particular aspects of performance. Second, performance measures must be defined so that the individuals held responsible for various controllable aspects of performance know the basis of evaluation. Finally, the organization must have a means of rewarding appropriate control actions and penalizing inappropriate control actions.

Ascertaining the Degree of Control

Coordinating the evaluation of individual decision makers with the degree of control they exert over shared processes is difficult because no scientific means of ascertaining the degree of control for shared processes exist. Hence, to eliminate the arbitrary allocation of responsibility, those individuals or groups that share control should be evaluated as a unit (functional unitization[6] as opposed to departmentalization).

Specifying Performance Measures

A responsibility accounting system must have an evaluation focus—e.g., profit. However, once the evaluation focus has been chosen, any number of performance statistics related to the evaluation focus may be used to evaluate performance (see Question 7-2). For example, in the case of a profit evaluation focus, performance statistics related to profitability may be developed from input, process, or output measures. Therefore, if the responsibility accounting system is to elicit effective and efficient management of the organization's resources, decision makers held responsible for various aspects of performance must know (1) which measures of performance are considered important by the managers of the institution, and (2) which departmental performance goals are considered important in achieving institutional goals (see Question 7-7).

Relating the Responsibility Accounting System to the Evaluation of Managerial Performance

If a responsibility accounting system is to be effective in controlling resources, the organization must have a reward/penalty system that is sensitive to performance deviations so that decision makers can be made aware of how the organization evaluates their control actions. In the case of unfavorable performance deviations, the resultant penalty may be as simple as a memo from the controller indicating the importance of monitoring performance to keep the results of activity at a desirable level. At the other extreme, repeated failure to keep performance under control may result in dismissal.

Factors Important in Operationalizing a Responsibility Accounting System

Developing and maintaining an effective responsibility accounting system is a difficult organizational task. Given the above discussion, the following factors must be considered if organizational decision makers are to effect resource control through a responsibility accounting system.

1. One individual must be accountable for the performance of a specific set of activities. The actions taken by this individual to control performance must be evaluated in conjunction with the control actions taken by other accountable individuals, and the results of that evaluation must be communicated to the individual being evaluated (feedback).
2. Individuals who have control over the performance of the activities for which they are accountable must be able to effect changes in the statistics (cost or profit) used to describe the performance of these activities. Control is present when the individual accountable for the performance of specific activities may take actions which are effective in directly reorienting such performance in a timely manner. However, the existence of control is not sufficient to imply that control actions are desirable. For example, as shall be discussed in the general medical clinic case study, controlling allocated variable costs by reducing the service of the unit may be inconsistent with the goals of the institution. Therefore, not only must control actions be feasible, they also must be consistent with the explicit performance goals of the institution.

3a. Evaluation Statistics: Cost statistics which are used as a basis of performance evaluation must consist of costs that can be changed effectively by the actions of the departmental manager. Figure 7-9 illustrates the general relationship between the cost control potential of responsibility accounting systems and various types of cost. As illustrated, responsibility accounting systems generally are most effective in promoting cost control when the cost activities to be controlled are direct and variable. As costs become fixed and indirect, the effectiveness of responsibility accounting systems in providing cost control diminishes.

3b. Evaluation Statistics: Revenue and Profit statistics also may be used as a basis of performance evaluation. The nature of these performance evaluation statistics in relation to organizational resource control (as opposed to departmental resource control) is a complex issue. This subject is discussed in detail in Chapter 8.

In conclusion, "responsibility accounting" is only a term for the systematic control of performance on a particular evaluation dimension. Responsi-

Figure 7-9 Cost Categorization as Related to the Effectiveness of Responsibility Accounting Systems in Controlling Costs.

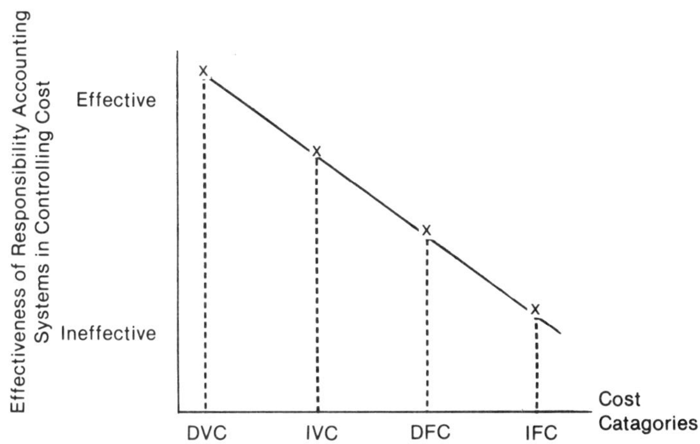

bility accounting is actually a philosophy of control, rather than a special technique which exists independent of the many other performance planning and control systems used in the organization. The following case study examines the concepts of responsibility accounting discussed in this chapter.

THE GENERAL MEDICAL CLINIC: A STUDY OF THE EFFECT OF COST CONTROLLABILITY ON PROFIT RESPONSIBILITY ACCOUNTING SYSTEMS

This case illustrates a process whereby the reasonability of evaluating a general medical clinic as an independent profit responsibility center may be ascertained. The relationship between the classifications of the clinic's costs and management's ability to take effective and desirable (i.e., consistent with the goals of the institution) control actions is of particular interest. The cost classifications are discussed in detail in the first part of the case. Then the clinic's revenue sources are described so that the break-even volume of the clinic may be computed. The case concludes with an evaluation of the clinic as an independent responsibility center and a discussion of the propriety of a profit responsibility accounting system in units like the general medical clinic.

Description of the Costs Associated with the General Medical Clinic (GMC)

The cost data reported and derived for the operation of the General Medical Clinic (one of the outpatient department clinics) for the period July 1, 19X1, to June 30, 19X2, are presented in Table 7-5. This information was prepared and compiled by the hospital controller's office. Descriptions of the various direct and indirect costs, including methods and bases of allocation are provided in the following paragraphs. In subsequent

Table 7-5 General Medical Clinic Cost Statement for the Year Ending June 30, 19X2

Item	Allocation Base	Cost
DIRECT COSTS		
Department of Medicine (DOM) Salaries		$ 37,000
Direct Salaries		21,925
Nursing Salaries		19,137
Other Costs		4,174
Total Direct Costs		$ 82,236
INDIRECT COSTS		
Other Salaries	PV	$ 17,576
Building and Equipment Depreciation	SF	6,262
Administrative and General	GS	7,909
Employee Health and Welfare	GS	7,210
Operation of Plant	SF	9,444
Maintenance of Plant	SF	4,647
Laundry and Linen	PV	551
Housekeeping	SF	3,185
Cafeteria	Empl	626
Nursing Service Administration	PV	1,393
Medical Supplies	PV	201
Medical Records	PV	13,066
Social Service	PV	8,710
Nursing School	PV	6,644
Interns and Residents	PV	41,945
Total Indirect Costs		$129,369
Total Costs		$211,605

COST ALLOCATION BASES:
PV = Patient Visit
GS = Gross Salaries
SF = Square Footage
Empl = Number of Employees

sections, these costs are categorized into controllable and uncontrollable, fixed and variable costs.

Total Direct Costs: $82,236

Department of Medicine Salaries. This category includes the salaries of the chief of the clinic, other faculty and nonfaculty physicians, and a part time secretary. The physician's salaries are allocated from the Department of Medicine because the primary appointment of the clinic physicians is the department of medicine.

Direct Salaries. This category includes the salaries of a clerical supervisor and two clerks assigned to the GMC.

Nursing Salaries. Two nurses, an RN and an LPN, are assigned full time to the GMC. The salary figure shown includes overtime paid to these individuals, as well as the full time nursing salaries.

Other Costs. This account includes miscellaneous expenses incurred by the GMC.

Total Indirect Costs: $129,369

Indirect costs are those costs allocated to various departments on some logical basis. The most important criterion for selecting a basis of allocation for indirect costs is that the basis used to assign costs must be logically related to the incurrance of the assigned costs. The following paragraphs discuss the bases of allocation selected for the various indirect costs in the GMC.

Other Salaries. This category includes a portion of the salaries of administrative personnel assigned to the outpatient department (OPD). These salaries are allocated to the GMC on the basis of patient visits because they represent patient-related clerical and administrative costs within the OPD.

Building and Equipment Depreciation. These costs are allocated among all departments based upon the square footage occupied by each department. The square footage in a department is directly related to the portion of the building utilized by that department and is, therefore, appropriate as an allocation base for building depreciation. The square footage occupied by each department is used as the basis for allocating equipment depreciation too.

Administrative and General. The basis of allocation used for these costs is gross salaries. Since 62 percent of the hospital's operating expenses are salaries, most of the administrative costs are related to employee activities.

Therefore, the gross salaries in each department should be proportional to the general and administrative costs expended for that department.

Employee Health and Welfare. Since these costs vary with respect to individual salary levels, gross salaries are used as a basis of allocation for employee health and welfare costs.

Operation of Plant. This category includes the costs incurred to maintain the hospital's operations. Since expenses such as fuel and electricity are accumulated in this account, square footage is selected as the basis of allocation.

Maintenance of Plant. These costs are incurred in the maintenance and upkeep of the physical properties of the hospital and are allocated on the basis of square footage.

Laundry and Linen. These costs represent the cleaning and replacement of linens used in the GMC. The basis used to allocate these laundry and linen expenses is patient visits.

Housekeeping. The basis used to allocate these expenses is square footage.

Cafeteria. This account represents the expenses incurred to provide cafeteria service to the hospital employees. Hence, the number of employees in each department is used as a basis for allocating these cafeteria costs.

Nursing Service Administration. This account represents the administrative expenses necessary to provide the nursing service. The base used to allocate these costs is patient visits.

Medical Supplies. Since medical supply usage varies proportionately with the number of patients, medical supplies expense is allocated to the GMC according to the number of patient visits.

Medical Records. This account represents both the costs incurred in setting up and updating the patient's medical history records and the costs incurred in making these records available to each clinic and department. Since the number of medical records varies directly with the number of patients, patient visits are the basis used to allocate medical records costs.

Social Service. This account represents the expenses incurred to provide social services to patients in various hospital clinics and departments. The cost of the social service is a function of the number of patients in the clinics and departments. Therefore, patient visits are the basis for allocating social service costs.

Nursing School. This account represents the expenses incurred by the nursing school. The service provided by the nursing school to various clinics and departments varies with the number of patients visits, which form the basis for allocating these costs.

Interns and Residents. This account represents the salaries of interns and residents who render service in the clinic. These costs are allocated according to the number of patient visits in the clinic. The number of visits has always been used as a surrogate for the time spent by the interns and residents in each of the hospital's departments.

These 15 cost categories were formulated by the hospital. The bases for allocating indirect costs (which were developed by the hospital controller) were investigated and deemed reasonable. Having gathered this information, the direct variable costs (DVC), direct fixed costs (DFC), indirect variable costs (IVC), and the indirect fixed costs (IFC) incurred by the GMC must be divided into controllable and uncontrollable categories.

Analysis of Cost Controllability

Table 7-6 categorizes the GMC costs listed in Table 7-5 in a 2 × 2 matrix of controllable and uncontrollable fixed and variable costs. The breakdown of costs was prepared by the head of the GMC. The following discussion describes the rationale underlying the assignment of each of these costs to their respective cells in the matrix.

Controllable Direct Variable Costs (DVC)

The GMC does not presently categorize any costs as controllable direct variable costs because the costs perceived as being variable are allocated to the GMC on the basis of patient visits. Therefore, the director of the GMC can reduce the size of the variable cost allocation only by reducing the number of visits. (Recall the responsibility accounting discussion on p. 252). Since no direct desirable managerial action can be taken to reduce variable costs and leave the patient volume unaffected, all of the variable costs allocated on the basis of patient visits are categorized as uncontrollable.

Controllable Direct Fixed Costs (DFC)[7]

The basic unit of activity for the GMC is patient visits. The direct salaries, representing medical and clerical personnel costs, are controllable in the long run, i.e. they may be increased or decreased appropriately with significant changes in the volume of activity over the long run. However, within a given accounting period (one year), the direct salaries are fixed over the estimated range of activity for that period.

Table 7-6 Grouping of Direct Fixed, Indirect Fixed, and Indirect Variable Costs into Controllable and Uncontrollable Categories

Cost

	VARIABLE			FIXED		
CONTROLLABLE	*Direct*			*Direct*		
				Direct Salaries	$21,925	(DFC)
				Nursing Salaries	19,137	(DFC)
				DOM Salaries	37,000	(DFC)
				Other Costs	4,174	(DFC)
			I	II	$82,236	
UNCONTROLLABLE	*Indirect*		III	IV *Indirect*		
	Laundry & Linen	$ 551	(IVC)	Building Depreciation	$ 5,747	(IFC)
	Nursing Service Administration	1,393	(IVC)	Equipment Depreciation	515	(IFC)
	Medical Supplies	201	(IVC)	Administrative & General	7,909	(IFC)
	Medical Records	13,066	(IVC)	Employee Health & Welfare	7,210	(IFC)
	Social Service	8,710	(IVC)	Operation of Plant	9,444	(IFC)
	Nursing School	6,644	(IVC)	Maintenance of Plant	4,647	(IFC)
	Interns & Residents	41,945	(IVC)	Housekeeping	3,185	(IFC)
	Other Salaries	17,576	(IVC)	Cafeteria	626	(IFC)
		$90,086			$39,283	

Uncontrollable Indirect Variable Costs (IVC)

The costs listed in cell three (III) of the matrix are uncontrollable because they are all allocated costs based upon patient visits. Therefore, the only control action which may be taken to alter costs is to reduce patient volume. As suggested, this is not an appropriate control action.

Uncontrollable Indirect Fixed Costs (IFC)

The costs listed in cell four (IV) of the matrix also are uncontrollable because they are allocated costs, and the basis of allocation for each cost is fixed for a particular accounting period. Administrative and general costs and employee health and welfare costs are fixed due to their primary dependence upon the fixed portion of gross salaries (those listed in the second cell (II)). Cafeteria costs also are fixed because their level depends upon the number of GMC employees which, in most cases, is fixed for a given period. The remaining costs listed in this cell are fixed due to their basis of allocation (square footage).

Categorizing the costs incurred by the GMC yields only half of the information necessary to establish the clinic as a profit center. To operate as a profit center, the sources, nature, and magnitude of revenue associated with the GMC must be identified.

Ascertaining the Revenue Earned by the General Medical Clinic

The method of analysis used to isolate GMC revenues consisted of identifying the various payment plans which reimburse the clinic, describing the distribution of payment liability between the plan and the patient, defining the total payment liability expected by the clinic, and computing the percentage of patients falling within each plan. With this information, a patient revenue profile was generated for the clinic to calculate the clinic revenue expected during the year.

A sample of 840 patients (approximately 15 percent) was taken from the active patient file of the GMC. According to this sample, the primary payment plans encountered at the clinic are self-payment by the patient (20 percent), an Indigent Outpatient Assistance Program (IOAP) (18.2 percent), Medicare and Medicaid (25.4 percent), and a State Health Care Program (33.6 percent).[8] Given this patient revenue profile for the clinic, the average revenue computed for the first 8,000 patients entering the GMC in any given period is \$7.72 per patient. After 8,000 patients, however, IOAP usually is exhausted. Hence, for each patient beyond 8,000 patients, the average revenue falls to \$6.97 per patient.

Break-Even Analysis

Given the GMC patient revenue profile and the costs categorized and reported in Table 7-6, the break-even volume may be computed for the GMC. Fixed costs from Table 7-6 are \$121,519 and variable costs are \$90,086. Since patient volume has averaged 16,800 patient visits over the last few years, the variable cost per patient and the average revenue per patient may be computed as follows:

$$\text{Variable Cost Per Patient} = \frac{\$90{,}086}{16{,}800}$$

$$= \$5.36$$

$$\text{Average Revenue per Patient} = \frac{(\$8{,}000 \times \$7.72) + (8{,}800 \times \$6.97)}{16{,}800}$$

$$= \$7.33.$$

Hence, the break-even point for the GMC is:

$$\hat{X} = \frac{c_F}{b_R - b_V}$$

$$= \frac{\$121,519}{\$7.33 - \$5.36}$$

$$= 61{,}685 \text{ patients.}$$

This computed break-even volume is so high that the GMC could never treat enough patients to break even. However, if the break-even volume for the clinic could be reduced through managerial action, the GMC might be able to succeed as a profit responsibility center (see Question 7-9). Unfortunately, given the breakdown of controllable and uncontrollable costs, management cannot take desirable corrective actions to reduce the GMC costs and thereby lower the break-even volume.

Profit Responsibility Center

The reasonability of developing the GMC as a profit responsibility center is related to the impact that desirable control actions might have on the GMC costs. In this case, within a relevant range of activity, the clinic director cannot reduce the controllable fixed costs significantly. In addition, the clinic director does not have the authority to reduce uncontrollable variable costs on a short-term basis. Hence, there is not a sufficient degree of cost control to warrant evaluating the GMC as a profit responsibility center.

The lack of cost control is primarily due to the fact that many costs are incurred from functional areas not under the control of the director of the GMC. Hence, the only viable alternative in effecting decentralized cost control is to extend the responsibility accounting concept to functional units.

In summary, when developing or implementing a responsibility accounting system within the institution, the primary administrative concern should be to determine the cost and revenue structure of operating each function (functional unitization). Then the costs of each function can be divided into controllable and uncontrollable, fixed and variable costs. Underlying this concept is the assumption that in contrast to the cost classifications in the GMC, most costs within each functional area generally will be controllable. If empirical evidence supports this assumption, establishing a profit responsibility center within each functional area could enhance cost control.

NOTES

1. The solution to this problem is simplified by using the quadratic formula:

$$X = \frac{-b \pm \sqrt{b^2 - 4ac}}{2a},$$

where a, b, and c are the coefficients and X is the variable in the general quadratic equation $aX^2 + bX + c = 0$. In this case, the equation $a_R\hat{X}^2 + b_R\hat{X} = a_V\hat{X}^2 + b_V\hat{X} + c_F$ may be rewritten as: $(a_R - a_V)\hat{X}^2 + (b_R - b_V)\hat{X} - c_F = 0$, so that $a = a_R - a_V$, $b = b_R - b_V$, $c = -c_F$ and $X = \hat{X}$.
2. Given any set of points, regression analysis may be used to develop linear, quadratic, or polynominal equations of any order. In order to ascertain the appropriateness of the order of the regression equation, one often evaluates the R^2 (see Problem 7-3).
3. In this equation, $\Delta c_F > 0$ and has, therefore, been subtracted from c_F. To be consistent, $\Delta\hat{X}$ has been subtracted from $\hat{X}$. However, the sign of $\Delta\hat{X}$ has not been determined.
4. In this equation, $\Delta b_V > 0$ and is, therefore, subtracted from b_V. Again, for consistency, $\Delta\hat{X}$ is subtracted from $\hat{X}$, but the sign of $\Delta\hat{X}$ has not been determined.
5. Note that a revenue increase of \$.53 per patient would have the same effect as a variable cost decrease of \$.53 per patient. However, such a revenue increase may cause a reduction in patient volume of indeterminable magnitude (see the management of accounts receivable, Chapter 3).
6. Functional unitization is discussed briefly in the general medical clinic case in this chapter.
7. This categorization was prepared after considerable discussion with the head of the GMC. More than a reasonable doubt still exists regarding the controllability of these fixed costs in the long run. Therefore, all of the costs incurred by the GMC may be uncontrollable.
8. The sum of the percentages listed is 97.2. The remaining 2.8 percent of the sampled files were those of hospital employees receiving free care.

Questions and Problems

Question 7-1. Discuss the following statement: Break-even analyses, traditionally concerned with the point at which total costs equal total revenue, can cause serious systems dysfunctions if one considers that the purpose of hospitals has nothing to do with profitability. Relate your discussion to the desirability of particular control actions.

Question 7-2. In this chapter, profit has been used as the focus of the responsibility accounting system. However, responsibility accounting systems with multiple foci can be developed. Suggest another focus not related directly to profit and show how the responsibility accounting system could be used to evaluate performance.

Question 7-3. In Figures 7-7 and 7-8, the linear and quadratic cases for the revenue and the total cost functions were presented. State the likely economic circumstances which would lead to:

a. a linear variable cost function,
b. a quadratic variable cost function,
c. a linear revenue function, and
d. a quadratic revenue function.

Question 7-4. Consider the following graph.

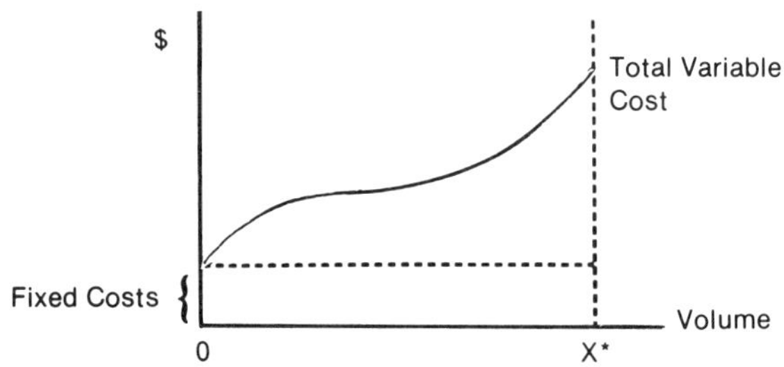

a. What is the general form of the total cost equation from 0 to X*?
b. What is the general form of the marginal cost equation from 0 to X* (i.e. the domain of X)?
c. Give an economic interpretation to the total and marginal cost equations over the domain.

Question 7-5. Consider the following graph.

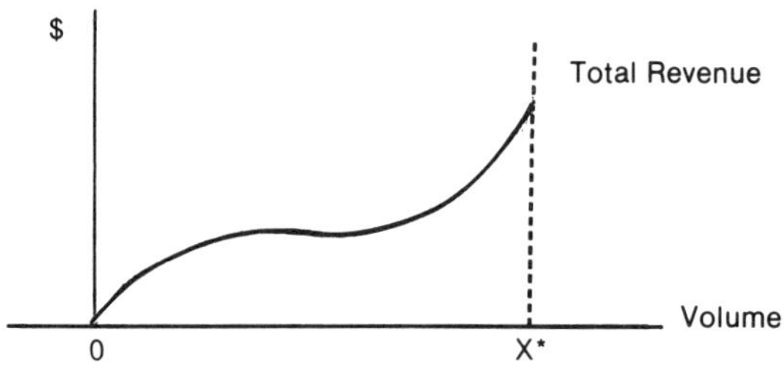

a. What is the general form of the total revenue function from 0 to X*?
b. What is the general form of the marginal revenue equation from 0 to X*?

c. Give an economic interpretation to the total and marginal revenue equations over the domain.

Question 7-6. Given the general form of the total cost and total revenue functions in questions 7-4 and 7-5, what condition will lead to:

a. break-even?
b. profit maximization? (Profit is maximized when $MC = MR$, where $MC = dTC/dX$ and $MR = dTR/dX$.
c. Assume that the equations represented in Questions 7-4 and 7-5 are actual cost and revenue functions. Discuss the control problems created if linear regression equations are used as estimates of the nonlinear equations represented in Questions 7-4 and 7-5.

Question 7-7. How would the manager of a particular department ascertain if control actions were consistent with the goals of the institution? Be specific in answering this question.

Question 7-8. Assume that data in the interval $[A, B]$ is used to estimate a linear regression function. If the coefficient of determination of the regression equation is 1.0 (see Appendix B) what will the standard error or the estimate (S_e) be:

a. for any interpolation, i.e. any regression estimation in the interval $[A, B]$?
b. for any extrapolation, i.e. any regression estimate not in the internal $[A, B]$?
c. Discuss the control implications of regression interpolations and extrapolations. Relate this discussion to Figure 7-3.

Question 7-9. Assume the material discussed in the GMC case is presented to the controller of the hospital. After considering this information the controller sends the following memo to the medical director of the GMC:

MEMO

From: Controller
To: Medical Director—GMC
Subject: Break-Even Analysis of the GMC

I agree that there is very little opportunity to take effective managerial actions which would reduce costs. However, why bother with reducing costs? Increase the number of patients seen. This will reduce unit costs and everything can be worked out from there.

Required: Discuss this memo.

Question 7-10. Discuss the planning and control information which may be derived from a break-even analysis.

Question 7-11. Assume that the manager of a department sets a profit goal for the department. If the fixed costs, variable costs per unit, and revenue per unit are c_F, b_V, and b_R respectively, and the profit goal is $\hat{\pi}$ (a total dollar amount), at what volume will the department attain the profit goal? Discuss the relationship between break-even analysis and profitability analysis.

Question 7-12. The square of the difference between the regression estimate and the actual revenue for month 2, Table 7-2, is:

$$[(-210.24 + 24.66(1462) - 26{,}552]^2 = 86{,}316{,}735.$$

The average of the square of the differences between the regression estimate and the actual revenues for the other 14 months is 467,594. The range, the highest and lowest values, for the other 14 months is 137,923 and 852,003.

a. What does this information imply?
b. What effect does the actual value in Table 7-2 for month 2 have on:
   i. the regression equation?
   ii. the values of R and R^2? and
   iii. the standard error of the estimate?

Question 7-13. Consider the example of the radiology department on page 232 and assume the cost of making a fixed cost alteration is $1,150, but is only incurred once, rather that annually. Further assume that the benefit (a reduction in fixed costs of 12 percent) is expected to be realized each year for three years and that the institution can earn eight percent on invested capital. In this case, using the present value criterion, which alternative has the largest economic benefit? Discuss the implications of your analysis.

Problem 7-1. Given the following functions:

	Cost	Revenue
i.	$8{,}400 + 9.83X$	$10{,}813 + 6.47X$
ii.	$73 - 12.34X + .73X^2$	$9.72X - .17X^2$

a. Derive the respective profit functions.
b. What are the break-even points for these profit functions?
c. Using the information developed in (b), determine the optimal number of units (X^*).

d. Verify your answer in (c) with calculus.
e. Where possible, interpret the coefficients of the profit functions developed in (a).

Problem 7-2. a. Derive the break-even point given the following functions:

Fixed cost:	$a_F + b_F X$
Variable cost:	$a_V + b_V X$
Revenue:	$a_R + b_R X$

b. Given the break-even formula, Equation 7-2, discuss the effect of changes in each parameter on the break-even point.
c. What is the economic interpretation of b_F, a_R, and a_V not equal to zero?

Problem 7-3. Assume the hospital administrator analyzes the daily EKG volume and the related costs using regression analysis. The following cost function is generated using a linear regression:

Total Cost: $c(X) = 436.8 + 12.3X$

$R^2 = .93$ (see Appendix B).

Using a nonlinear regression, the following cost and revenue functions are generated:

Total Cost: $\hat{c}(X) = 735.7 - 3.4X + .2X^2$

$R^2 = .07$

Total Revenue: $r(X) = 326.0 + 39.3X - .2X^2$

$R^2 = .96$

Required:

a. Graph $c(X), \hat{c}(X), r(X)$.
b. Construct the profit functions which may be used to determine the break-even points.
c. What are the roots of the profit functions?
d. Graph the profit functions.
e. What is the relevant break-even point found using $\{c(X), r(X)\}$?; using $\{\hat{c}(X), r(X)\}$?
f. At what point is profit maximized using $\{c(X), r(X)\}$?; using $\{\hat{c}(X), r(X)\}$?

g. How should the hospital administrator use the coefficient of determination information?

Problem 7-4. Assume the profitability of laboratory procedures may be described with the following function:

$$\pi(X) = -9{,}653.84 + 1.3X.$$

The function which describes the behavior of laboratory cost is:

$$c(X) = 10{,}973.84 + 8.3X.$$

Required:

(a) What is the revenue function?

(b) The hospital administrator wishes to increase the net income of the laboratory by \$5,000. Either one of two actions (A_1 and A_2) may be taken:

A_1 = will reduce fixed costs by \$6,834.16

A_2 = will reduce variable costs by \$3.06 per procedure.

Assuming the break-even volume before the actions is attainable, what cost of action 1 *and* what cost of action 2 will make the hospital administrator indifferent between the two actions, A_1 and A_2?

Problem 7-5. Assume the following cost function $\hat{C}(X) = C + BX + AX^2$, $C, B, A > 0$; and revenue function $R(X) = \alpha C(X)$; where $\alpha > 1$, describe the costs and revenues of an institution.

Required:

a. Show that no reasonable root exists for the profit function. What does this mean?

b. What are the implications for cost plus contracts?

c. Is there a profit where $\alpha < 1$? Why?

Problem 7-6. In the text (p. 250), the manager of the radiology department chose to alter variable costs because the net economic benefit of altering variable costs was greater than the net economic benefit of altering the fixed costs. Determine at what patient volume the manager would be indifferent to altering the fixed costs or altering the variable costs. Also determine at what patient volume the manager would choose to alter fixed costs. Can you generalize these results in terms of break-even analysis? In the radiology case, why will the manager choose neither a fixed cost alteration nor a variable cost alteration at the point of indifference?

Problem 7-7. The administrator of a prepaid medical group is considering the construction of an addition to the main building to accommodate an anticipated increased patient load. The current facility is capable of processing a patient load of 48,612 patients per year. The facility and its equipment cost $297,411. The variable treatment costs are $4.73 per patient visit. The maximum capacity of the new addition will be 25,000 patients per year. The construction firm indicates that the addition will cost $637,000. The administrator wishes to have the total per patient cost remain the same as before the addition. Is this possible given the patient capacity of the new facility? How many patients must be seen in the new facility for the total per unit costs to remain the same as they were before the new facility was constructed? (Assume the variable cost per patient remains the same.)

Chapter 8

Profit Responsibility Accounting: Its Pricing Aspects

You can't always get what you want; but if you try sometime, you might find you get what you need.

M. Jagger and K. Richard

Responsibility accounting systems are designed to control the acquisition and use of organizational resources. To control these resources effectively, the organization's responsibility accounting system must have an evaluation focus, such as profit or efficiency of performance, that is associated with the organizational goals and objectives. In addition, effective responsibility accounting systems must use performance measures, such as maximizing profit per period or minimizing cost per service, that accurately reflect a manager's performance in controlling resources and hence in attaining organizational goals. A responsibility accounting system that has an inappropriate evaluation focus or uses inappropriate performance measures misallocates the organization's resources and creates an illusion of control, while in fact the organization continues to operate in an uncontrolled manner.

Profit responsibility accounting systems, or responsibility accounting systems that have profit as the evaluation focus and use the maximization of periodic profit as the performance measure, require the organization's managers to attempt to minimize costs and maximize revenues. Since the fundamentals of effective cost control were discussed in the previous chapter, this chapter deals solely with the revenue, or pricing, aspects of profit responsibility accounting systems. The first section discusses the pricing aspects of such systems in profit making organizations. The applicability of these systems in nonprofit health care organizations is discussed in the second section. The chapter concludes with a case study that illustrates a health care organization's difficulty in evaluating departmental performance in terms of departmental profit.

PROFIT RESPONSIBILITY ACCOUNTING IN PROFIT MAKING ORGANIZATIONS

The fundamental goal of profit making organizations is to maximize the wealth of the owners. Hence, these organizations traditionally have developed responsibility accounting systems that focus on profit as the basis of evaluation and measure managerial performance in terms of departmental profit. The premise underlying this approach is that if each department in the organization endeavors to maximize departmental profit, the net result will be the maximization of total organizational profit.[1]

Methods of Interdepartmental Pricing

When an organization is operating under a profit responsibility accounting system, the manager in each department attempts to minimize the unit cost and maximize the unit price of departmental output. However, in vertically integrated organizations, including many health care institutions, the price charged by one department is a cost incurred by another department (see Figure 8-1). Hence, interdepartmental conflicts arise as the "seller" department tries to maximize revenues and the "buyer" department tries to minimize costs.

These interdepartmental conflicts have caused profit making organizations to seek objective prices that can be used interdepartmentally. The six objective prices most commonly suggested for estimating the appropriate interdepartmental price are (1) market price, (2) marginal cost, (3) average accounting cost, (4) full cost, (5) a negotiated price, and (6) a price determined by central management. The rationale underlying the selection of each of these transfer prices is discussed in the following sections.

Market Price as the Interdepartmental Price

The market price, as found in price lists of other organizations that sell products or provide services similar to the seller department's output, is the simplest and most objective interdepartmental price. The argument for selecting the market price as the interdepartmental price is that the market price tends to simulate the market conditions that the seller department would face if it were a separate economic entity, rather than an integral part of the organizational network. However, market price may not be fair for internal pricing and evaluation because the seller department usually has a captive market and does not have to incur the selling and administrative expenses of external sellers. In fact, evidence exists that the market price can inflate the buyer department's cost to such an extent that the buyer department is unable to market its output economically.

Figure 8-1 Pricing and Cost Schematic: Two Departments

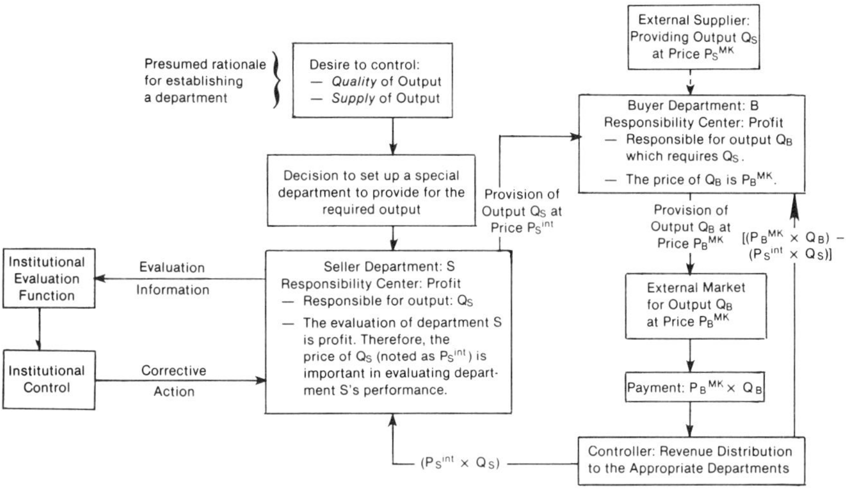

Marginal Cost as the Interdepartmental Price

The marginal cost of a unit of output is the additional cost that must be incurred to produce that unit of output. Hence, to compute the marginal cost of the ith unit of output, the total cost of producing i-1 units must be subtracted from the total cost of producing i units. Since diminishing returns of additional units of input occur after a specific output is reached, the marginal cost of each additional unit of output generally should be expected to increase. However, economies of scale are sometimes evidenced in the initial stages of production, resulting in decreasing marginal cost for the first several units of output. Therefore, the marginal cost for a particular product or service often is graphically depicted as a curve that declines at first and then bends upward (see Figure 8-2).

Since marginal cost varies inversely and then directly with the level of output, marginal cost should be less than the market price within some range of output[2] (e.g., the range between output levels i and k), and should be minimized at some production level within this range (e.g., the production level of j units). However, within other ranges of output, the marginal cost may be greater than the market price (the range between output levels 0 and i and the range above output level k). Consequently, if marginal cost is used as the interdepartmental price, the evaluations of the buyer and seller departments will depend on the seller department's level of output.

Figure 8-2 Marginal Cost and the Market Price at Various Levels of Output

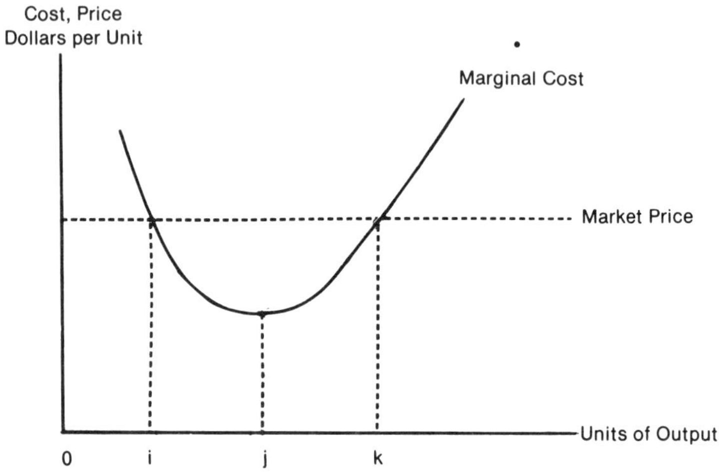

Of course, marginal cost is seldom, if ever, used as the interdepartmental price because, in the short run, marginal costs cannot be measured precisely (see Question 8-1). However, in the long run, the marginal cost of the seller department generally tends to be less than or equal to the market price because departments that operate at a level where the marginal cost is greater than the market price will be undersold by external suppliers if interdepartmental prices are set equal to marginal cost, or will realize losses if interdepartmental prices are set equal to the market price. Therefore, in subsequent discussions in this chapter, the marginal cost will be assumed to be less than the market price.

Average Accounting Cost as the Interdepartmental Price

The average accounting cost (AAC) of a department's output also can be used as the interdepartmental price. To compute the average accounting cost, the estimated total cost for the department must be divided by the estimated number of units of departmental output as follows.

$$\text{AAC} = \frac{\text{Estimated Total Cost (Direct and Indirect)}}{\text{Estimated Number of Units of Output}}$$

Generally, the total cost and the units of output estimates are based on the previous year's activities. Of course, these estimates must be accurate if the average accounting cost is to be a valid interdepartmental price.

For example, overestimating total cost will inflate the average accounting cost, resulting in an unfair interdepartmental price for the buyer department, while underestimating the total cost will deflate the average accounting cost and result in an unfair price for the seller department. Similar problems can arise from inaccurately estimating the number of units of output. Furthermore, the average accounting cost is an unfair price for the seller department unless the average accounting cost contains a profit element.

Full Cost as the Interdepartmental Price

For interdepartmental pricing purposes, the full cost (C_F) of a unit of departmental output is defined as the average accounting cost of that unit plus a reasonable profit element, or

$$C_F = AAC + \pi$$

where: π is the economic profit per unit that provides a reasonable economic return to the seller department.

The problems with using full cost as a surrogate for the interdepartmental price are similar to the problems associated with the average accounting cost except that in the full cost case, the profit element has not been disregarded. However, although one problem has been eliminated by including this profit element, other problems are encountered in attempting to estimate the profit element accurately.

Negotiated Interdepartmental Prices

The most common means of selecting interdepartmental prices is negotiation between the buyer and seller departments. This process sometimes produces a fair interdepartmental price for both the seller and buyer department because a negotiated price usually reflects cost recoupment plus an element of "profit." However, the size of the profit element sometimes depends on the political power of the managers in the respective departments (see Question 8-5). Hence, using the negotiated price as the interdepartmental price could in some cases lead to invalid conclusions regarding periodic managerial performance.

Centrally Determined Interdepartmental Prices

Interdepartmental prices also can be selected and enforced by the organization's central management. This method removes all traces of pricing autonomy at the departmental level. However, it allows the central management, which presumably has superior knowledge of the market, to direct all departments toward an overall "best" result. Unfortunately, by eliminating a portion of departmental autonomy, this pricing method simultaneously eliminates a portion of the department managers' control over departmental profit.

Interdepartmental Pricing in Profit Making Organizations

Given the set of alternative pricing schemes, the seller department, in an attempt to maximize revenues, will opt for the pricing scheme that yields the highest possible price for its output, while the buyer department, in an attempt to minimize costs, will prefer the pricing scheme that yields the lowest possible price for the seller department's output. When a competitive external market exists for the seller department's output, the maximum price that this department can charge for its output is a price equal to the market price because if the interdepartmental price exceeds the market price, the buyer department will buy elsewhere. On the other hand, the minimum price that the seller department can charge for its output without incurring losses is the marginal cost price associated with the volume of output at which the seller department's average total costs are minimized. Figures 8-3 and 8-4 illustrate how the respective departments would react to each of these pricing schemes.

Figure 8-3 shows how a market price interdepartmental pricing scheme and how a "minimal" marginal cost interdepartmental pricing scheme would affect operations in the seller department. The MC_S curve and the ATC_S curve represent the marginal costs and the average total costs, respectively, at various levels of output in the seller department, when this output is sold to the buyer department. The seller department must be able to estimate the magnitude of these costs at various levels of output[3] because, given a specific interdepartmental price, an optimal level of output exists at which the profits derived from interdepartmental sales at that price are maximized. This level is the volume of output at which the marginal cost of the seller department equals the interdepartmental price. More fundamentally, the seller department is able to avoid losses only by making sure that the average total cost of the output to be sold to the buyer department is less than or equal to the interdepartmental price.

Since the seller department only avoids losses when the interdepartmental price is greater than or equal to the average total cost at a specified level of output, the lowest price that the seller department should accept for its output is a price equal to the minimum average total cost. This price is designated as $\hat{P}_S^{MC}$ in Figure 8-3, and can occur only if the buyer department demands $\hat{Q}_S$ units of the seller department's output. Given this price

Figure 8-3 Effects of Interdepartmental Pricing Schemes on the Seller Department: Marginal Cost and Market Price

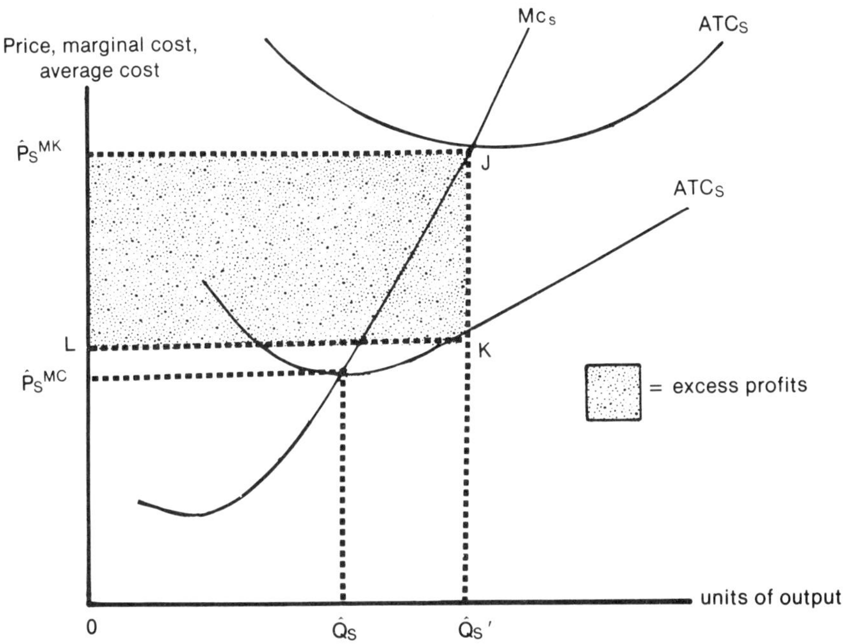

and volume, the seller department will break even. However, at the price $\hat{P}_S^{MC}$, $\hat{Q}_S$ is also the volume of profit maximization because the marginal cost of $\hat{Q}_S$ units of output is equal to the interdepartmental price, $\hat{P}_S^{MC}$. Furthermore, neither increasing nor decreasing volume, given the price $\hat{P}_S^{MC}$, can increase the seller department's profit.

The probability that the buyer department would demand exactly $\hat{Q}_S$ units at the price $\hat{P}_S^{MC}$ is unlikely. The probability that the seller department actually would accept the price $\hat{P}_S^{MC}$ is even more unlikely because the buyer department's only alternative source of the seller department's output is the external market. Hence, the seller department can raise the price above $\hat{P}_S^{MC}$ and reap the excess profits associated with the higher price.

Of course, the seller department would like to raise the interdepartmental price to equal the market price, $\hat{P}_S^{MK}$ in Figure 8-3. At this price, the seller department could maximize its profits by producing $\hat{Q}_S'$ units (see Question 8-5). Given this price and volume, if this seller department can sell all of its output to the buyer department, the excess profits will be equal to the area of the shaded rectangle, $JKL\hat{P}_S^{MK}$ in Figure 8-3.[4]

Figure 8-4 Effects of Interdepartmental Pricing Schemes on the Buyer Department: Marginal Cost and Market Price

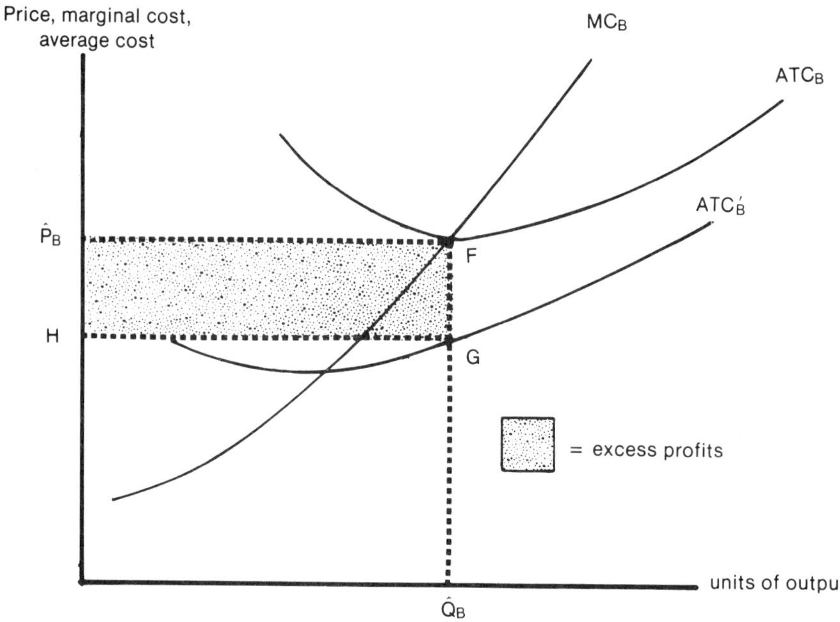

However, the probability that the buyer department would accept an interdepartmental price equal to the market price is very unlikely. The buyer department knows that the seller department is earning excess profits because the market price provides for the recoupment of the normal selling costs associated with external sales, and the seller department is not incurring these costs. Furthermore, the buyer department knows that if the seller department had to sell its output in the external market, the costs associated with the external sales would shift average total costs of the seller department to approximately ATC_S'.[5] Given the costs represented by this curve, the seller department could, at best, only break even. This fact, coupled with the fact that the buyer department would be indifferent to buying in the market or buying from the seller department at the market price, gives the buyer department the bargaining power to reduce the interdepartmental price below the market price.

Of course, a lower interdepartmental price means higher excess profits for the buyer department. If the interdepartmental price is equal to the market price, the buyer department's marginal costs and average total costs are represented by the MC_B curve and the ATC_B curve, respectively, in Figure 8-4. Since the market price of the buyer department's output is $\hat{P}_B$, given the costs represented by the MC_B and ATC_B curves, the buyer department's optimal level of output is $\hat{Q}_B$, the economic break-even point. On the other hand, if the interdepartmental price is equal to the minimal marginal cost price, $\hat{P}_S^{MC}$ in Figure 8-3, the buyer department's average total costs shift to $ATC_B{}'$. Given these costs, the buyer department again maximizes profits by operating at the volume $\hat{Q}_B$. However, the reduced average total costs give rise to excess profits equal to the area of the shaded rectangle, $FGH\hat{P}_B$. Hence, the buyer department would prefer the lower interdepartmental price.

As shown, the higher the interdepartmental price, the greater the excess profits in the seller department, and the lower the interdepartmental price, the greater the excess profits in the buyer department. Since the buyer and the seller departments have opposing perspectives on interdepartmental pricing, in profit making organizations the interdepartmental price is usually a negotiated price that is less than the market price, but greater than the minimal marginal cost price. The actual value of the interdepartmental price usually depends on the organizational political power of the managers in the negotiating departments.

Summary

Profit responsibility accounting systems are effective in controlling the acquisition and usage of resources in profit making organizations because the focus of evaluation in profit responsibility accounting systems is congruent with the goals and objectives of profit making organizations. In addition, the performance measures of profit responsibility accounting systems accurately reflect managerial performance in profit making organizations because these organizations sell their output to a market of aggressive buyers who are seeking comparable products and services at the lowest price. Therefore, the buyer department, which sells all of its output to this market of aggressive buyers, also must act as an aggressive buyer when purchasing inputs so that its output can be competitively priced in the market. Furthermore, since the buyer department seeks products and services at the lowest price, if the seller department acquires expensive or inefficient equipment or assumes a disproportionately large share of organizational overhead, the interdepartmental price of the seller department's output may exceed the market price and the buyer department may seek to obtain similar output at a lower price elsewhere. Of course, if the interdepartmental price of the seller department's output cannot exceed the market price, the seller department also must act as an aggressive buyer when purchasing inputs because failure to do so will reduce departmental profits. In conclusion, profit responsibility accounting systems are effective in controlling the acquisition and usage of resources in profit making organizations because an efficient market of aggressive buyers effectively controls the price of organizational output, thus requiring organizational managers to control costs by controlling the acquisition and usage of resources.

PROFIT RESPONSIBILITY ACCOUNTING SYSTEMS IN NONPROFIT ORGANIZATIONS

Profit responsibility accounting systems often are used to control the acquisition and usage of resources in nonprofit organizations. Using a profit responsibility accounting system avoids the difficult task of specifying a comprehensive set of nonprofit evaluation criteria. Furthermore, the departments within these organizations all have measurable costs, even though the costs may be arbitrarily assigned, and usually the services provided by each department must be priced for billing purposes. Therefore, profit (revenue less cost) appears to be a simple and efficient means of evaluating departmental performance and hence controlling the acquisition and usage of resources in nonprofit organizations. However, as discussed previously, an effective responsibility accounting system must have an evaluation focus that is congruent with the organization's goals and objectives and uses performance measures that accurately reflect managerial performance. Therefore, although a responsibility accounting system that focuses on profit may be simple to administer in a health care institution, this type of responsibility accounting system may not provide an effective means of controlling the acquisition and usage of the institution's resources.

In fact, since the goals and objectives of most health care institutions center on the humanitarian principles of improving the community health care delivery system or providing for patient welfare, a responsibility accounting system that uses profit as an evaluation focus is not likely to aid the institution in achieving its goals. On the contrary, a profit responsibility accounting system may misdirect the institution toward undesired goals. In addition, the performance measures of profit responsibility accounting systems usually cannot reflect managerial performance in health care institutions accurately. These institutions sell services to a market of passive buyers who are willing to accept the services at almost any price since the principal burden of payment usually is on a third party (see Question 8-2). Although the third party payers attempt to limit these payments to the reimbursement of the "reasonable costs" of providing the service, the cost ceilings that specify the upper limit on reasonable costs generally are well above the market price of comparable services and thus provide no real incentive to control service costs (see Problem 8-4). Consequently, treatment departments are willing to use the services of the service departments, even though the interdepartmental price of these services may exceed the market price, because the excessive cost will be reimbursed by the third party payer. Similarly, the service departments have no incentive to limit their costs because the interdepartmental price can exceed the market price without consequence. Therefore, profit responsibility accounting systems are ineffective in controlling the acquisition and usage of resources in health care institutions because regardless of managerial performance in controlling resources, the departments or the institution can achieve the economic break-even point.

The result of ineffective profit responsibility accounting systems is that some of the institutions' resources are consumed in creating an illusion of control, while in fact, the institution continues to operate in an uncontrolled manner. Managerial performance evaluations are inaccurate because the presumed relationship between the evaluation focus and effective management does not exist. In addition, the institution may be motivated to create internal reimbursement subsidies by allocating disproportionately large shares of overhead to revenue-producing service departments because these departments can incorporate these excess overhead costs in the interdepartmental price (see Question 8-3). Finally, departments within the institution may acquire excessive, expensive, or inefficient equipment because the resultant increase in operating costs can be defrayed partially by including a recoupment percentage in the interdepartmental price. Hence, as illustrated in the following case, resource management in a health care institution operating under an ineffective profit responsibility accounting system will be similar to resource management in health care institutions operating in the absence of systematic resource control.

ELECTROCARDIOGRAM COSTING CASE STUDY

This case examines the cost and price structure of the electrocardiogram (EKG) activity in the cardiovascular (CV) unit in a large urban hospital. The institutional overhead allocated to the EKG activity and the CV unit's ability to incorporate these overhead charges in the price of an EKG are of particular interest. The first section of the case delineates the cost components of the EKG activity. The overhead cost component is compared with the total cost of an EKG in the second section. The third section includes a break-even analysis for the EKG activity. Finally, the case concludes with a discussion of ineffective resource management in health care institutions.

Delineation of EKG Cost Components

The CV unit renders EKG services to several different patient groups within the hospital. The number of EKGs supplied to these patient groups in the months of July through December, as well as the average number of EKGs rendered per month, are shown in Table 8-1.

Four distinct and identifiable types of cost are associated with the EKG activity: (1) overhead costs, (2) reading costs, (3) personnel costs, and (4) machine and supplies costs. Each component is discussed and the average value of each cost component per EKG is computed in the following paragraphs. These average values are useful in calculating the average cost of an EKG and in evaluating the allocation of overhead to the EKG activity.

Overhead Costs

The overhead costs assigned to the EKG activity are variable and are a function of the price charged to the patient group receiving the EKG. Where reimbursements are received, a percentage of the EKG price is deducted by the hospital for overhead costs allocated to the CV unit. The overhead rate varies, depending on the patient group serviced (see Table 8-2).

To compute the average monthly overhead cost of the EKG activity, the numbers in the "Average" column of Table 8-1 are substituted for the respective variables in the "Number of EKGs Rendered" column in Table 8-2. Hence, the average monthly overhead cost is:

$$\begin{aligned}\text{Average Monthly Overhead Cost} &= \$4.00 \times 1350 + \$20.00 \times 452 \\ &\quad + \$20.00 \times 191 + \$0.00 \times 221 \\ &\quad + \$14.00 \times 100 + \$15.00 \times 15 \\ &\quad + \$10.00 \times 8 + \$20.00 \times 97 \\ &= \underline{\underline{\$21{,}905}}\,.\end{aligned}$$

Then, the average overhead cost per EKG can be computed by dividing the average monthly overhead cost by the average number of EKGs processed per month. In this case, the average overhead cost per EKG is:

$$\begin{aligned}\text{Average Overhead Cost per EKG} &= \frac{\$21{,}905}{2{,}434} \\ &= \underline{\underline{\$9.00}}\,.\end{aligned}$$

Table 8-1 Total EKGs Processed

Patient Group	July	August	September	October	November	December	Total	Average
Private and Semiprivate	1,407	1,386	1,321	1,342	1,355	1,289	8,100	1,350
Ward	463	471	432	425	457	464	2,712	452
Outpatient Clinic	168	163	209	225	191	188	1,144	191
Private Outpatient	183	197	251	262	219	215	1,327	221
Diagnostic Clinic	121	106	101	113	119	129	689	115
Clinical Research Center	10	12	4	9	8	5	48	8
Receiving Ward	96	103	92	105	96	90	582	97
TOTAL	2,448	2,438	2,410	2,481	2,445	2,380	14,602	2,434

Table 8-2 EKG Price and Overhead Cost Information by Patient Group

Patient Group Serviced	Number of EKGs Rendered	Charge per EKG	Overhead Rate*	Overhead Cost per EKG
Private and Semiprivate	E_{psp}	\$20.00	20%	\$ 4.00
Ward	E_{w}	20.00	100	20.00
Outpatient Clinic	E_{opc}	20.00	100	20.00
Private Outpatient	E_{pop}	20.00	0	0.00
Diagnostic Clinic	E_{dc}	20.00	70 ($E_{dc} \leq 100$)	14.00
			75 ($E_{dc} > 100$)	15.00
Clinical Research Center	E_{crc}	20.00	50	10.00
Receiving Ward	E_{rw}	20.00	100	20.00

*For the Diagnostic Clinic patients the overhead rate is 70% for the first 100 EKGs and 75% for all subsequent EKGs.

Reading Costs

The costs to interpret an EKG are also variable. When the EKGs are read by staff doctors, the reading cost is 40 percent of cost. However, some preoperative EKGs are read by medical residents. In this case, the reading cost incurred by the CV unit is \$3 per private or semiprivate patient EKG. The ward patient EKGS are read at no charge. The reading cost information is summarized in Table 8-3.

To compute the average monthly reading cost of the EKG activity, the numbers from the "Average" column of Table 8-1 are substituted for the respective variables in the "Number of EKGs Read" column of Table 8-3. The average number of private and semiprivate patient EKGs read by medical residents each month is computed in Table 8-4. Hence, the average monthly reading cost is computed as:

$$\begin{aligned}\text{Average Monthly Reading Cost} &= \$3.00 \times 195 + \$6.40 \times (1350 - 195) \\ &\quad + \$0.00 \times 452 + \$0.00 \times 191 \\ &\quad + \$8.00 \times 221 + \$2.40 \times 100 \\ &\quad + \$2.00 \times 15 + \$4.00 \times 8 \\ &\quad + \$0.00 \times 97 \\ &= \underline{\underline{\$10,047}}\,.\end{aligned}$$

Then, the average reading cost per EKG is computed by dividing the average monthly reading cost by the average number of EKGs read each month. In this case, the average reading cost per EKG is:

$$\begin{aligned}\text{Average Reading Cost per EKG} &= \frac{\$10,047}{2,434} \\ &= \underline{\underline{\$4.13}}\,.\end{aligned}$$

Personnel Costs

The personnel costs incurred by the EKG activity have a fixed component, administrative personnel costs, and two variable components, personnel costs associated with operating the EKG machines and personnel costs associated with processing EKGs. Information regarding the administrative personnel costs is given in Table 8-5. The personnel costs associated with operating the EKG machines, on the other hand, must be com-

Table 8-3 EKG Reading Cost Information by Patient Group

Patient Group Serviced	Number of EKGs Read	Net Price per EKG (Price − Overhead Cost)	Reading Cost Percentage	Reading Cost per EKG
Private and Semiprivate	E_r*	$16.00	—	$3.00
	$E_{psp} - E_r$	16.00	40%	6.40
Ward	E_w	0.00	—	0.00
Outpatient Clinic	E_{opc}	0.00	40	0.00
Private Outpatient	E_{pop}	20.00	40	8.00
Diagnostic Clinic	E_{dc}	6.00 ($E_{dc} \leq 100$)	40	2.40
		5.00 ($E_{dc} > 100$)	40	2.00
Clinical Research Center	E_{crc}	10.00	40	4.00
Receiving Ward	E_{rw}	0.00	—	$0.00

*E_r indicates the number of private and semiprivate patient EKGs read by medical residents.

Table 8-4 Medical Resident EKG Reading

Month	Payment	Number of Private and Semiprivate Patient EKGs Read
February	$618	206
March	675	225
April	432	144
May	399	133
June	603	201
July	564	188
August	615	205
September	609	203
October	552	184
November	693	231
December	435	145
January	807	269
TOTAL		2334

$$\text{Average number read per month by residents} = \frac{2334 \text{ readings/year}}{12 \text{ month/year}}$$

$$= 195 \text{ readings/month}$$

Table 8-5 EKG Administrative Personnel Cost Information

Name	Yearly Salary	Percent of Time Related to EKG Unit	Yearly Cost Related to Unit	Monthly Cost Related to Unit
Administrative Employee:				
1	$7,900	100%	$ 7,900.00	658.33
2	6,350	25	1,587.50	132.29
3	6,250	0	0	0
4	6,050	50	3,025.00	252.08
5	6,000	50	3,000.00	250.00
6	5,600	100	5,600.00	466.67
7	5,550	100	5,550.00	462.50
8	5,300	100	5,300.00	441.67
9	5,250	100	5,250.00	437.50
10	1,800	0	0	0
TOTAL			$37,212.50	$3,101.04

puted because EKG technicians both operate machines and process EKGs. Consequently, their salaries (see Table 8-6) must be divided into personnel costs associated with each of these two functions. An efficiency study showed that 25 percent of the technicians' time was spent operating EKG machines. Hence, 25 percent of the technicians' salaries should be allocated to the number of EKGs taken by the EKG technicians. This number is less than the number of EKGs rendered by the CV unit because hospital personnel outside the CV unit sometimes operate the EKG machines. Information regarding the number of EKGs taken by EKG technicians is given in Table 8-7. Finally, the personnel costs associated with processing EKGs include 75 percent of the EKG technicians' salaries and 100 percent of the wages of part time personnel hired to process EKGs (see Table 8-8).

To compute the average monthly personnel cost of the EKG activity, the average monthly administrative personnel cost, the average monthly

Table 8-6 EKG Technicians' Salaries

Name	Yearly Salary	Monthly Salary
Employee:		
1	$ 5,500	$ 458.33
2	4,775	397.92
3	4,400	366.67
4	4,400	366.67
5	4,400	366.67
6	4,400	366.67
7	4,200	350.00
8	4,200	350.00
TOTAL	$36,275	$3,022.93

Table 8-7 EKG Machine Operation Information by Patient Group

Patient Group Serviced	Number of EKGs Rendered	Percent Taken by EKG Technicians
Private and Semiprivate	E_{psp}	100
Ward	E_{w}	90
Outpatient Clinic	E_{pop}	100
Private Outpatient	E_{opc}	100
Diagnostic Clinic	E_{dc}	0
Clinical Research Center	E_{crc}	100
Receiving Ward	E_{rw}	0

Table 8-8 EKG Part Time Employees Wage Information

For the eight-month period between July 1 and February 28, the total part time payroll was $10,118.00. This yields an average monthly payroll of $1,264.75.

personnel cost associated with operating EKG machines and the average monthly personnel cost associated with processing EKGs must be summed. The average monthly administrative personnel cost is $3,101.04, as shown in Table 8-5. The average monthly cost associated with operating EKG machines is 25 percent of the average monthly technicians' salaries, or:

$$\text{Average Monthly Personnel Cost of Machine Operation} = 25\% \times \$3{,}022.93 = \underline{\underline{\$755.73}}\,.$$

Finally, the average monthly cost of processing EKGs is 75 percent of the average monthly technicians' salaries plus 100 percent of the average monthly part time employees' payroll, or:

$$\begin{aligned}\text{Average Monthly Personnel}\\ \text{Cost for EKG Processing} &= 75\% \times \$3{,}022.93 + 100\% \times \$1{,}264.75\\ &= \underline{\underline{\$3{,}531.95}}\,.\end{aligned}$$

Therefore, the average monthly personnel cost is:

$$\begin{aligned}\text{Average Monthly Personnel Cost} &= \$3{,}101.04 + \$755.73 + \$3{,}531.95\\ &= \underline{\underline{\$7{,}388.72}}\,.\end{aligned}$$

To compute the average personnel cost per EKG, each component of the average monthly personnel cost must be divided by the number of EKGs to which it relates, and then, the average component costs must be summed. Since the average monthly administrative personnel cost relates to the average number of EKGs rendered by the CV unit each month, the following computation must be made:

$$\begin{aligned}\text{Average Administrative Personnel Cost per EKG} &= \frac{\$3{,}101.04}{2434}\\ &= \underline{\underline{\$1.27}}\,.\end{aligned}$$

The average monthly personnel cost of machine operation, on the other hand, only relates to the number of EKGs actually taken by EKG technicians. To compute this number, the numbers from the "Average" column of Table 8-1 must be substituted for the respective variables in the "Number of EKGs Rendered" column in Table 8-7. Hence, the average number of EKGs taken by EKG technicians each month is:

$$\begin{aligned}\text{Average Monthly EKGs Taken by EKG Technicians} &= 100\% \times 1350 + 90\% \times 452 \\ &\quad + 100\% \times 191 + 100\% \times 221 \\ &\quad + 0\% \times 115 + 100\% \times 8 \\ &\quad + 0\% \times 97 \\ &= \underline{\underline{2{,}177}}\,,\end{aligned}$$

and the average personnel cost per EKG for machine operation is:

$$\begin{aligned}\text{Average Personnel Cost per EKG for Machine Operation} &= \frac{\$755.73}{2{,}177} \\ &= \underline{\underline{\$.35}}\,.\end{aligned}$$

Finally, the average monthly personnel cost for EKG processing relates to the average number of EKGs rendered by the EKG unit each month so that the average personnel cost per EKG for processing is computed as:

$$\begin{aligned}\text{Average Personnel Cost per EKG for Processing} &= \frac{\$3{,}531.95}{2434} \\ &= \underline{\underline{\$1.45}}\,.\end{aligned}$$

Therefore, the average personnel cost per EKG is:

$$\begin{aligned}\text{Average Personnel Cost per EKG} &= \$1.27 + \$.35 + \$1.45 \\ &= \underline{\underline{\$3.07}}\,.\end{aligned}$$

Machine and Supplies Costs

The machine and supplies costs incurred by the EKG activity have a fixed element, depreciation allowed on the EKG machines, and a variable element, the cost of Perma paper, professional paper towels, tape, redox paste, mounting sheets, and photocopying. The CV unit has 11 EKG machines that were purchased for an average price of $1,000. Each machine has an estimated useful life of eight years and an average scrap value of $40. Hence, the average monthly cost of the EKG machines is computed as:

$$\text{Average Monthly Cost of EKG Machines} = \frac{11 \times (\$1000 - \$40)}{8} \times \frac{1}{12}$$

$$= \underline{\underline{\$110.00}}\,.$$

The average monthly cost of the EKG supplies, on the other hand, is calculated to be $1,195.23. Therefore, the average monthly machine and supplies cost is:

$$\text{Average Monthly Machine and Supplies Cost} = \$110.00 + \$1{,}195.23$$

$$= \underline{\underline{\$1{,}305.23}}\,.$$

The average machine and supplies cost per EKG can then be computed by dividing the average monthly machine and supplies cost by the average number of EKGs rendered each month. In this case, the average machine and supplies cost per EKG is:

$$\text{Average Machine and Supplies Cost per EKG} = \frac{\$1{,}305.23}{2434}$$

$$= \underline{\underline{\$.54}}\,.$$

Overhead Analysis

The cost and revenue information for the EKG activity is summarized in Table 8-9. Note that overhead costs comprise more than 50 percent of the cost of an EKG. However, the CV unit is able to cover this high overhead cost, charge an interdepartmental price of $20.00 per EKG, and realize a profit of $3.26 per EKG. The profit margin yields an average monthly profit of $7,934.84 and an average annual profit of $95,218.08. To examine this profit margin more closely, a break-even analysis for the EKG activity is presented in the next section.

Break-Even Analysis

The monthly break-even volume of the EKG activity is computed as:[6]

$$\hat{X} = \frac{c_F}{b_R - b_V} \tag{7-2}$$

where: $\hat{X}$ is the monthly break-even volume;
c_F is the average monthly fixed cost;
b_R is the price of an EKG; and
b_V is the average variable cost per EKG.

The fixed costs associated with the EKG activity include administrative personnel costs of \$3,101.04 per month and machine depreciation costs of \$110 per month. The price of an EKG is \$20 and the average variable cost per EKG includes overhead costs of \$9 per EKG, reading costs of \$4.13 per EKG, personnel costs associated with machine operation and with processing EKGs amounting to \$1.80 per EKG, and supplies costs of \$.49 per EKG. Hence, the monthly break-even volume of the EKG activity would be:

$$\hat{X} = \frac{c_F}{b_R - b_V}$$

$$= \frac{\$3{,}101.04 + \$110.00}{\$20.00 - (\$9.00 + \$4.13 + \$1.80 + \$.49)}$$

$$= \frac{\$3{,}211.04}{\$20.00 - \$15.42}$$

$$= 701 \text{ patients.}$$

This break-even analysis shows that the \$4.58 (\$20.00−\$15.42) marginal contribution of each EKG to revenue is large enough to cause the break-even volume of the EKG activity to be very low. This low break-even volume means that the CV unit is able to earn substantial profits from EKGs.

Case Discussion

This case study illustrates that a profit responsibility accounting system that uses departmental profitability as a performance measure may fail

Table 8-9 Cost and Revenue Information for EKG Activity

Cost Component	Average Cost per Month	Unit Cost	Percentage
Overhead	$21,905.00	$ 9.00	53.8
Reading	10,047.00	4.13	24.7
Personnel	7,388.72	3.07	18.3
Machine & Supplies	1,305.23	.54	3.2
TOTAL	$40,645.95	$16.74	100.0
Price per EKG	$20.00	Profit Margin per EKG	$3.26
Average Revenue per Month	$48,680.00	Average Profit per Month	$7,934.84

to effect systematic economic control over departmental resources in nonprofit institutions. For example, in this case, the director of the CV unit is able to realize a considerable profit from the EKG activity without taking managerial actions to control costs. The overhead analysis shows that an inordinate amount of institutional overhead is borne by the EKG activity. However, the CV unit is able to recoup these overhead costs through an arbitrarily established interdepartmental price.[7] The break-even analysis further illustrates how profit responsibility accounting systems fail in nonprofit institutions. For example, the managers of the departments serviced by the CV unit accept the arbitrary interdepartmental price of an EKG and continue to use the service at a volume well above the break-even volume because higher departmental costs arising from high interdepartmental prices can be recouped through higher market prices with apparently no reduction in demand (see Question 8-3). Hence, the management of the CV unit does not have the incentive to (1) control direct costs (see Question 8-4) or (2) demand a more equitable allocation of institutional overhead.

Conclusion

Given the various problems associated with implementing a profit responsibility accounting system in a health care institution, the prospect for accurate departmental evaluations based on profit certainly does not look promising. Consequently, to evaluate managerial performance in health care institutions, nonprofit measures of performance must be developed. A process for developing these nonprofit performance measures will be discussed in Chapter 9.

NOTES

1. Although this premise has intuitive appeal, extensive research has shown that in many cases, the assumptions underlying the premise are naive and oversimplify the effect that positive and negative externalities have on institutional performance.
2. The market price could be less than the marginal costs over the entire range of output. However, departments operating under these conditions probably will discontinue operations.
3. Similarly, the buyer department should be acquainted with its marginal and average total cost curves.
4. The magnitude of this profit is calculated by taking the difference between total revenue and total cost. Since total revenue is equal to the price per unit multiplied by the number of units sold, total revenue would be represented by the rectangle $J\hat{Q}_s{}'O\hat{P}_s{}^{MK}$. On the other hand, since total cost is equal to the average total cost per unit multiplied by the number of units sold, total cost would be represented by the rectangle $K\hat{Q}_S{}'OL$. Hence, profit is equal to the area of the rectangle $JKL\hat{P}_S{}^{MK}$.
5. Of course, the exact magnitude of the cost shift would not be known by the buyer department because the two departments are presumed to be autonomous decision making units.
6. See Chapter 7 for the derivation of this formula.
7. As far as could be determined during the study, the price charged for EKGs, $20, was not established after a careful analysis of costs and revenues for the EKG activity. The head of the cardiology department, who was concerned about the possible findings of an impending third party audit, initiated the study reported in the text. During the initial meeting, he stated that he had no idea how much profit was generated by the EKG activity. He mentioned that he thought the cardiology department benefitted greatly from the EKG activity; however, he hoped that this study would show that a price increase would not be unreasonable. When asked how the $20 EKG price was selected, he replied that he was not sure, but that price seemed reasonable given the charges of other institutions.

Questions and Problems

Question 8-1. Discuss the problems inherent in measuring (a) the profit of a department within an institution, (b) the total cost of operations of a department, (c) the cost of a particular procedure in a department, and (d) the profit of a particular procedure in a department.

Question 8-2. Consider the following table:

	Third Party Payers or Patients with No Insurance Coverage			
Department Delivering Service	Market Price	Minimal Marginal Cost	Direct Variable Cost	Total Variable Cost
	Direct Fixed Cost	Total Fixed Cost	Average Accounting Cost	Full Cost
	Negotiated Price	Regionally Imposed Price	Nationally Imposed Price	Full Cost plus $\gamma\ \pi$, $\gamma > 0$

a. Assume that each entry in this table represents a possible per procedure charge made by the department delivering the service. Discuss the preferences of each group (department delivering the service and third party payers or self-paying patients) for each of the 12 possible charges.

b. Replace the third party payers or patients group with "department requesting service or patients with insurance coverage" and conduct a similar preference analysis. Discuss the implications of the preference differences between the two analyses.

Question 8-3. a. With respect to the EKG costing study reported in the chapter, how would the administrator of the hospital attempt to make the CV unit cost conscious?

b. Assume that the administrator formulates these suggestions into a formal proposal and delivers it to the chief of cardiology. After some period of time, the chief of cardiology requests a meeting with the administrator. In the meeting, the chief of cardiology makes the following statement: "Your proposal is interesting, but let's be reasonable. Overhead loading benefits more than it costs. For example, our maternal and infant care and VD clinics are supported through our overhead apportionment to profitable departments, not to mention our various research programs, for which DHEW seed money has stopped. Also, it enables our fixed resource base to be large, which attracts some of the best medical teachers and researchers in the country. This large fixed resource base will be important if the Carter administration ever acts on the regionalization proposals. Further, it keeps revenue less costs at a reasonable figure. We both know if it gets too high, Blue Cross starts getting nervous. So why don't we shelve or restudy your proposal for awhile, say, until the economic climate changes 'dramatically'." How would you argue—point by point—for your proposal?

Question 8-4. Prepare a table similar to Table 7-6 for the costs reported in the EKG case discussed in this chapter. Discuss the appropriateness of a profit responsibility accounting system from the standpoint of cost and revenue controllability.

Question 8-5. In this chapter, political considerations are assumed to play an important part in establishing the interdepartmental price. Economists would argue that, when possible, goods produced and used internally should be priced at the marginal cost of the producer. They would suggest that to do otherwise is to misallocate the institution's resources.

Required:

a. Discuss the marginal cost pricing rule from a resource allocation perspective.
b. Discuss the marginal cost pricing rule from a measurement perspective.

Problem 8-1. The following information pertains to the laboratory service of the Riverside Memorial Hospital for the year 19X1. During the year the direct fixed costs of the laboratory were $82,000.00 and the controller calculated that the average direct variable cost was $.437 per laboratory procedure. The indirect variable costs vary seasonally. During May, June, July, and August, 9,600 laboratory procedures were performed and the indirect (allocated) variable cost was $.195 per laboratory procedure. During the other eight months, the indirect variable cost was twice the direct variable cost. The allocated fixed costs were $2,000 per month. The average market price for the type of services provided by the laboratory was $7.50. The interdepartmental price charged by the laboratory was 108 percent of this market price, which included transportation and advertising expenses of approximately eight percent. The profit factor in the $7.50 market price was 18 percent. During the year, 19X2, laboratory volume is expected to be 130 percent of the break-even volume in 19X1. All costs, direct and variable, are expected to increase by nine percent during 19X2. During 19X1, the volume of laboratory procedures for May, June, July, and August was twice that of the other months. These volumes relationships are assumed to hold for 19X2.

Required:

From this information, compute a transfer price based upon market price, average accounting cost, and full cost for 19X2.

Problem 8-2. Assume the Collins Clinic, a prepaid group practice, maintains a special service unit for the diagnostic testing of patients. The average direct variable cost for the clinic is $AVC_c = \$13.00 + \$.01X$, where X is a variable representing patient volume. The average direct variable cost for the service unit is: $AVC_{SU} = \$5$. The price charged by the Collins Clinic for each patient tested by the service unit is \$25. This charge also covers the cost of services rendered in the clinic before the patient is sent to the service clinic. The fixed costs of the service unit and the clinic are \$100 each. The allocated costs are \$100 to the clinic and \$350 to the service unit. All patients serviced in the service unit are serviced first in the clinic before they are sent to the service unit. The clinic and the service unit are profit responsibility centers. Even though the clinic maintains the service unit, the service unit is an autonomous decision-making entity.

Required:

a. What is the optimal number of patients for the clinic to send to the service unit? (See note.)
b. Considering the clinic and the service unit together, rather than as separate entities, what would the profit be if the optimal number of patients is referred to the service unit?
c. If you were the administrator of the clinic, how much would you offer to the service unit for each patient referred from the clinic? Note: the service unit is paid by the clinic for each patient tested. The service unit does not bill patients.
d. If you were the administrator of the service unit, how much would you demand from the clinic for each patient tested?
e. If the administrator of the clinic offers to pay the service unit the marginal cost of testing each patient and this price is accepted by the administrator of the service unit, what is the optimum number of patients to be referred to the service unit? Does this differ from (a) above? Why?
f. What is the profit for the clinic alone if marginal cost is paid to the service unit for each patient seen?
g. Discuss the usefulness of profit as the focus of the responsibility accounting system in this case.
h. What important decision-making information may be derived from this analysis?

Note: where MC = MR, the organization maximizes its profit. Also, if VC (X) represents variable cost, then total variable cost is [VC(X)]X. Finally, if TC (X) represents total cost, then MC = dTC(X)/dX.

Problem 8-3. Assume the facts as they are represented for the Collins Clinic in Problem 8-2, except that the clinic and the service unit now has no fixed costs and the average direct variable cost of the service unit is $AVC_{SU} = \$2. + \$.01X$.

Required:

a. What is the optimal number of patients to send to the service unit?
b. Graph the marginal cost of the service unit.
c. What is the income of the clinic and service unit as a whole if the optimal number of patients are seen?
d. If the clinic offers to pay the service unit the marginal cost of testing an additional patient at the optimal referral level computed in (a) and this price is accepted by the service unit, what will the optimal number of patients be? How does this compare with the answer derived in (a)?
e. Discuss the usefulness of profit responsibility accounting in this case.

Problem 8-4. You are the chairperson of a committee charged to investigate the reasonableness of prices charged by hospitals for internally supported services. You engage a consultant to gather information relevant to the committee's charge. The consultant's report contains the following information:

Contrast of Selected Services
Market and Hospital Charges
(Authors' note: This information represents the results of an actual sample.)

Service or Test	Market (n = 4)		Hospital Charge (n = 4)		Computed	$t_{6.05}$
	$\overline{X}$	s	$\overline{X}$	s	t	= 2.44
Glucose Serum	\$2.49	\$ .792	\$ 7.69	\$3.48	3.04	S
CO_2	5.85	2.37	8.78	3.58	1.56	NS
Sodium	2.95	.184	10.22	3.51	4.25	S
SMA-12	7.73	.965	24.94	6.83	7.26	S
Routine Urine	2.63	.855	5.69	.834	3.04	S
Alkaline Phosphate	3.48	.618	9.55	3.68	2.99	S
TB Culture	9.89	2.90	21.69	4.11	5.36	S

$\overline{X}$ represents the mean;
s represents the standard deviation;
S indicates that there was a significant difference at the $\alpha \leq .05$ level of confidence between the hospital and market charges; and
NS indicates that there was not a significant difference between the hospital and market charges at the $\alpha \leq .05$ level of confidence.

Details of Sampling Process

The hospital sample consisted of four urban hospitals. The market sample was controlled for comparability and was drawn from four firms servicing the same city from which the hospital sample was drawn.

Other Information Abstracted from the Consultant's Report

Comparison of hospital charges to market charges for comparable services must be made subject to the following condition: market must reflect the price resulting from economic bargaining and negotiation between supplier and purchaser. Side payments (kickbacks and fraud) which affect the reported market price should be considered in determining the real economic market price.

According to the Special Committee on Aging (Chairman F. Moss (D-Utah)), urban laboratory markets may be characterized as supporting a significant volume of unnecessary and fraudulent service claims on Medicaid resources which often materially mask the true market price. The kickback behavior may result from the economic conditions which exist between the market demand for laboratory services and the suppliers of that service. Specifically, if a fixed reimbursement price exists for Medicaid laboratory services and this price does not provide an economic return at specific volumes, the laboratory must either raise prices or reduce costs. Cost reduction may take the form of increasing efficiency or increasing volume, with the latter being the most accessible means of reducing costs. On the other hand, in regard to raising prices, evidence exists that the Medicaid reimbursement system is so poorly administered that the price charged to Medicaid often exceeds specific charge ceilings. For example, F. Holstein,* Executive Director of the New Jersey State Com-

---

*Testimony given to the Senate Committee on Aging.

mission of Investigation, pointed out that the "shortcomings and loopholes which had developed in the New Jersey Medicaid program present a virtual open door to those laboratory owners to profiteer at the taxpayers' expense." Holstein cited one instance where seven parts of a test performed by a New Jersey corporation were performed at a cost of $3.40 and billed to Medicaid at $58.00, where the maximum allowed by Medicaid was $12.50.

Both behaviors, increasing volumes through kickback arrangements and raising prices in excess of allowable limits, seem to exist. Generalizations regarding the market effect of this behavior are not possible. In one set of circumstances, one may predict that the market price is inflated by charging prices in excess of specific reimbursement ceilings, but for other tests and services the market price may be deflated by interorganization volume subsidies. However, one conclusion does seem warranted: the market for laboratory services is so loosely controlled that, regarding Medicaid services, a clear and apparent opportunity for profiteering exists.

Required:

a. Evaluate this information relative to the charge of your committee.
b. What other information would you desire? Why?

Problem 8-5. Figure 8-3 illustrates the case where the demand for service is insensitive to price changes. This may be rationalized given a centralized pricing policy and a high degree of centralized control over the use of alternative service markets. Relax this assumption and assume that the demand for services behaves as depicted in the following graph:

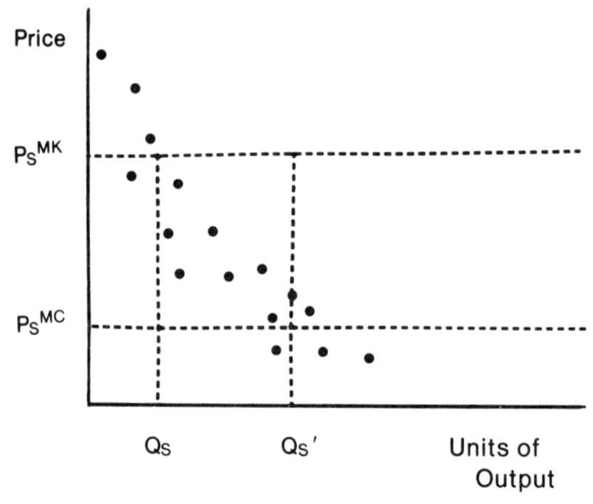

where: Each of the 16 points represents a quarterly historical relationship adjusted for price inflation.

Required:

Discuss the interdepartmental pricing implications of the relationship represented in the above figure.

Chapter 9

Budgeting and Control

Forethought we may have, undoubtedly, but not foresight.
Napoleon

Managers often believe that organizational control can be effected merely by maintaining a budgeting system. However, budgeting and control actually are two separate, but related, activities. Budgeting is the process by which decision makers allocate resources to effect a particular organizational plan for the ensuing period. In contrast, control is the process by which actual performance is compared with budgeted performance and the necessary corrective actions are taken to modify or reorient actual performance to planned performance. Hence, budgeting is required to effect control, but control will not be effected merely by maintaining a budgeting system.

This chapter examines two types of budgeting systems that are instrumental in planning organizational performance. Tactical budgeting systems, including traditional tactical budgets and planning, programing, budgeting systems, are the subject of the first section of the chapter. The second section of the chapter deals with the control aspects of tactical budgeting systems. In the third section, capital budgeting systems and the selection of investment alternatives are discussed.

TACTICAL BUDGETING

A tactical budget delineates the organization's operating plans for the ensuing period. The desired or expected volume of operations, revenues, and costs to be incurred are specified by each department within the organization. By authorizing departments to incur certain costs at particular volumes of activity and specifying the allocation of organizational resources to departments, the tactical budget outlines an operating plan that directs departmental activities toward organizational goals and objectives.

This chapter does not deal with the derivation of the various elements in a tactical budget because these elements are derived from a complex network of decision inputs that are unique to each organization. What has been delineated is both an organizational framework that would facilitate effective tactical budgeting and the technical requirements of both traditional tactical budgeting systems and planning, programing, budgeting systems.[1] In addition, the problems encountered in developing and implementing an effective tactical budgeting system in a health care institution are discussed.

Conditions for an Effective Tactical Budgeting System

Tactical budgeting systems are most effective in organizations that have a management structure which permits and encourages responsibility accounting because managers are most likely to perform in compliance with the budget if they know that their performance will be evaluated. Furthermore, organizations operating under responsibility accounting systems usually can develop (1) a system of rewards and penalties that encourage efficient resource management and (2) performance standards or expectations that define efficient management in terms of the minimum amount of input required to produce an output of a specific quality. The organization may use these standards or expectations to develop the tactical budget and the control information useful in directing the organization to particular performance goals.

Traditional Tactical Budgets

Traditional tactical budgeting systems have three technical requirements. First, the relationship between the results of activity (i.e., output) and the organizational goals must be defined explicitly so that a tactical plan can be devised that will direct organizational activities toward the proper goals.[2] Second, the departments within the organization must have a means for specifying and justifying departmental needs for costly resources so that these needs can be evaluated and possibly incorporated in the budget. Third, the organization must have a chief financial officer or budgeting committee with the authority and the responsibility (1) to evaluate departmental needs for resources with respect to the relationship between departmental output and organizational goals, (2) to approve the organization's tactical plan, and (3) to allocate resources so that the tactical plan can be realized (see Figure 9-1).[3] If the organization can meet these technical requirements, a traditional tac-

Figure 9-1 Traditional Tactical Budgeting and Control Functions

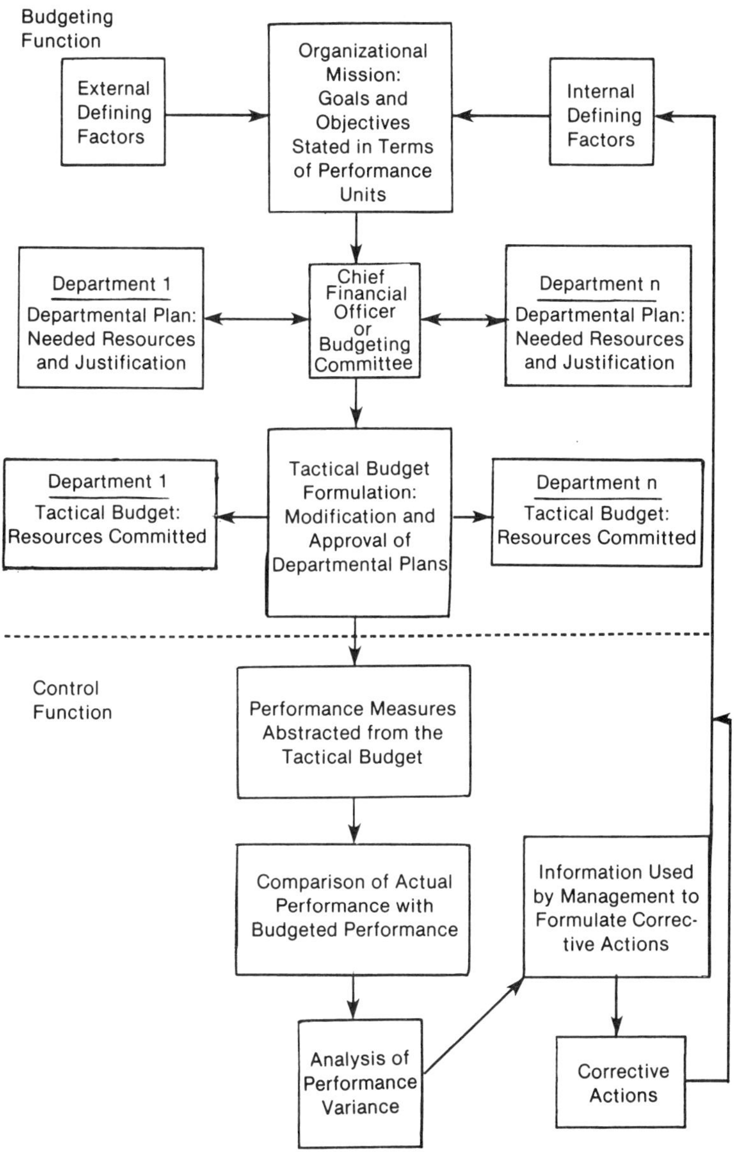

tical budgeting system will form the basis for both efficient resources utilization and the achievement of organizational goals.

Unfortunately, health care institutions usually do not meet the technical requirements of a traditional tactical budgeting system. The first problem arises in trying to specify a relationship between institutional output and organizational goals. Health care institutions often are unable or unwilling to measure either institutional or departmental output. In addition, even if the institution measures performance in terms of the processing of departmental inputs, developing a relationship between this measure and the organizational goals is a most difficult task. Furthermore, since some departments within health care organizations are highly autonomous[4] and can not be integrated into the institution's budgeting system readily, the chief financial officer or budgeting committee may not be able to allocate resources in a manner that will achieve the tactical plan. Therefore, tactical budgeting systems rarely achieve their potential in health care institutions. Despite this fact, traditional tactical budgeting systems are used in many health care institutions and resources are routinely allocated. However, the allocation of resources may reflect political satisfaction rather than optimal resource utilization.

The Program Budgeting Alternative

An alternative to the tactical budgeting system is the planning, programing, budgeting system. Planning, programing, budgeting system (PPBS) was developed and first used by Robert MacNamara, who successfully implemented PPBS in the Department of Defense (DOD). The success of PPBS in the DOD caused President Johnson to advise all federal agencies to adopt the "very new and very revolutionary system of planning and programing and budgeting" that would help to find "new ways to do jobs faster, to do jobs better and to do jobs less expensively."[5] Many state and local agencies, including some health care institutions, also adopted PPBS. However, few of these agencies realized the same measure of success with PPBS that had been experienced in the DOD. In fact, most health care institutions even have problems satisfying the technical requirements of PPBS.

Technical Requirements of PPBS

Planning, programing, budgeting systems have four technical requirements. First, the relationship between the program efforts and the organizational goals must be defined explicitly so that a tactical plan can be developed which will coordinate the program efforts with the organizational goals. Second, the program directors must be able to specify program needs for costly resources, justifying these needs with a summary of the expected long-range effects of the program, including both the direct and indirect costs and the performance externalities, so that these needs can be evaluated fully. Third, the institution must have a chief financial officer or budgeting committee with the authority and the responsibility to (1) evaluate program needs for resources with respect to the long-range effects of the program and the organizational goals and objectives, (2) approve the tactical plan, and (3) appropriate resources to the programs so that the tactical plan can be realized. Lastly, each program within the organization must have a director who is responsible for executing the tactical plan specified, and allocating the appropriated resources to the departments that support program activities (see Figure 9-2). Each of these requirements must be satisfied if PPBS is to reach its full potential.

Problems in Implementing PPBS in Health Care Institutions

The technical requirements of PPBS present the same basic problems to health care institutions as the technical requirements of traditional tactical budgeting systems. The only important difference is that the traditional budgeting approach assumes that specific departments can be evaluated on criteria particular to their operation and that a relationship exists between departmental output and organizational goals; the PPBS approach assumes that various departments totally or partially support various programs which exist because they contribute to the mission of the organization.

Although the difference between the two types of tactical budgeting systems is profoundly important in motivating the allocation of resources,[6] it does not provide the means for solving problems encountered in implementing a tactical budgeting system in a health care organization. Specifying the relationship between program output and organizational goals is as difficult as specifying the relationship between departmental output and organizational goals. Lacking the specification of this relationship, the chief financial officer or budgeting committee again cannot evaluate program needs objectively. In addition, largely autonomous programs still may prohibit the appropriation of resources in a manner that will achieve the tactical plan. Furthermore, program directors may face problems similar to those encountered by the chief financial officer or budgeting committee when evaluating the needs of supporting departments and allocating resources to them. Consequently, implementing a PPBS in a health care organization may be more complex than implementing a traditional tactical budgeting system and, in fact, PPBS is seldom used in health care institutions.

Figure 9-2 Program Budgeting and Control Functions

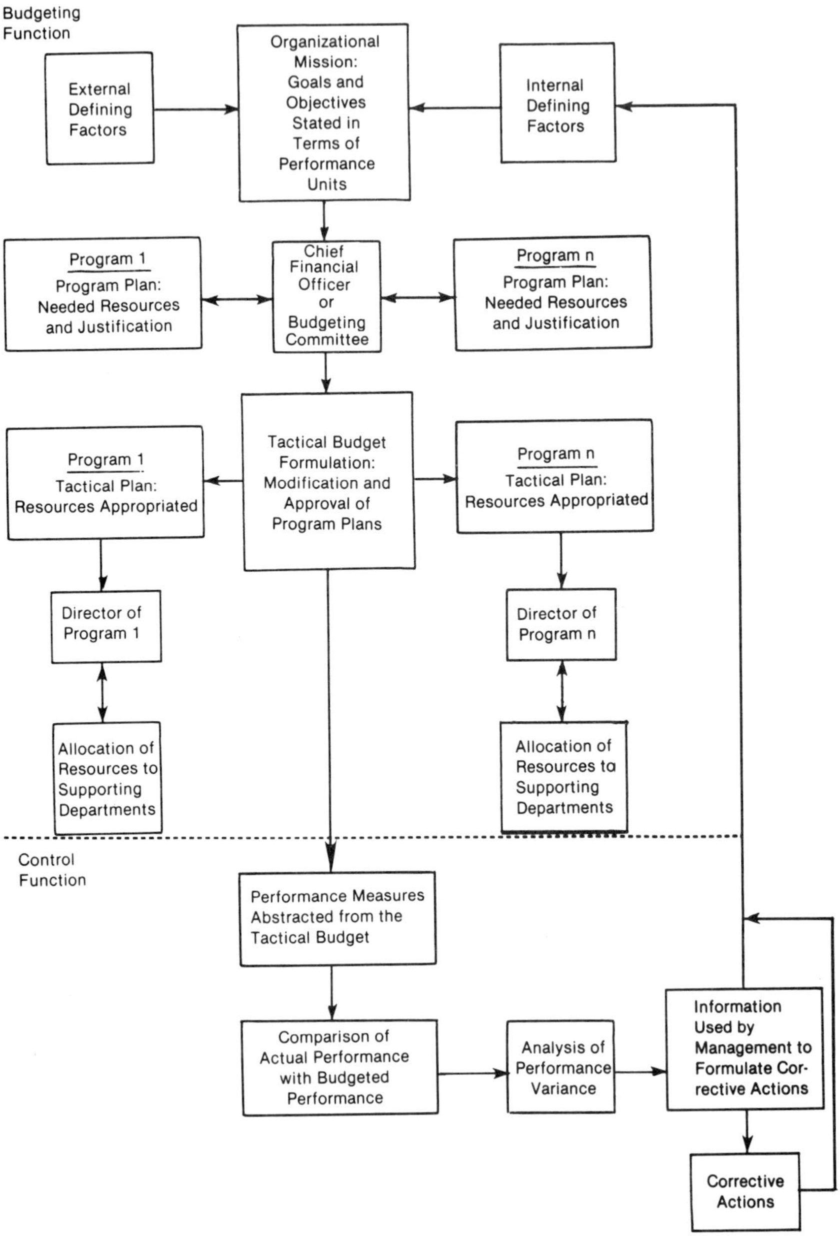

Additional Problems in Implementing Tactical Budgeting Systems in Health Care Organizations

Many problems are encountered as health care institutions attempt to satisfy the technical requirements of either a traditional tactical budgeting or a planning, programing, budgeting system. These institutions cannot meet the technical requirements of tactical budgeting systems because tactical budgeting systems are most effective in organizations that (1) permit and encourage responsibility accounting, (2) administer rewards and punishments based on managerial performance, and (3) develop performance standards related to output. Unfortunately, health care institutions can rarely satisfy these conditions.

Health care institutions generally do not provide an environment conducive to responsibility accounting (see Chapters 7 and 8). Administrators encounter many difficulties in trying to control the activities of medical personnel. In addition, the departmental organization, as opposed to a unit structure, in these institutions does not provide a direct line of responsibility among the individuals associated with specific treatment plans, thus making managerial evaluation a difficult task. The fact that the accounting departments in health care institutions place a higher priority on the demands of third party reimbursers than on those of internal management also inhibits effective responsibility accounting by placing a major constraint on the prompt and accurate reporting of managerially relevant information. Furthermore, since the development of useful performance standards is dependent on the organization's ability to measure output, health care institutions generally do not develop these standards and, hence generally have no objective basis on which to judge managerial performance. All of these failings combine to make the establishment of a rational system of rewards and penalties most difficult.

In summary, numerous problems impair the ability of health care institutions to implement successful traditional tactical budgeting or planning, programing, budgeting systems. However, health care institutions routinely develop tactical plans and allocate resources according to those plans by relaxing the technical definitional and measurement requirements. Therefore, tactical budgeting systems can and do exist in health care institutions, but their form, development, and implementation are peculiar to the specific institutions in which they exist.

Controlling the Tactical Budget

Most health care institutions currently have some means of generating periodic tactical budgets. However, as previously suggested, budgeting alone is not sufficient to effect the control of tactical resources. In fact, tactical budgeting systems that exist without an explicitly associated control function (and tactical budgeting systems that only have apparent control functions) may direct the organization toward undesired goals. Effective tactical control implies organizational movement toward the desired mission (i.e., desired goals and objectives of the organization). To accomplish effective tactical control, the organization must have some systematic means of relating output to the organizational mission so that periodic performance can be evaluated and, therefore, controlled. Thus, to effect tactical control, health care institutions must define the organizational goals and objectives and develop useful performance measures that are related to these goals and objectives.

Unfortunately, health care institutions often encounter difficulties in specifying the actual organizational mission. The first and most important problem occurs because while different coalitions within the institution have different organizational performance expectations, the actual organizational mission usually is not known explicitly. Consequently, each coalition develops a different concept of the organizational mission that reflects its own desired goals and objectives. This is a fundamental problem that may cause serious planning and control dysfunctions as each coalition tries to achieve different and often conflicting goals and objectives. Although this problem has no simple solution, a process that can aid in deriving the actual organizational mission will be discussed in subsequent sections.

The second problem encountered in specifying the organizational mission occurs because individuals perceive the same actual mission from different points of view. This problem usually is not critical because it presupposes that the mission is known explicitly to some individuals. Therefore, this problem may be corrected through information systems procedures that enable all individuals in the organization to perceive the intent of processing organizational inputs.

Given that a health care organization has an explicit statement of the organizational mission, tactical control still is complicated by the problems that arise in trying to develop useful performance measures that are related to the mission. The purpose of tactical control systems is to assure that the organizational mission is being achieved through the most efficient use of tactical resources (see Problem 9-1). Since tactical resources combine to produce organizational output, which in turn is produced to achieve the organizational mission, output controls simultaneously can be used to monitor resource usage and assure achievement of the mission. Hence, useful performance measures should require information that describes the effect of processing inputs in terms of some relevant scale of measured output.

Unfortunately, as suggested, most health care institutions have great difficulty in measuring output. Therefore, these institutions must use performance measures that control the processing of inputs rather than output. However, this process orientation can focus control at an inappropriate level, yielding performance measures that (1) reflect process goals which are not important in achieving the organizational mission, or (2) cause managers to focus on some aspects of the organizational mission while neglecting others.

For example, a nursing agency may select "skilled nursing costs" as a performance measure that will relate efficient resource utilization with the organizational mission of improving the health of the community. If information collected on this performance measure is used in such a way that skilled nursing personnel spend less, but more productive time with each patient, "skilled nursing costs" is a useful performance measure. If, on the other hand, this performance measure causes skilled nursing personnel (1) to spend an inadequate amount of time with each patient, (2) to see fewer patients, or (3) to employ lower salaried, less experienced, and inappropriate personnel who adversely affect patient welfare, then "skilled nursing costs" is not an appropriate performance measure and should be augmented by other measures of performance (see Chapter 10).

Developing a System for Tactical Evaluation and Control

Effective tactical evaluation and control systems require performance measures that describe the effect of processing inputs in terms of some relevant scale of measured output. The development of a relevant output measure is a process which involves three phases: (1) specification of the organizational mission, (2) development of reasonable evaluation and control questions, and (3) selection or development of output measures that aid in answering the evaluation and control questions. In the following sections, systems procedures are suggested that can help health care institutions to accomplish each of these steps.

Phase I: Specifying the Mission

Since the various coalitions within the organization may have different organizational expectations, a number of steps are helpful in developing an explicit statement of the organizational mission. The first step in the process is:

> Require each decision maker within the organization to develop a short written statement specifying what the organizational mission should be.

These individual statements, in aggregate, should represent the organizational expectations of all of the coalitions within the organization. Then, the second step in the mission specification process can be undertaken.

> Distribute the individual mission specifications among all of the decision makers and schedule a meeting so that these decision makers can develop a group statement of the desired organizational mission.

This desired organizational mission should reflect the consensus regarding the organization's projected goals and objectives.

Once the desired mission has been defined, the organization's ability to achieve this mission, given the evaluation and control information currently collected, must be ascertained. The first step in this process is:

> Require the decision makers to specify in short, simple statements the information currently collected to evaluate the performance of subordinates.

Care should be taken to include all informational inputs to the current evaluation and control system, because all of these inputs presumably are relevant in directing the organization toward the mission. These informational inputs must be related to the desired mission in the next step.

> Require decision makers to define explicitly the relationship between the desired organizational mission and the information currently collected to evaluate performance.

Generally, this step is quite difficult because, due to the lack of output measures, the evaluation information currently collected may focus only on process control. Therefore, only a vague relationship may exist between the evaluation information (process-oriented) and the desired organizational mission (output-oriented). However, as the decision makers attempt to define these relationships, and as their efforts are reviewed and more precise definitions are required, they realize that some of the evaluation information currently collected is not relevant in coordinating performance control with the achievement of the desired organizational mission.

Phase II: Developing Reasonable Evaluation and Control Questions

Before the decision makers are required to develop evaluation and control questions coordinated with the desired mission, they should assess the actual mission toward which the current evaluation information is directing the organization. Therefore, the first step in Phase II of the analysis should be:

> Require the decision makers (1) to specify the organizational mission that best seems to fit the evaluation information currently collected, and (2) to define explicitly the relationship between this actual mission and the evaluation information.

This step is important because the actual mission usually differs significantly from the desired mission and, thus, the decision makers become aware of how inappropriate evaluation information can direct the organization toward inappropriate goals and objectives.

Once the differences between the actual and desired missions have been assessed, the decision makers are ready to develop new evaluation and control questions. To begin this process:

> Require each decision maker to specify the information that could aid them in evaluating and controlling subordinate performance so that effective corrective actions could be taken at the appropriate times to reorient the organization to the tactical plan (presumably documented in the tactical budget) and achieve the desired mission.

The resultant list of evaluation and control questions probably will be both lengthy and partially irrelevant. Therefore, the organization should:

> Solicit expert opinions regarding the ability of each evaluation and control question to provide information that will be useful in evaluating and controlling subordinate performance.

These expert opinions should reduce the list of evaluation and control questions to a reasonable list by eliminating redundant and other irrelevant questions that might provide such an excess of information that the evaluation and control process would be rendered ineffective.

The final step in this phase of the analysis involves judging the feasibility of utilizing the set of reasonable evaluation and control questions.

> Management must judge the feasibility of answering the set of reasonable evaluation and control questions with information that is or could be collected currently.

If most of the evaluation and control questions can be answered with information that is collected currently, then the organization should be able to control the tactical plan adequately and achieve the desired organizational mission. On the other hand, if a considerable number of the reasonable evaluation and control questions cannot be answered with information currently collected (because the currently collected information is process-oriented, while the new evaluation and control questions are output-oriented), then new measures must be developed that can relate the processing of inputs to output and, hence, to the desired mission.

Phase III: Selecting or Developing Output Measures

The selection and development of output measures is the most complex phase in the analysis. The output measures which are developed must use an explicit scale(s) by which the processing of inputs can be judged according to their contribution to the desired organizational mission. Therefore, Phases I and II, which develop a statement of the desired organizational mission and a statement of the informational inputs needed to evaluate the effect of tactical performance on the desired mission are fundamental to the selection and development of output measures.

Once the desired organizational mission and the evaluation and control questions have been specified:

> Management must ascertain how the intervention of the organization's service or the generation of the organization's output makes a difference relative to the desired mission.

Then, to evaluate the intervention of service or the generation of output with respect to the desired organizational mission:

> Management must select or develop output measures that will reflect subordinate performance in achieving the desired mission and will allow management to take corrective actions when performance deviates from the tactical plan as documented in the periodic budget.

This step completes the analysis because at this point, the organization has developed performance measures that describe the effect of processing inputs in terms of some relevant scale of measured output. Therefore, the organization has the information to design and implement an effective tactical budgeting and control system such as those represented in Figures 9-1 and 9-2 (see Problem 9-2).

Case Study: Developing a Nursing Evaluation and Control System

This case describes the efforts of a Community Nursing Agency (CNA) to develop a nursing management information system. The CNA used the systems procedures discussed in the preceding sections, and the information developed in Phases I, II, and III are examined in the paragraphs that follow. After discussing the development of the management and control system, the case concludes with a discussion of the benefits derived from undergoing the three-phased systems analysis even when explicit output measures cannot be developed.

Phase I

During Phase I of the analysis, which took approximately six months to complete, the CNA personnel involved in establishing and implementing policy were asked to develop individual statements specifying what the organizational mission should be. These mission statements were compiled and distributed to the group, which then met to develop a joint statement of the desired organizational mission. The following statement was developed after a number of meetings.

Desired Mission: The nursing intervention sponsored by the agency will facilitate the movement of an individual or a family unit from a dependent health status to an independent health status.

In the second part of Phase I, the same individuals were asked to compile a list of questions that were being used currently to evaluate subordinate performance. A list of 108 questions was compiled, including the following examples.

- What are the number of not at home visits made by the agency?
- How many visits are made by nurses in particular health districts?
- What are the insurance coverage situations of the individuals requesting service?

The agency personnel spent a good deal of time attempting to show how the 108 evaluation and control questions related to the desired mission. After a number of verbal and written attempts, these individuals suggested that the evaluation and control questions were not related to the desired mission explicitly, and that developing new evaluation and control questions might be useful.

Phase II

During Phase II of the analysis, which consumed approximately three months of very intense introspection, the agency policy makers were asked to develop a mission that best seemed to fit the evaluation and control questions that were being used to evaluate subordinate performance. The resultant actual mission was specified as follows.

Actual Mission: The nursing agency will allocate resources in a manner that enables the agency to continue to compete successfully for health resources and to be economically viable.

The agency personnel noted that the actual mission seemed to focus on the economics rather than the effectiveness of delivering the service. This realization reinforced the agency's commitment to developing an evaluation and control system that would direct the CNA toward the desired mission.

The agency personnel then began to develop new evaluation and control questions. The consultants who were assisting in the development of the nursing management information system judged 78 of the new questions as reasonable. Some of these questions follow.

- Is there a significant relationship between the uncontrolled input, population characteristics, and the ability of the agency to reach its selected objective? How strong are the relationships between various population characteristics and patient outcome, as measured by the functional health status of the serviced population upon discharge?
- What percentage of the patients known to the CNA are a hazard to others at first assessment and at discharge assessment?
- What percentage of the patients known to the field and clinic staffs show no progression of their illness? Is this percentage different in the risk populations?
- What percentage of the patients exhibit physical or psychosocial functional dependence upon discharge? Why are these functionally dependent patients discharged?
- Is the service delivered in accordance with standards of practice? Is the appropriateness of care by practice standards less evident in those patients or families with no change in health status? How strong is the relationship between services delivered in accordance with standards of practice and the ability of the agency to meet (or not meet) the selected objectives?

The agency personnel assessed the feasibility of answering these questions and decided that this information could be collected if new output measures were developed.

Phase III

Having developed a statement of the desired organizational mission and a set of reasonable evaluation and control questions, the staff was ready to develop output measures for judging the processing of inputs in terms of their contribution to the desired organizational mission. The agency personnel ascertained that the intervention of the nursing service should enable patients or families to care for themselves on a daily basis. Therefore, the Activity of Daily Living (ADL) index,[7] a scale that evaluates an individual's ability to perform functions required in daily life, was selected as an output measure.

The ADL activity set selected by the CNA personnel was bathing, dressing, toileting, transfer, continence and feeding. Patients or families could be judged as either dependent or independent with respect to each of these activities and formal definitions of functional dependence and independence were developed for each activity. For example, the definition of independence and of dependence suggested by the agency for bathing (sponge, shower or tub) were:

Independent: Adult—Requires assistance only in bathing a single part (back or disabled extremity) or bathes self completely.
Child—Requires only general assistance by six years of age.

Dependent: Requires assistance in bathing more than one part of the body; requires assistance in getting in or out of the tub; or cannot bathe self.

To test the applicability of the ADL index and gain insights regarding the control possibilities of this output measure, the CNA conducted a survey of 130 patients. Each patient was judged as functionally dependent or independent at the time of admission and discharge. Functional dependence was presumed to exist if the patient was dependent respecting at least one of the activities of daily living. Functional independence, on the other hand, was presumed to exist if the patient was independent respecting all of the activities of daily living. The information collected on these 130 patients is summarized in Table 9-1.

A χ^2 test performed on the information in Table 9-1 showed that the changes in the number of dependent and independent patients were statistically significant at a confidence level less than .01 (i.e., $\alpha \leq .01$). Hence, the intervention of the nursing service appears to be an important

Table 9-1 Number and Percentage of Patients Admitted to the CNA Program with Physical or Psychosocial Dependency and Discharged with Physical or Psychosocial Independency: Last Quarter, Fiscal Year 19X5

	Patients Admitted		Patients Discharged	
Functional Health Status	No.	%	No.	%
Dependent	85	65.4	6*	4.6
Independent	45	34.6	124	95.4
Total	130	100.0	130	100.0

* One patient was admitted as functionally independent, but discharged as functionally dependent.

factor in moving individuals from a dependent to an independent health status, and the ADL index seems to reflect the effects of the nursing service adequately. However, to provide more conclusive evidence, the CNA should conduct other surveys that include proper control groups and that judge patient dependence and patient independence more scientifically.

Conclusion

In the CNA case, the organization was successful in developing output measures that could describe the effect of processing inputs. However, even if an organization is unable to complete Phase III of the analysis and construct useful or meaningful output measures, the insights provided in Phases I and II can aid in refining the organization's tactical budgeting and control processes. For example, Phase I develops a statement of the desired organizational mission which, at least, provides a basis for resource allocation. Furthermore, the analysis of the current evaluation and control questions and the development of the actual organizational mission can be useful in redirecting organizational efforts. Finally, the new evaluation and control questions developed in Phase II of the analysis should indicate what types of information the organization should be gathering to evaluate performance and, hence, may lead to more valuable process-oriented performance measures. Therefore, the systems analysis described in this section can aid in the development of better budgeting and control processes, even if explicit output measures cannot be developed.

CAPITAL BUDGETING

A capital budget delineates the organization's plans for investing in various capital or program alternatives that will have a long-range impact on the generation of the organization's output. The purpose of a capital budget is to control the number and type of investments undertaken by the organization so that (1) investment costs do not exceed the available financing, (2) current investments prepare the organization for future operational demands, and (3) the selected investments are coordinated with the goals and objectives of the organization.

Technical Requirements of a Capital Budgeting System

Capital budgeting systems have four technical requirements. First, the organization must forecast its future environment, including patient mix, departmental use, and technology required and available, so that the future demands on the organization can be estimated.[8] Second, the available sources and amounts of capital financing must be delineated so that the ability to finance various investments can be ascertained.[9] Third, the departments must have a means of specifying and justifying investment proposals on objective criteria so that these proposals can be evaluated. Finally, the organization must have a chief financial officer or a planning committee responsible for selecting investment alternatives that enable the organization to achieve its mission (see Figure 9-3).

Given an objective means of ascertaining the relationship between the organization's capital investment criteria and its mission (see Chapter 11), the implementation of an effective capital budgeting system can be a straightforward task because (1) a number of techniques can be used to forecast the institution's future environment, although more sophisticated techniques may require the expertise of a consultant; (2) the advantages and disadvantages of the available financing alternatives can be delineated with the help of an investment banker; and (3) departments usually are able to justify investment proposals by preparing a document which contains the basic purchasing information as well as the other planning information required to evaluate the investment. However, if the institution has not, or cannot, define the organizational mission explicitly, departmental activities cannot be interrelated, budgeted, evaluated, or controlled using a common set of objective performance criteria, and the investment selection process can become complicated.

In the absence of an explicit statement of the organizational mission, each department may believe that its activities form the rationale for the existence of the institution. Hence, each may operate as an autonomous unit with its

Figure 9-3 Selection of Capital Investment Alternatives

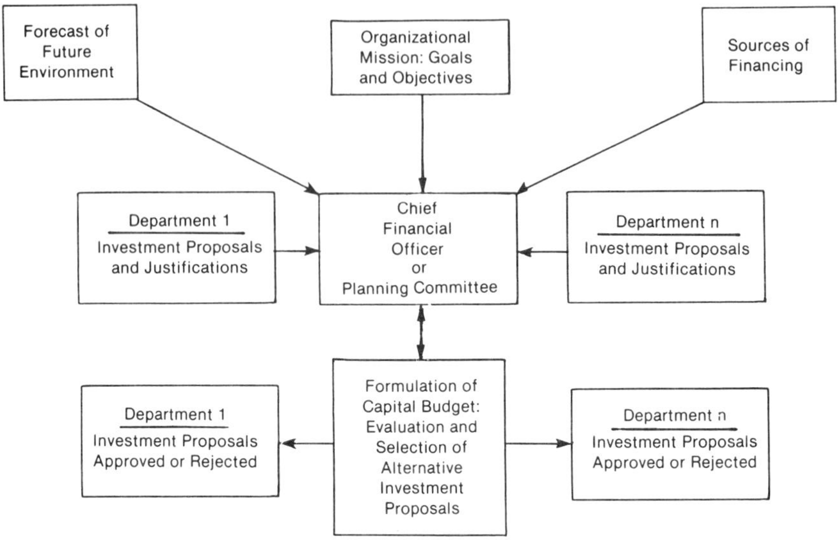

own set of goals and objectives. Then, if highly autonomous departments are able to generate sufficient funds, they may finance investments that are not related to the organizational mission. Consequently, an explicit statement of the organizational mission is important in evaluating investment alternatives and developing the capital budget.

Simple Planning Information

The chief financial officer or planning committee needs a variety of information to evaluate the submitted investment proposals. Some of this information is supplied by the departments making the investment proposals. For example, a department proposing an investment should be required to prepare a document that specifies the cost and benefits of the investment, the terms of the investment contract, and the timing of the investment. In addition, the department should estimate the costs of replacing the investment and the indirect costs associated with undertaking the investment, and provide information verifying the suggested benefits. These informational inputs are all important in the capital budgeting process.

The means for deriving the department's capital budgeting information inputs, including investment benefit validation, investment replacement costs, and indirect investment costs, are delineated in the following sections.

Although these departmental inputs to the capital evaluation process are not coordinated with the organizational goals and objectives systematically, they are related. To evaluate the various investment proposals with respect to the goals and objectives of the organization, the chief financial officer or planning committee must evaluate the institution's planning criteria with respect to the organization's mission, and also must evaluate each investment with respect to each planning criterion. (A description of this evaluation process and alternatives selection is given in Chapter 11.)

Validating Investment Benefits

In the past, managers in health care institutions had little incentive to analyze and evaluate investment benefits comprehensively because these benefits had little impact on investment selection. Departments proposing investments often justified their proposals with vague and unquantifiable benefits that were not easily incorporated in the investment evaluation process. In addition, even when investment benefits could be quantified, management's evaluation of the benefits often was superficial because the investment selection process was subjective and usually based solely on political considerations. This type of investment selection was fostered by the availability of philanthropic funds and the willingness of most third party payers to support comprehensive coverage without reimbursement ceilings.

However, given the current economic environment, philanthropy is no longer a factor in generating investment capital. Furthermore, third party payers have imposed reimbursement ceilings and limited their coverages. Therefore, health care organizations have had to become more selective in evaluating and undertaking investments. To improve the evaluation and selection process, these organizations have attempted to justify investment costs in terms of investment benefits. Unfortunately, this justification process can improve the investment selection process only if the investment benefits are valid. Therefore, a means of validating investment benefits is necessary to provide information useful to an objective evaluation of investment alternatives.

The major problem of investment benefit validation is estimating the probability of attaining the benefits that should affect an investment's funding priority significantly (i.e., the critical benefits). To assist management in ascertaining the probability of attaining the critical benefits, the following three-step process is suggested. The first step involves delineating investment evaluation categories that are related to the goals and objectives of the organization.[10] The second involves isolating the benefits of a particular investment alternative that affect one or more of these categories and then associating them with the appropriate categories. The final step involves collecting the data necessary to validate the critical benefits identified in the second step. Hence, investment benefit specifications must be stated explicitly so that relevant validation information can be collected. By following these procedures, health care institutions often can improve their investment selection process significantly.

For example, assume that the director of a hospital's outpatient department wants to reduce the department's "no show" rate by implementing a computer scheduling system that will reduce the patient appointment interval (i.e., the interval between the time that the individual calls for an appointment and the time it is scheduled). Further assume that reducing this rate would improve the hospital's health care delivery system—one of the organizational goals. In this case, reducing the no show rate would be a critical benefit of the computer scheduling system. In addition, if the hospital conducts a study to ascertain the probability that the critical benefit will be attained and finds, for example, that in 85 percent of the test cases the no show rate rises when the appointment interval is reduced (see Question 9-12), then no resources should be committed to implementing the computer scheduling system. Hence, in this case, the elementary benefit validation procedure would keep the hospital from selecting the investment alternative because the critical benefit is not likely to be realized.

Investment Replacement Costs

Once a health care institution undertakes an investment, the services provided as a result of that investment usually become a permanent part of the institution's health care delivery system. Consequently, when the assets associated with that investment become physically deteriorated or obsolete, new assets must be purchased so that the associated service can be continued. These future asset replacement or renewal costs should be considered in the initial investment evaluation because these costs could significantly affect the institution's ability to undertake other investments in the future.

Some of the investment replacement costs are recouped through the periodic depreciation of the assets associated with the investment because while asset depreciation does not require a cash outlay, depreciation expense is reimbursed. Hence, during each period the institution should be able to save an amount of cash equal to the depreciation expense. Furthermore, these savings can be invested at some institutional or bank interest rate, i. Therefore, if the asset has a life of n periods and a salvage value, S, and if the depreciation expense in a particular period is A, the resources available for reinvestment (RAR) at the end of the life of the asset would be computed as follows:[11]

$$\text{RAR} = \frac{A[(1 + i)^n - 1]}{i} + S \qquad (9\text{-}1)$$

Of course, if the asset is replaced before or after the end of its depreciable life, n in equation (9-1) would reflect the proper number of years until replacement (see Problem 9-4).

The RAR represents the amount of resources that can be generated through the depreciation of an asset by the time that asset is expected to be replaced. This amount should be compared with the expected replacement cost (ERC) when evaluating the investment so that the institution can estimate future financing needs. The ERC can be computed as:

$$\text{ERC} = C(1 + r + b)^n \times \gamma \tag{9-2}$$

where: C represents the original cost of the asset;
r represents the expected annual inflation rate (r is negative if deflation is expected);
b represents the expected annual rate of cost increase due to technological innovation (b is negative if technological improvements are expected to decrease costs);
n represents the number of years until replacement; and
γ represents the probability of replacing the investment[12] (i.e., $0 \leq \gamma \leq 1$).

The difference between the ERC and RAR will be referred to as the investment renewal differential (IRD) and is formulated as follows:

$$\text{IRD} = \text{ERC} - \text{RAR} \tag{9-3}$$

If the IRD is positive, the institution will have a financing requirement at the time the investment is renewed. If it is negative, the resources generated through depreciation will exceed the amount needed to renew the investment. Therefore, the institution will have additional resources to finance other investment alternatives.

The amount of the IRD and the timing of the investment replacement are important inputs to the planning process regarding the institution's future financing needs. For example, if $150,000 is expected to be generated through debt financing in 19X5 and the institution currently is maintaining an investment that will have to be renewed in 19X5 at a cost of $100,000, any new investment alternative under consideration that is due for renewal in 19X5 at a cost exceeding $50,000 will have to be rejected unless some additional sources of financing are found. Accordingly, investment alternatives currently under consideration that will be due for renewal in 19X5 at costs of $50,000 or less are viable options for the institution.

Another measure that may be valuable in comparing current investment alternatives is the value of the annuity, VA_{IRD}, that must be invested at interest rate i so that the institution will have available funds equal to the IRD when the investment must be replaced. The VA_{IRD} can be calculated as follows:

(9-4) $$VA_{IRD} = \frac{IRD}{[(1+i)^n - 1]/i}$$

where: i represents the annual interest rate that can be earned on monies invested; and
n represents the number of years until the investment is to be replaced.

This measure is useful in comparing investment alternatives that are due for renewal at different times. The smaller the annuity (i.e., the smaller the amount of cash that would have to be invested at interest rate i each year), the more likely it is that the institution will be able to replace the investment without constricting external financing alternatives. The following example illustrates the usefulness of this measure in addition to the other computations required to evaluate investment replacement costs.

Assume that a hospital has two investment alternatives. The first requires an initial investment of $100,000. This investment has a salvage value of $10,000 and definitely will be replaced ($\gamma = 1.0$) at the end of five years. The second alternative also requires an initial investment of $100,000. It, however, has a salvage value of $5,000 and an 80 percent chance of being replaced at the end of ten years. To evaluate these two investments, the hospital management decides to compute the investment replacement costs.

Management estimates that cash investments will earn eight percent over the foreseeable future. Therefore, the two investment alternatives will have the following resources available for reinvestment when the original investments must be replaced.[13]

Investment 1

$$RAR_1 = \frac{A_1[(1+i)^{n_1} - 1]}{i} + S_1$$

$$= \frac{\$18{,}000[(1+.08)^5 - 1]}{.08} + \$10{,}000$$

$$= \$115{,}599$$

Investment 2

$$\text{RAR}_2 = \frac{A_2[(1+i)^{n2}-1]}{i} + S_2$$

$$= \frac{\$9{,}500[(1+.08)^{10}-1]}{.08} + \$5{,}000$$

$$= \$142{,}622$$

Furthermore, the management estimates that the inflation rate will continue at nine percent per year over the next ten years, and that health care costs will increase by an additional five percent as a result of technological innovation. This information is used to compute the expected replacement cost of each investment alternative as follows.

Investment 1

$$\text{ERC}_1 = \text{C}_1(1+r+b)^{n1} \times \gamma_1$$

$$= \$100{,}000\,(1+.09+.05)^5 \times 1.0$$

$$= \$192{,}541$$

Investment 2

$$\text{ERC}_2 = \text{C}_2(1+r+b)^{n_2} \times \gamma_2$$

$$= \$100{,}000\,(1+.09+.05)^{10} \times .8$$

$$= \$296{,}578$$

Once these preliminary calculations have been performed, the investment renewal differential for each investment alternative can be computed.

Investment 1

$$\text{IRD}_1 = \text{ERC}_1 - \text{RAR}_1$$

$$= \$192{,}541 - \$115{,}599$$

$$= \$76{,}942$$

Investment 2

$$\text{IRD}_2 = \text{ERC}_2 - \text{RAR}_2$$

$$= \$296{,}578 - \$142{,}622$$

$$= \$153{,}956$$

These IRD computations show that each investment would require some form of financing at the time of renewal. Furthermore, the annual deficit would be $15,388 ($76,942/5) for the first alternative and $15,396 ($153,956/10) for the second. Since both investments require an initial investment of $100,000 and the annual deficits are approximately equal, choosing between them could be difficult, particularly if no other financial complications exist.

Assume that future financing and investing activities will not be affected when the hospital has to replace either one of the two investments. Further assume that the hospital can obtain only $100,000 of financing this year, and therefore must choose between the two investments. In this case, the VA_{IRD} can be helpful in selecting one of the two alternatives. The VA_{IRD} for each investment alternative would be calculated as follows.

$$VA_{IRD_1} = \frac{IRD_1}{[(1 + i)^{n_1} - 1]/i}$$

$$= \frac{\$76,942}{[(1 + .08)^5 - 1]/.08}$$

$$= \$13,115$$

$$VA_{IRD_2} = \frac{IRD_2}{[(1 + i)^{n_2} - 1]/i}$$

$$= \frac{\$153,956}{[(1 + .08)^{10} - 1]/.08}$$

$$= \$10,628$$

Since the VA_{IRD} of the second investment alternative is less than that of the first, only the second investment alternative would be able to be renewed if the cash available for reinvestment is between $10,628 and $13,115 annually (see Question 9-14 and Problem 9-11). However, it is important to remember that other criteria must be considered before a final decision is made (see Chapter 11).

Indirect Investment Costs

The services provided by health care institutions generally are interrelated, and consequently, investments in almost any technology or program will have an indirect effect on the cost structure of the institution. For example, a technological modernization of a hospital's outpatient facility may increase the number of outpatient department (OPD) visits. Since some proportion of outpatients become inpatients, the increase in the OPD volume probably will affect the inpatient utilization of the hospital. If the patients admitted to the hospital through the OPD usually generate unreimbursed service losses because of the high proportion of indigent OPD patients, then these losses are indirect costs of the OPD modernization and should be estimated and included in the investment evaluation. These indirect investment costs, in addition to the investment renewal differential and the investment benefit validation information, are important in evaluating and selecting capital investment alternatives. This information usually can be derived on a cost-efficient basis by most institutions and should be used to evaluate investment proposals.

NOTES

1. Numerous budgeting techniques or specific organization heuristics are used to prepare the budget, disseminate the budgeting information, generate control information, measure periodic performance variances, and select particular control actions. These various techniques or heuristics have many labels, including zero-based budgeting, flexible budgeting, target analysis, and program budgeting. The purpose of this chapter is to consider a general context within which all of the various approaches to using the tactical budget may be related.
2. Management usually states the performance for the coming period in *standard units* (i.e., the desired output of the departments, given the resources committed to them) or *expected units* (i.e., what management expects the departmental output to be, given the resources committed to them). The choice between these two alternatives are discussed in Chapter 10.
3. The role of the chief financial officer varies considerably across institutions. In this text the chief financial officer assumed to be in a position of real authority consistent with primary responsibility for the institution's planning and control functions. When this responsibility is not vested in one organizational position, a budgeting or planning committee is usually formed.
4. Autonomy is defined as ability to set output levels, incur debt, and spend accumulated earnings without the approval of central management. In most hospitals, departments of medicine and cardiology are autonomous.
5. Commission on the Organization of the Executive Branch of the Government. *Budgeting and Accounting* (Washington, D.C.: U.S. Government Printing Office, 1969), p. 8.
6. Recall that in a planning, programing, budgeting system, resources are appropriated on a program basis. Once this appropriation has been approved, the resources are allocated to the various departments that support the programs.
7. See S. Katz et al., "Studies of Illness in the Aged: The Index of ADL, A Standardized Measure of Biological and Physiological Function," *Journal of the American Medical Association*, and S. Katz et al., *Effects of Continued Care: A Study of Chronic Illness in the Home.*
8. For an excellent presentation and discussion of various forecasting models, see R. S. Pindyck and D. L. Rubinfeld (1976).
9. In this chapter, the organization is assumed to be evaluating purchase alternatives. See Appendix 9-A for a discussion of the leasing alternative.
10. One such category which is related to the functional objectives of the institution is: Providing for Excellence in Teaching, Research, and Health Care Delivery (see Chapter 11).
11. To simplify the various computations, i is assumed to be constant over time. However, in reality, i changes over time, which means that solving for the RAR is a formidable computation.

12. Note that the concept of estimating the likelihood of replacement is relevant to developing an expectation of the funding requirements over future years for a number of assets, investments, or projects. However, a particular investment alternative will either be renewed ($\gamma = 1.0$) or not renewed ($\gamma = 0$).
13. The annual depreciation on each investment is calculated on a straight line basis. Therefore, $A = (C - S)/n$ (see Problem 9-12).

Appendix 9-A

Leasing: An Alternative to Direct Asset Acquisition

In addition to selecting among various investment alternatives based upon their ability to facilitate achievement of the organization's mission, the capital budgeting process involves evaluating the alternative means of financing proposed investments. Two primary financing alternatives are direct purchase or leasing (see Question 9-10 and Problems 9-7 and 9-10). Leasing opportunities should be considered carefully because different types of lease contracts require different methods of accounting, and may, therefore, have different effects on institutional reimbursement. This Appendix defines two basic types of lease contracts and examines the accounting and reimbursement implications of each.

OPERATING AND CAPITAL LEASES

From the lessee's point of view, two basic types of leases exist: operating leases and capital leases. The fundamental difference between these two types of leases involves the types of benefits and risks assumed by the lessee in the leased property. Under a capital lease, the lessee is presumed to assume a major portion of the benefits and risks incident to ownership of the leased property. Under an operating lease, on the other hand, the majority of the benefits and risks incident to owning the leased property are not transferred to the lessee. The Financial Accounting Standards Board (FASB) Statement No. 13 specifies the criteria used to distinguish an operating lease from a capital lease.

According to FASB Statement No. 13, "if at its inception a lease meets one or more of the following four criteria, the lease shall be capitalized as a capital lease by the lessee.

a. The lease transfers ownership of the property to the lessee by the end of the lease term.
b. The lease contains a bargain purchase option.[1]
c. The lease term is equal to 75 percent or more of the estimated economic life of the leased property. However, if the beginning of the lease term falls within the last 25 percent of the total estimated economic life of the leased property, including earlier years of use, this criterion shall not be used for purposes classifying the lease.
d. The present value at the beginning of the lease term of the minimum lease payments, excluding that portion of the payments representing executory costs such as insurance, maintenance, and taxes to be paid by the lessor, including any profit thereon, equals or exceeds 90 percent of the excess of the fair value of the leased property to the lessor at the inception of the lease over any related investment tax credit retained by the lessor and expected to be realized by him. However, if the beginning of the lease term falls within the last 25 percent of the total estimated economic life of the leased property, including earlier years of use, this criterion shall not be used for purposes of classifying the lease. A lessor shall compute the present value of the minimum lease payments using the interest rate implicit in the lease. A lessee shall compute the present value of the minimum lease payments using his incremental borrowing rate, unless (i) it is practicable for him to learn the implicit rate computed by the lessor and (ii) the implicit rate computed by the lessor is less than the lessee's incremental borrowing rate. If both of those conditions are met, the lessee shall use the implicit rate."

Unless a lease can be classified as a capital lease under the provisions of FASB Statement No. 13, the lease is considered to be an operating lease. Such a lease is an executory contract that requires continued performance on the part of the lessor and the lessee over the life of the lease.

Accounting Considerations

The nature of the difference between capital and operating leases necessitates different accounting treatment. Under a capital lease, the property should be capitalized as an asset, and the lease obligation should be recorded as a liability. FASB Statement No. 13 stipulates that the amount at which the asset and the related liability are recorded should be equal to the lesser of the fair market value of the leased property at the inception of the lease or "the present value[2] at the beginning of the lease term of minimum lease payments[3] during the lease term, excluding that portion of the payments representing executory costs such as insurance, maintenance, and taxes to be paid by the lessor, together with any profit thereon." These amounts should be classified properly, but identified separately from other assets and liabilities in the organization's balance sheet. The statement also stipulates that the asset should be depreciated over its useful life if at the inception of the lease the lessee is reasonably assured of attaining ownership of the property by the end of the term. On the other hand, if the lessee is not reasonably assured of eventual ownership, the asset should be depreciated over the term of the lease. Furthermore, the statement specifies that each minimum lease payment should be allocated between a reduction of the lease obligation and an interest expense so as to produce a constant periodic rate of interest on the remaining balance of the obligation.

Under an operating lease, the leased property is not capitalized. Hence, this type of lease has no impact on the assets or liabilities of the organization. However, the rental should be charged to expense over the lease term. In addition, to avoid the issuance of misleading information to the users of the institution's financial statements, FASB Statement No. 13 requires that pertinent noncapitalized lease information be disclosed in the footnotes to the institution's published financial statements.

Reimbursement Implications

Reimbursement policies regarding leases are fairly straightforward.[4] The institution is reimbursed for the reasonable costs incurred under the lease contract. Therefore, the lease payments under an operating lease would be included in reimbursable costs. Under a capital lease, the institution's reimbursement would include the allowable depreciation on the capitalized property, the interest expense on the current portion of the lease,[5] any maintenance costs, and insurance or tax expenses included in the lease. The following example illustrates the reimbursement differences of an operating lease, a capital lease with the implicit interest rate not specified, and a capital lease with the implicit interest rate specified.

Assume that Memorial Hospital leases radiology equipment with a fair market value of $7,750 and a depreciable life of 15 years for $1,200 per year. Further assume that the lease agreement cannot be canceled for ten years and includes no provisions for renewing the lease or for purchasing the leased radiology equipment. In addition, all insurance, maintenance, and taxes associated with the equipment, amounting to $45 per year, are paid by the lessor. The hospital's incremental borrowing rate is 11 percent. In this case, the lease would be classified as an operating lease, and the hospital would be reimbursed $1,200 per year (see Table 9-1A), providing that it could not obtain a similar lease for the same equipment at substantially lower rental rates.

On the other hand, assume that Memorial Hospital leases the radiology equipment for $1,200 per year and that the lease contract permits the hospital to purchase the equipment for a nominal fee at the end of the ten years. Again, assume that the $45 annual cost of insurance, maintenance, and taxes is paid by the lessor, and that no interest rate is specified in the lease contract. In this case, the contract would be classified as a capital lease, and the hospital would be required to capitalize the asset. Third party payers would reimburse the hospital for (1) depreciation, (2) insurance, maintenance, and tax expenses, and (3) imputed interest expenses associated with the contract.

Since no interest rate is specified in the lease contract, the third party payers would require the hospital to capitalize the asset as if the hospital and the lessor were one. Hence, the hospital would be required to capitalize the radiology equipment at its fair market value of $7,750, and the

Table 9-1A Reimbursed Expenses and Lease Payment under an Operating Lease

Year	Lease Payments	Reimbursable Expenses	Net Cash Inflow (Outflow)*
1	$ 1,200	$ 1,200	$0
2	1,200	1,200	0
3	1,200	1,200	0
4	1,200	1,200	0
5	1,200	1,200	0
6	1,200	1,200	0
7	1,200	1,200	0
8	1,200	1,200	0
9	1,200	1,200	0
10	1,200	1,200	0
Total	$12,000	$12,000	$0

*Assuming that the lease payments are reimbursed in the same fiscal year in which they are made.

third party payers would impute the interest rate implicit in the lease by solving for i in the following equation:[6]

$$\text{CV} = \text{LP} \times \text{PV}(i, n) \qquad \text{(9A-1)}$$

where: CV represents the capitalized value of the asset (when i is not specified, CV is assumed to be equal to the fair market value so that the value of i may be computed uniquely);
LP represents the minimum lease payment required under the lease; and
PV(i, n) represents the present value of an annuity for n periods at interest rate i. $\text{PV}(i, n) = (1 - (1 + i)^{-n})/i$.[7]

In this case, CV = \$7,750; LP = \$1,155; and $n = 10$; so that i is determined to be 8 percent. The reimbursable expenses for the term of the lease, the lease payments, and net cash flow are represented in Table 9-2A (see Problem 9-9).

If the interest rate implicit in the lease is specified in the lease contract, equation (9A-1) may be used to solve for the value at which the leased equipment should be capitalized for reimbursement purposes. Assuming that the interest rate specified in the lease contract is 12 percent, the capitalized value of the radiology equipment for reimbursement purposes would be:[8]

$$\text{CV} = \text{LP} \times \text{PV}(i, n)$$

$$\text{CV} = \$1{,}155 \times (1 - (1 + .12)^{-10})/.12$$

$$= \$6{,}526.$$

The reimbursable expenses for the term of the lease, the lease payments, and the net cash flow are represented in Table 9-3A.

Comparing the information in Tables 9-1A, 9-2A, and 9-3A, the most economically desirable lease contract would be the operating lease of Table 9-1A. However, if Memorial Hospital were to select a capital lease, the most economically desirable alternative would be the lease that specifies the interest rate (see Question 9-7). Of course, general advantages and disadvantages of leasing must be considered before selecting a specific type of lease.

MAJOR ADVANTAGES OF LEASING

The primary advantage of leasing is that it provides a hedge against technological obsolescence because the term of the lease may be fixed by

Table 9-2A Reimbursed Expenses and Lease Payments under a Financing Lease: Imputed Interest at Eight Percent

Year	Imputed Interest Expense (8%)	Depreciation Expense	Insurance, Maintenance, and Tax Expenses	Total Reimbursable Expenses	Minimum Lease Payments ($1,200 − $45)	Cash Inflow (Outflow)
1	$ 620	$ 517	$ 45	$1,182	$ 1,155	$ 27
2	577	517	45	1,139	1,155	(16)
3	531	517	45	1,093	1,155	(62)
4	481	517	45	1,043	1,155	(112)
5	427	517	45	989	1,155	(166)
6	369	517	45	931	1,155	(224)
7	306	517	45	868	1,155	(287)
8	238	517	45	800	1,155	(355)
9	165	517	45	727	1,155	(428)
10	86	517	45	648	1,155	(507)
Total	$3,800	$5,170	$450	$9,420	$11,550	$(2,130)

Table 9-3A Reimbursed Expenses under a Financing Lease: Stated Interest at 12 Percent

Year	Interest Expense (12%)	Depreciation Expense	Insurance, Maintenance, and Tax Expense	Total Reimbursable Expenses	Minimum Lease Payments ($1200 − $45)	Cash Inflow (Outflow)
1	$ 783	$ 435	$ 45	$1,263	$ 1,155	$ 108
2	738	435	45	1,218	1,155	63
3	688	435	45	1,168	1,155	13
4	632	435	45	1,112	1,155	(43)
5	570	435	45	1,050	1,155	(105)
6	499	435	45	979	1,155	(176)
7	421	435	45	901	1,155	(254)
8	333	435	45	813	1,155	(342)
9	234	435	45	714	1,155	(441)
10	126	435	45	606	1,155	(549)
Total	$5,024	$4,350	$450	$9,824	$11,550	$(1,726)

management's estimation of the asset's technological life. However, since the lessor usually will charge a rate of interest greater than that charged by a bank to borrow the funds to purchase the asset, the cost of leasing usually will be higher than that of purchasing. A secondary benefit afforded by leasing is that the debt structure of the institution is unaffected if the lease is classified as an operating lease (see Question 9-11).

APPENDIX 9-A NOTES

1. FASB Statement No. 13 defines a bargain purchase option as follows: "A provision allowing the lessee, at his option, to purchase the leased property for a price which is sufficiently lower than the expected fair value of the property at the date the option becomes exercisable that exercise of the option appears, at the inception of the lease, to be reasonably assured."
2. This present value should be computed using (1) the lessee's incremental borrowing rate (i.e., the interest rate that the lessee would have incurred at the inception of the lease to borrow over a similar term the funds necessary to purchase the leased asset), or if known, (2) the implicit rate computed by the lessor, providing that this rate is less than the lessee's incremental borrowing rate. (See paragraph 10 of FASB Statement No. 13.)
3. Minimum lease payments include (1) the minimum rental payments, (2) payment required by a bargain purchase option, (3) any guarantee by the lessee of the residual value at the expiration of the term of the lease, and (4) any payment that the lessee must make or can be required to make upon failure to renew or extend the lease at the end of the term. However, minimum lease payments do not include (1) a guarantee by the lessee of the lessor's debt, and (2) executory costs such as insurance, maintenance, and taxes in connection with the leased property. (See paragraph 5 (*j*(*i*)) of FASB Statement No. 13.)
4. The current Medicare regulations, adopted in December 1974, were written with Accounting Principles Board (APB) Opinion No. 5 as a point of reference. FASB Statement No. 13 supercedes APB Opinion No. 5. However, the information regarding operating and capital leases (referred to in the Medicare regulations as a virtual purchase) provided by FASB Statement No. 13 is not inconsistent with the information contained in APB Opinion No. 5.
5. If the interest rate is not specified in the lease contract, it is imputed by the third party payers to determine the interest expense associated with the lease contract.
6. This computation would be required for reimbursement purposes. However, if the financial statements are to be certified by an independent certified public accountant, the hospital's incremental borrowing rate (11 percent) should be substituted for i in the given equation, and the capitalized value of the asset should be computed.
7. Computing the present value of an annuity as:

$$PV(i, n) = (1 - (1 - i)^{-n})/i$$

implies that the annuity is paid in arrears. However, if the lease requires annuity payments in advance, the appropriate present value formula would be:

$$PV(i, n) = [(1 - (1 - i)^{-(n-1)})/i] + 1.$$

8. If the financial statements are subject to a certified audit in this case, the capitalized value of the asset must be computed using the 11 percent incremental borrowing rate because the implicit interest rate is greater than the incremental borrowing rate. (See Paragraph 10, FASB Statement No. 13.)

Questions and Problems

Question 9-1. Analyze and discuss the following statement: Performance measures must relate to the institution's output if tactical budgeting and control systems are to be effective in relating corrective actions to achievement of the organization's mission.

Question 9-2. How should standards of performance be used to develop the tactical budget? Does this differ for performance expectations?

Question 9-3. What are some of the difficulties involved in formulating control measures for nonprofit organizations? How does the three-phased analysis mitigate or eliminate these difficulties?

Question 9-4. How might the organization be affected if process, rather than output, measures were used to generate control information? Under what circumstances are process measures acceptable for generating relevant control information?

Question 9-5. What are the benefits derived by going through a process such as the one described in this chapter for specifying the desired and actual organizational mission? What problems might the organization create in conducting such a process?

Question 9-6. Consider the following statement: In the for-profit sector, important negative externalities exist which make the single-minded pursuit of maximum profit unattractive. Is there an analogous statement for the nonprofit sector? Discuss its control implications.

Question 9-7. If a lease contract does not specify the interest rate, the third party must impute the interest rate in order to ascertain the reimbursable interest expense. Assume that equation (9A-1) is used to impute the interest rate which in part determines the institution's reimbursement. As the controller of an institution, would you want an interest rate to be specified in the lease contract or would you allow a third party to impute the interest rate? Rationalize your answer.

Question 9-8. The federal income tax regulations prohibit a firm in the business of leasing assets to take (or pass) the investment tax credit if the lessee uses that leased asset in operations which generate nontaxable income. Discuss the possible reason for this federal income tax regulation.

Question 9-9. Calculate the total cash dispensed over the life of the radiology equipment leased by the Memorial Hospital (Appendix 9-A) under the operating lease, the capital lease with an imputed interest rate, and the capital lease with a stated interest rate.

Question 9-10. Suggest a method for evaluating the following two alternatives:

Alternative 1: Purchase a specific asset.
Alternative 2: Lease a specific asset.

In developing an answer to this question, it is recommended that the reader follow the method suggested by Ofer (1976). Also see Problem 9-7.

Question 9-11. Discuss the working capital implications of a capital asset purchase financed by a bond sale, an operating lease, and a capital lease with interest rate specified.

Question 9-12. The example discussed on pages 321–322 regarding the implementation of a computer scheduling system was abstracted from an actual case. List two reasons why the no-show rate increased when the appointment interval was reduced.

Question 9-13. Discuss the implications of the following proposal on insurance premiums, health care delivery costs, and the quality of care: The annual allowable depreciation on capital investments may be increased so that the VA_{IRD} equals zero.

Question 9-14. After reviewing the IRD and VA_{IRD} computations, the controller makes the following observation:

> If two investments have equal *yearly* investment renewal differentials, the investment with the longer useful life will have a lower VA_{IRD}. This means that investments with longer lives will be selected over investments with shorter lives.

Discuss this observation.

Problem 9-1. In Figure 9-1, the traditional tactical budgeting process is outlined and the control function represented. In controlling the execution of the organization's tactical plan as represented by the budget, performance will be contrasted with what was budgeted to occur. If the budget represents what is expected to happen during the period of time over which performance must be monitored, how should management react to a performance variance between what was expected and what actually happened? Would your answer change if what was represented in the tactical budget was the desirable or standard occurrence? Does your answer to either question change if the budgeting system is a PPBS system (Figure 9-2)?

Problem 9-2. In this chapter the terms "tactical budget," "tactical evaluation," and "tactical control" all have been related to the movement of the organization toward its goals. With Figure 9-1 as a reference point, construct a diagram for a hospital which explicitly relates budgeting, evaluation, and control to the concept of responsibility accounting where the focus of the accounting system is profit. Construct a similar diagram where the focus is patient welfare. Assume measures of patient welfare exist which may be used by the institution.

Problem 9-3. Suggest a process by which the various informational elements developed in Phases I, II, and III may be used to develop a tactical budgeting system and to control the execution of the tactical budget.

Problem 9-4. Assume that the W. Russell Clinic, a tax-paying entity, purchases an asset which has a cost of $250,000 and a salvage value of $43,000. The useful life of the asset is estimated to be seven years. The tax rate is 48 percent and is expected to be constant. The organization earns 11 percent on invested capital. Management's intention is to replace the asset at the beginning of the eleventh year. The rate of inflation (r) during these ten years is estimated to be: conservatively four percent; liberally, 12 percent. The rate of cost changes due to technological innovation (b) is estimated to be: conservatively a decrease of two percent; liberally, an increase of four percent.

Required:

a. Compute the IRD using both the conservative and liberal estimates of r and b, assuming straight line depreciation is used for both tax and reimbursement purposes.
b. How is the IRD affected if the clinic were to qualify as a tax-exempt organization?
c. Assume that the actual market value of the asset to be replaced is expected to increase at the rate of eight percent per year. How would this fact affect your analysis in (a) and (b)?

Problem 9-5. Assume a nursing agency is considering an investment in a mobile diagnostic unit. The cost of the unit is $137,000, and if properly maintained, the unit would have a useful life of eight years and a salvage value of $15,000. The maintenance costs are expected to be $4,000 in the first year and are expected to increase by ten percent per year (the expected inflation rate (r)). Maintenance costs are reimbursed in the year paid. Health care cost increases due to technological innovation are expected to be 150 percent of the inflation rate. The agency earns 15 percent on its invested capital.

a. With this information, compute the IRD_{MDU} assuming $\gamma = 1.0$.
b. Determine the value of γ which makes the $\text{IRD}_{\text{MDU}} = 0$. What managerial significance can be attached to this information?

Problem 9-6. Assume the nursing agency in Problem 9-5 also is considering an investment in maternal and infant care (MIC) equipment which costs $140,000. This equipment is estimated to have a salvage value of $15,000 and will be replaced at the end of six years. The rate of cost increases due to technological innovation (b) for this equipment is estimated to be eight percent.

a. Compute the IRD_{MDU} assuming a 50 percent chance that management will replace the mobile van at the end of its useful life.
b. Compute the IRD_{MIC} assuming $\gamma = 1$.
c. Based upon a comparison of IRD_{MDU} and IRD_{MIC}, which investment will be selected?
d. Compute the $\text{VA}_{\text{IRD MDU}}$ and $\text{VA}_{\text{IRD MIC}}$. Does this change your investment selection? Rationalize your answer.
e. How would the organization use other planning criteria (see Figure 9-3) to augment the simple planning information (i.e., the IRD and VA_{IRD})?

Problem 9-7. The administrator of a hospital is evaluating an asset which may either be purchased or leased. The lease contract can be written as a capital or an operating lease. The administrator also has gathered the information needed to compute the IRD and the VA_{IRD} and wishes to evaluate the following:

Alternative 1:	*Purchase the asset.* The asset is described by the IRD and the VA_{IRD}.	or	*Lease the asset.* Capital lease with interest rate specified.
Alternative 2:	*Purchase the asset.* The asset is described by the IRD and the VA_{IRD}.	or	*Lease the asset.* Operating lease.

The administrator is having difficulty relating the information so that a decision can be made. For alternative 1, the information developed for the asset purchase and the lease are almost identical if the present value criteria is applied to the lease. For alternative 2, no basis of comparability seems to exist.

Required:

a. Discuss the problems the administrator is having. Relate your discussion to Question 9-10.

b. Develop a simple example which illustrates these problems (also see Problem 9-10).

Problem 9-8. Reproduced below is an excerpt from the Medicare Regulations (12-74; Depreciation, p. 108.2, Section 110).

110. SALE AND LEASEBACK AND LEASE-PURCHASE AGREEMENTS (MEDICARE)

A. *Sale and Leaseback Agreements—Rental Charges.* Where a provider enters into a sale and leaseback agreement with a non-related purchaser involving plant facilities or equipment the incurred rental specified in the agreement is includable in allowable costs if the following conditions are met:

1. The rental charges are reasonable based on consideration of rental charges of comparable facilities and market conditions in the area; the type, expected life, condition and value of the facilities or equipment rented and other provisions of the rental agreements;
2. Adequate alternate facilities or equipment which would serve the purpose are not or were not available at lower cost; and
3. The leasing is based on economic and technical considerations.

If all these conditions are not met, the rental charge cannot exceed the amount which the provider would have included in reimbursable costs had he retained legal title to the facilities or equipment, such as interest on mortgage, taxes, depreciation, insurance and maintenance costs.

The medical director of your institution is considering a sale and lease-back arrangement for certain equipment with a corporation which will purchase the assets, be responsible for maintenance, insurance, and tax expenses, and lease the assets back to the institution. The equipment, which has been especially modified by a research physicist on the hospital's staff, is not available elsewhere. The leaseback agreement is expected to enhance the institution's cash position and increase borrowing capacity. Further, the lease is considered a justifiable hedge against technological obsolescence.

Required:

a. Under this sale and leaseback arrangement, will the lease payments be reimbursable by Medicare?
b. What documentation would you offer to the Medicare auditors to convince them that this sale and leaseback qualifies to have the rental changes reimbursed?

Problem 9-9. The solution to equation (9A-1) in the example in Appendix 9-A yields $i = .08$. Therefore, equation (9A-1) may be restated as:

$$\$7{,}750 = \$1{,}155 \times \left[\frac{1 - (1 + .08)^{-10}}{.08}\right].$$

If the imputed interest calculation is noted as:

$$\text{IIE} = \text{LPR} \times \text{IIR}$$

where: LPR represents the lease principle remaining;
IIR represents the imputed interest rate; and
IIE represents the imputed interest expense,

the imputed interest in the first year of the lease would be (see Table 9-2A):

$$\text{IIE} = \$7{,}750 \times .08$$
$$= \$620.$$

Required:

Verify the imputed interest expense computations in Table 9-2A.

Problem 9-10. a. Assume Memorial Hospital may purchase the radiology equipment discussed in Appendix 9-A. If the organization earns 9.2 percent on invested capital and the combined rate of cost increases due to inflation and technological innovation is ten percent, compute the IRD and VA_{IRD} for the asset purchase assuming $\gamma = 1$.

b. Discuss the basis of comparison between the information represented in Tables 9-1A, 9-2A, and 9-3A and the information generated in (a). What additional information must be known to provide some reasonable basis of comparison between the lease and purchase alternatives?

Problem 9-11. Compute the IRD and the VA_{IRD} for the two investments described on page 325, assuming the probability of renewal for investment 1 is .8 and the probability of renewal for investment 2 is 1.0. Which investment minimizes the constriction of financing capital? Does your answer change if the probability of renewing both investments is 1.0? Which investment would be selected in each case if the cash available for reinvestment is \$10,000 annually. Defend your answer with computations.

Problem 9-12. Assume that the following investment is being considered:

Initial cash outlay	\$100,000
Interest which can be earned on invested capital (i)	7%
Salvage value	4,000
Yearly rate of inflation (r)	8%
Expected cost increase due to technological innovation (b)	3%
Expected useful life	5 years

a. Compute the IRD and the VA_{IRD} for the following three cases, assuming that the investment definitely will be replaced at the end of its useful life (i.e., $\Upsilon = 1.0$):

Case A

The straight line method of depreciation is used. The yearly straight line (SL) depreciation is as follows.

$$\text{SL} = \frac{\text{Initial Cash Outlay} - \text{Salvage Value}}{\text{Number of Years of Useful Life}}$$

Case B

The sum of the years' digits methods of depreciation is used to amortize the asset. The yearly sum of the years' digits (SYD) depreciation is:

$$\text{SYD}_{N-n} = (\text{Initial Cash Outlay} - \text{Salvage Value}) \times \frac{n + 1}{N(N + 1)/2}$$

where: n represents the number of years remaining in the useful life of the asset and

N represents the total number of years of useful life.

For example, the sum of the years digits depreciation for the third year would be:

$$SYD_3 = (\$100{,}000 - \$4{,}000) \times 3/15 = \$19{,}200.$$

Case C

The double declining balance method of depreciation is used to depreciate the asset. The yearly double declining balance depreciation (DDB_i) is:

$$DDB_i = (\text{Book Value}) \times 2/N.$$

For example, the double declining balance depreciation for the first and second year is:

$$DDB_1 = \$100{,}000 \times 2/5 = \$40{,}000.$$

$$DDB_2 = (\$100{,}000 - \$40{,}000) \times 2/5 = \$24{,}000.$$

Note: the book value of the asset cannot fall below the initial cash outlay less salvage value. Also, when using an accelerated method of depreciation, the organization has the option of switching to the straight line method of depreciation whenever it is economically advantageous.

b. Discuss the effect of accelerated depreciation on the IRD and the VA_{IRD}.

c. Why is the VA_{IRD} computed using DDB less than the other two methods?

Chapter 10

Tactical Cost Control: Its Operational Aspects

Self-conquest is the greatest of victories.

Plato

Efficient resource utilization is only one of a number of objectives that influence resource allocations in the not-for-profit sector. Other objectives—such as the maximization of positive externalities, minimization of negative externalities and equity considerations implicit in income redistribution—are also important determinants in the societal allocation of scarce resources. These multiple objectives often cause institutions to develop tactical budgets only to find that governmental agencies, with a system's view, are critical of the programs supported by the resource allocations documented in the tactical budgets. Hence, many states have empowered various agencies to oversee the activities of selected components of the health care delivery system to insure that their activities are coincidental with state and regional goals.

To deal (bargain) effectively with these governmental agencies, health care institutions must have systematic control procedures to document their ability to control their resource conversion processes. Institutions which are devoid of control systems exist at the pleasure of these agencies. Even though cost may not be the performance measure these agencies believe to be important, cost is nevertheless one objective performance statistic with both political and managerial control imperatives. For this reason, cost accounting systems are examined in this chapter.

COST ACCOUNTING CONTROL SYSTEMS

A cost accounting control system is a control system in which anticipated performance values are abstracted from the tactical budget and contrasted with actual performance during the control period so that corrective actions can be taken to reorient actual performance to comply with budgeted performance. Two types of cost accounting systems—standard and expected—are discussed in this chapter. Under a standard cost accounting system, the anticipated performance values abstracted from the tactical budget are stated in standard units (i.e., the values that management would like performance to attain at various times during the control period). Under an expected cost accounting system, the anticipated performance values abstracted from the tactical budget are stated in expected units (i.e., management's best estimates of the values that performance will attain at various times during the control period). The actual performance with which the anticipated values are contrasted is the measured result of processing inputs. As indicated in Chapter 9, the measurement or assignment of values for actual, expected, or standard performance must be stated in terms of organizational output if systematic cost control is to be effected. However, process or input measures may be used to value various aspects of performance as long as the selected measure is related to the organizational output explicitly (see the CNA case study, Chapter 9).

Isolation of the magnitude by which actual performance varies from standard or expected performance, referred to as the performance variance, is the end product of standard or expected cost accounting systems. The usefulness of this variance statistic depends upon the reasonableness of the anticipated performance values abstracted from the tactical budget.[1] For example, if the standards developed to prepare a standard cost tactical budget are reasonable, the proper investigation of performance variances should provide information which elicits an effective set of control actions, because these actions will reorient actual performance toward a reasonable set of desired performance statistics. On the other hand, if (1) expectations, (2) actual performance from previous periods, or (3) the performance of other comparable institutions are used to prepare the tactical budget, the control actions resulting from performance variances may not be effective because attaining expected, past, or comparable performance may be neither reasonable nor desirable.

Standard Cost Accounting Systems

The standard cost system used in many profit organizations develops performance variances for (1) direct materials used in resource conversion, (2) direct labor used in converting materials to units of output, and (3) overhead necessary to maintain the resource conversion process. These performance variances are simply the differences between the standard and the actual costs associated with direct materials, direct labor, and overhead. Variances occurring because actual performance is less costly than budgeted standard performance are said to be favorable. Conversely, variances occurring because actual performance is more costly than budgeted standard performance are said to be unfavorable.

Isolating Standard Cost Performance Variances

The performance variance in a standard cost system can be isolated by computing the difference between the budgeted performance indicated in the tactical budget and the actual performance recorded in the organization's accounting records as follows:

$$\text{(10-1)} \qquad \text{Performance Variance} = \text{Budgeted Performance} - \text{Actual Performance}$$

For example, to compute a direct labor performance variance, actual direct labor performance must be subtracted from budgeted direct labor performance. Budgeted direct labor performance can be derived by totalling the direct labor components of the tactical budget, while actual direct labor performance may be derived by totalling the direct labor wage expenses abstracted from the organization's general ledger. The difference between the two yields the direct labor performance variance.

However, the performance measures used to compute the total performance variance are products of two factors: budgeted performance is a product of (1) the standard unit cost of the input and (2) the standard number of units of input required to generate the output; actual performance is a product of (1) the actual unit cost of the input and (2) the actual number of units of input used to generate the output. Consequently, a performance variance could occur due to a difference between the budgeted and actual unit cost of the input, a difference between the budgeted and actual number of units of input required, or both. If the variance analysis is to provide information useful in taking corrective actions, the magnitude of the variance attributable to each of these differences must be isolated.

For example, in the case of a direct labor performance variance, the total variance could be stated as:

$$\text{(10-2)} \qquad \text{Direct Labor Performance Variance} = (SWR \times SH) - (AWR \times AH)$$

where: SWR represents the standard wage rate;
SH represents the standard number of direct labor hours required to generate the output;
AWR represents the actual wage rate; and
AH represents the actual number of direct labor hours used to generate the output.

This total variance is comprised of two parts:

(10-3) Direct Labor Rate Variance $= AH \times (SWR - AWR)$

and

(10-4) Direct Labor Efficiency Variance $= SWR \times (SH - AH)$.

The direct labor rate variance isolates the magnitude of the variance arising from differences between the budgeted and actual wage rate. The direct labor efficiency variance, on the other hand, isolates the magnitude of the variance arising from differences between the budgeted and actual direct labor hours required to generate the output. The sum of these two variances is equal to the total direct labor performance variance computed using equation (10-2), which is demonstrated as follows.

$$\begin{aligned}\text{Direct Labor Performance Variance}^{2} &= \text{Efficiency Variance} + \text{Rate Variance}\\ &= SWR \times (SH - AH) + AH \times (SWR - AWR)\\ &= SWR \times SH - SWR \times AH + SWR \times AH - AWR \times AH\\ &= (SWR \times SH) - (AWR \times AH)\end{aligned}$$

The information required to compute these variances is derived from a variety of sources. The actual number of direct labor hours used during the period and the actual wage rate per direct labor hour usually can be obtained from the payroll records. The standard wage rate may be established by a policy statement or through engineering studies. The standard number of direct labor hours that should be used during the period must be derived as the product of the number of direct labor hours required to complete one unit of output as derived through engineering studies, and the equivalent units of production for the period (EUP), computed as the number of whole units completed during the period, less the number of equivalent units in process at the beginning of the period, plus the number of equivalent units in process at the end of the period.[3] Once all of these measurements have been made, the respective direct labor performance variances can be isolated.

The isolation and the analysis of the performance variances for direct materials and overhead are similar to that for direct labor performance variances. In each case, measurements are needed for the actual unit cost of the input, the actual number of units of input used to generate the output, the standard unit cost of the input, and the standard number of units of input required to generate the output. These measurements are basic elements of a standard cost system.

Standard Cost Accounting Systems: A Health Care Emphasis

As discussed, standard cost systems require four basic measurements: the actual unit cost of the input, the actual number of units of input used, the standard unit cost of the input, and the standard number of units of input required to generate the output. Given the degree of sophistication of most health care accounting systems, some of these measurements may be tenuous, if they can be made at all. The measurability of these basic elements will be examined in the following example.

Consider the isolation of the labor variance illustrated in the previous section. This analysis requires the measurement of the actual wage rate, the actual number of direct labor hours used, the standard wage rate, and the standard number of direct labor hours that should be used. The measurement of the actual wage rate and the actual number of direct labor hours can be obtained from the institution's payroll records. The measurement of the standard wage rate can be established by a policy statement. However, the measurement of the standard number of direct labor hours used is the product of (1) the standard number of hours required to complete one unit of output, and (2) the equivalent units of service (EUS). Measuring these factors, while not impossible, is certainly subjective. In fact, the degree of uncertainty in making these measurements would probably preclude their use in an effective control system. In addition, effective standard cost accounting systems control output by monitoring the processing of inputs which have a defined relationship with output. However, as suggested, measuring the output of health care systems is problematic.

The problems inherent in measuring output and the subjectivity inherent in determining the standard number of units required cause similar problems in isolating performance variances for direct materials and overhead. These measurements are essential in standard cost accounting systems. The inability to make these measurements in a health care setting restricts the usefulness of the standard cost accounting system to those activities with well-defined output measures. For instance, various institutional service functions such as the laboratory may be amenable to control through information generated using a standard cost accounting system (see Problem 10-4). However, for most institutional activities, the standard cost system cannot be used to generate useful control information.

Expected Cost Accounting Systems

The operation of an expected cost system is similar to the operation of a standard cost system. The basic difference between the two is that under an expected cost system, performance variances are isolated by contrasting expected costs and actual costs, while standard costs and actual costs are used to isolate performance variances under the standard cost system. The development of variances under these two systems is illustrated schematically in Figure 10-1.

The sources of information used to develop performance expectations are different from those used to develop performance standards. For example, the expected wage rate can be estimated from the actual wage rate in prior periods and adjusted for inflation. The expected number of direct labor hours used during the period is, again, the product of the equivalent units of service and the expected number of direct labor hours needed to complete one unit of output. The equivalent units of service computation are the same under both the standard and expected cost systems. However, the expected number of direct labor hours needed to complete one unit of output is usually estimated from the average number of direct labor hours required to complete one unit of output in the prior period. Each of these measurements, in addition to the actual cost and unit measurements, is necessary for developing meaningful performance contrasts in an expected cost system.

As in the standard cost system, the inability to measure output in health care institutions is the central constraining factor inhibiting the implementation of an expected cost system. However, even if meaningful output measures could be defined, the subjectivity inherent in measuring the degree of completion of units (e.g., patients) in the system at the beginning and the end of the period may preclude the calculation of a useful measure of equivalent units of service (see Problem 10-4).

MEASUREMENT OF PERFORMANCE VARIANCES: A CASE EXAMPLE

The specification of standards and expectations is a complex undertaking, and even the measurement of actual performance may be difficult. In addition to the output measurement problems discussed in the previous section, behavioral problems evident in, but not unique to, health care institutions further complicate the institution's control process. The following case study provides a pertinent illustration of these measurement and behavioral problems.

Figure 10-1 Schematic of the Development of Performance Variances and Their Expected Managerial Use in a Standard or Expected Cost System

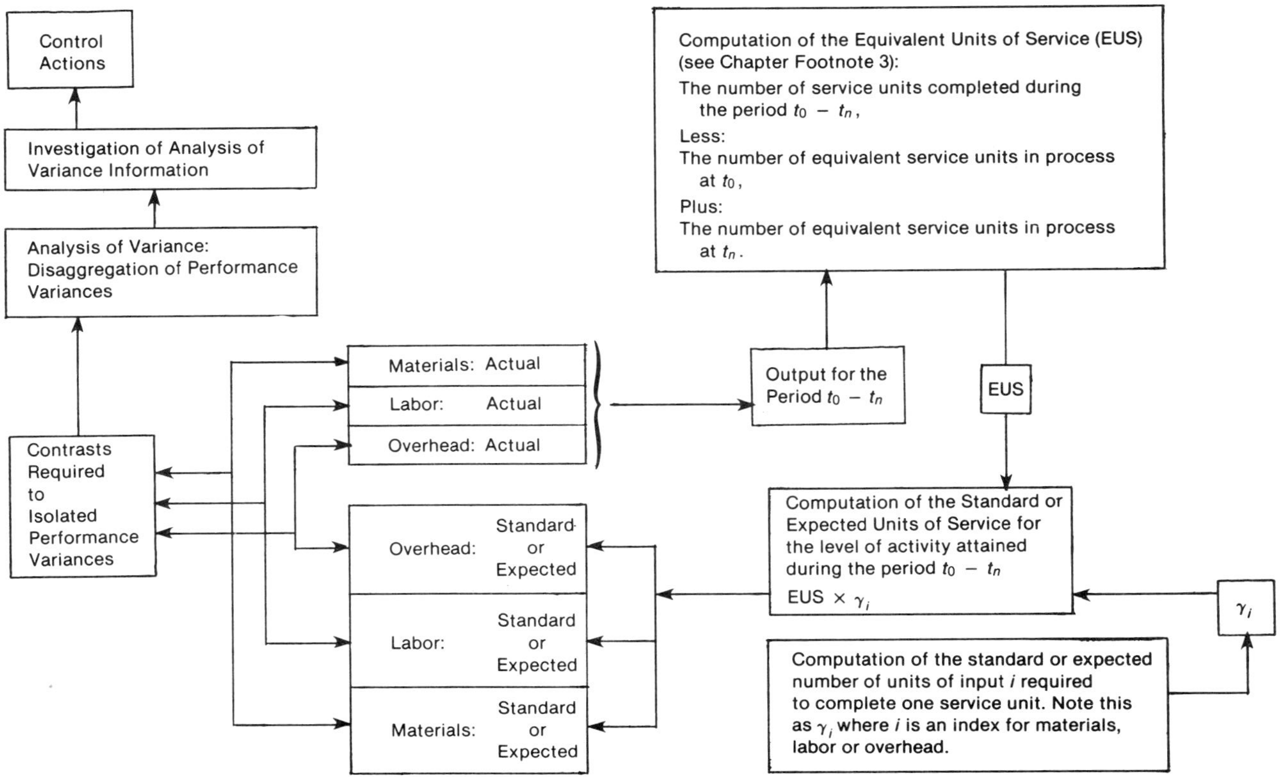

The study was conducted to review a hospital's cost control system, which seemed to be generating useless information. During the study, a number of individuals in the institution were interviewed. The following interview with the chief of radiology typifies the prevailing attitude in the hospital and indicates the behavioral and measurement problems encountered when specifying actual, expected, and standard performances.

Radiologist's Interview[4]

Consultant (Q) How do you specify standards of performance?

Radiologist (A) In this institution, and in the medical profession in general, we have not attempted to establish standards of medical practice. I agree with this practice for the following reasons: I believe that when specific standards are formulated for treatment plans, all physicians must adopt them as minimum defensible plans, even knowing that these standards are often erroneous because they actually should be associated with other treatment plans. Hence, the net effect of formulating standards is the escalation of treatment costs because no physician or institution can afford to do less, even if the standard is wrong, given the current malpractice climate. For example, in this institution, which is a teaching institution, we somehow have developed a principle of taking three films on each individual requiring x-rays. The new interns and teaching fellows, all seem to order three films. Now, I know that in most cases two films will give the physician the same diagnostic and treatment information as three films. However, suppose we try to save the third party payers or the patient a little money by taking two films and we miss a bone puncture of the lung. Let your imagination wander to a courtroom scene: the physician is being asked a question by the attorney prosecuting the malpractice case. "Would this bone fragment which ripped through my client's lung, impeding his God-given right to breathe nature's fresh air, have been located by taking another film?" The physician would have to answer, "Yes." What do you think the verdict would be as the attorney continues to press this point while waving a plastic lung with a pencil rammed through it in front of the jury? Well, you can see the problem. Therefore, medical standards are not likely to be developed, which I believe is how it should be.

Q: How do you formulate performance expectations for the coming year?

A: Let's look at film. We do almost the same thing for personnel, but film is more interesting. In fact, it opened my eyes to what this institution means by budgetary control. About six months before the end of our fiscal year, the controller's office sends down budget forms for capital acquisitions and for the current operating budget. One of the items I am supposed to include in the current operating budget is an estimate of the cost of film for the coming year. The first year I did this it was a disaster, because I submitted a request for the actual amount I expected to use. Unfortunately, I was unaware that the controller makes an across-the-board cut of about eight percent. I had real problems that year, particularly since film costs were higher toward the end of the year than I had anticipated. Since then, my procedure has been as follows. When I estimate the actual amount of film that I will need, I add a little extra to provide for the controller's annual cuts, which seem to range between five and 15 percent. Then I add a little more because I know that other departments are also adding a little bit. I hope that after cuts, this will give me the amount I really need for film. I have never been asked to support my computations, although that would be no real problem because I could fudge either the price or the anticipated volume. As a matter of fact, they probably never ask for support for the computations because they know there is no simple way to check the figures. Anyway, this system seems to work for me.

Q: Does the controller monitor performance by comparing actual volume with what you expect?

A: Yes, but the comparisons are meaningless. In fact, these comparisons make me operate less efficiently than I would if there were no checking.

Q: Could you be more specific?

A: You have to realize that if I am expected to use information to do something, it has to mean something. There are two problems with the cost control information that I get. First, I usually receive this information four to six weeks past the end of the month to which it relates. Mr. J, the person in charge of the computer system, says that billing is the first priority and cost control reports are second. But that's neither here nor there, because content is the second and biggest problem with the cost control information. Even if I had the information on time, I would be hard-pressed to figure out what it means. The way that they figure out how much I should use every month is to take the amount that the controller finally arrives at after cuts and negotiation and divide by 12. This is crazy because it presupposes that we don't have busy months. In reality, we have months where our volume is twice that of slower months. It is difficult for me to know what being over or under budget means if the amount against which my costs are compared is some average that never really happens.

Of course, this is bad enough, but the way they determine my actual film usage is insane. The controller decided that too much bookkeeping effort would have to be expended to actually keep track of the amount of film we shoot in a month. So, the amount of film that I order in a

> month is used as a surrogate for actual film usage. This information is obtained from the purchase orders that I submit monthly to the purchasing department.
>
> I'll never forget the first year I was in this position. I knew about a sale on film and I ordered a three-month's supply. When we finally got the IBM run which shows the difference between actual usage and expected usage for the month, we were shocked. We had a budget overrun of approximately 230 percent. Everybody was jumping up and down. It was a madhouse. Finally, the controller, who forgot how they were measuring actual film usage (he is a busy man, I guess), and I figured out that since the amount of film that I purchased was substituted for actual film usage in the cost control report and since I purchased more than a month's worth of film, the budget overrun was not real at all, but instead was related to the way the computations are made.
>
> The funny thing is that the same thing happened a year later and the budget overrun popped up on a management exception report, so that I had to write a memo explaining the difference. I don't like to say I am too busy to bother with all of this red tape, but I hate to write these meaningless memos explaining what happened with their system. So since then I actually just process monthly purchase orders to equal one-twelfth of the amount I am allocated during the year. Then, for the last month, I order what I need. If I have to write a memo ... well, one is better than 12. I am not doing this under the table either. I told the controller what I was going to do and he seems to think that it is all right. I guess he doesn't like to read memos any more than I like to write them.

This example illustrates four additional problems that may be encountered whenever a standard or expected cost system is implemented in a health care setting. One fundamental problem with far-reaching consequences is the inaccurate measurement of standard, expected, or actual performance. If performance measurements are not accurate, effective control actions can never result from the analysis of variance contrasts. Another problem that may arise is the untimely communication of variance information. If performance deviations are reported too late, managers may be unable to take corrective actions, or may take ineffective actions. On the other hand, if performance deviations are communicated too early, managers may take premature corrective actions that are ineffective. The third problem that may occur is the communication of meaningless information. If the manager receives too much, too little, or the wrong information, the manager's ability to take effective actions is diminished. Finally, if managers are not rewarded for taking appropriate actions or penalized for taking inappropriate actions, they may be encouraged to act unreasonably (for example, overstating budgetary needs or adopting uneconomical purchasing patterns as illustrated in the case of the radiologist).

Conditions for an Effecteve Standard or Expected Cost System

At this point, the seven conditions necessary for developing, implementing, or operationalizing an effective standard or expected cost may be summarized.

Measurement and Definition Conditions:

- A measurable and relevant unit of output must be specified.
- The equivalent units of production (EUP) or the equivalent units of service (EUS) must be computed.
- The standard or expected number of units (γ_i) of material, labor, and overhead necessary to complete one unit of output must be specified.

Management Information Systems Conditions:

- A means of accurately measuring standard, expected, and actual performance must exist.
- The information system must be capable of generating the appropriate control information on a timely basis (see Problem 10-5).
- A means of ascertaining what information will be useful and meaningful to decision makers must be available.
- A system must be established for rewarding managers for taking appropriate actions or penalizing them for taking inappropriate actions.

These seven conditions constrain the development of cost control systems to the extent that standard and expected cost systems currently are impractical for most activities in the health care environment. However, cost control is a managerial imperative. Hence, the managers in most health care institutions must opt for a third, more loosely defined method of cost control, which will be referred to as a cost finding system. A cost finding system is a systematic methodology by which total costs are identified and allocated to particular activities, yielding disaggregated cost information. A cost finding system is capable of providing information useful in controlling costs, and is the first step in the staged evolution of cost control in the health care industry from cost finding to cost control with expectations or standards.

COST FINDING SYSTEMS

Cost finding is the rudimentary aspect of cost control. Both the standard and the expected cost systems are dependent on cost finding systems (i.e., standard and expected cost systems require a cost finding rationale to develop useful performance variances). However, analysis of cost finding statistics does not presuppose the existence of standards or managerial expectations used to evaluate cost variances.

As suggested in Chapter 7, specific assignment assumptions usually are necessary for four types of costs: direct variable cost (DVC), indirect variable cost (IVC), direct fixed cost (DFC), and indirect fixed costs (IFC). The relationship between performance evaluation and cost assignment is illustrated in Figure 10-2. Although the technical aspects of the cost finding system are relatively simple, involving only the assignment of costs to specific activities, rationalizing the allocation assumptions often is very difficult.

Figure 10-2 indicates that the usefulness of the information provided by a cost finding system is dependent on the isolation and analysis of cost finding performance variances, and the specification of noncost measures of performance. Each of these aspects of a cost finding control system is discussed in the following sections. In addition, a case study is presented to illustrate the operationalization of a cost finding system in a health care setting.

Isolation of Performance Variances: A Cost Finding Perspective

In both the standard and the expected cost systems, the performance variances are developed as the difference between budgeted and actual costs. However, standards or managerial expectations are not fundamental to the development of performance variances. In fact, meaningful variances may be isolated whenever a difference occurs between two comparable measures of performance. Hence, if the current actual costs developed by the cost finding system can be contrasted with some other comparable costs, (i.e., other period costs or other institutional costs), a cost finding variance analysis can be performed.

For example, suppose the cardiac labor costs developed under a cost finding system in year i are:

(10-5)
$$CLC_i = AWR_i \times AH_i$$

where: CLC_i represents the total actual cardiac labor costs in year i;
AWR_i represents the actual wage rate for cardiac labor used in year i; and
AH_i represents the actual number of cardiac labor hours used in year i.

Figure 10-2 Cost Finding: The Generation of Performance Variances and the Evaluation of Analysis of Variance Information

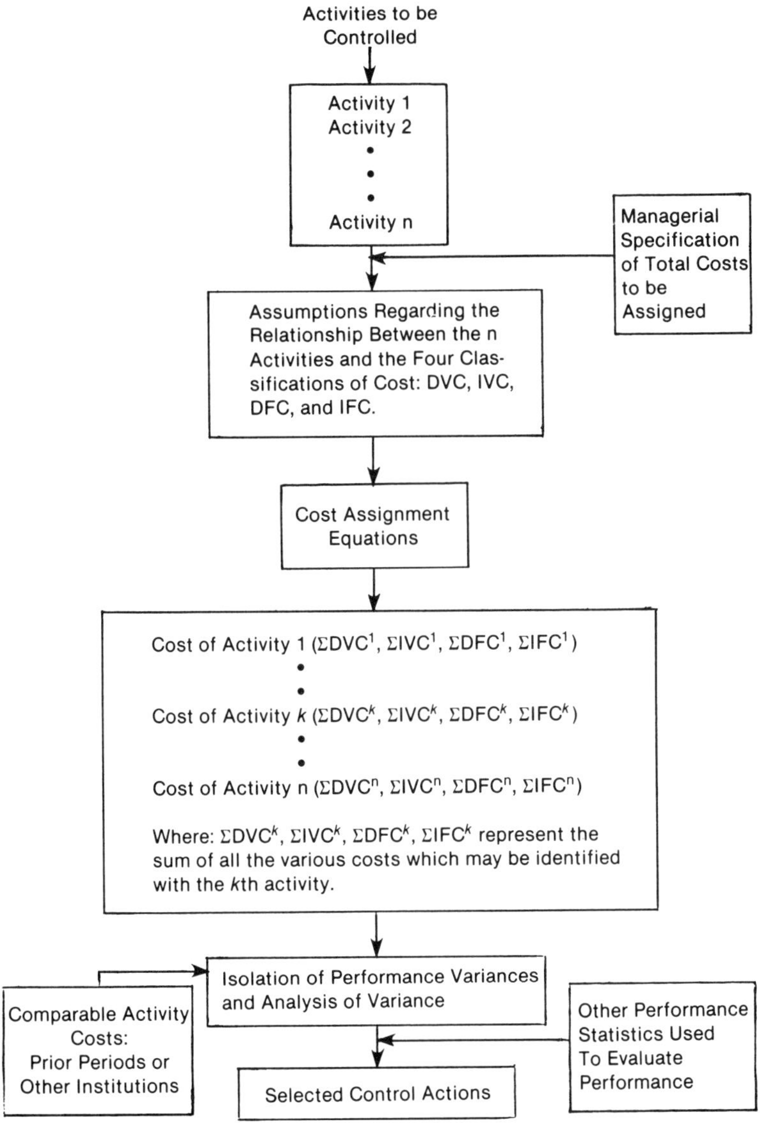

Given this computation, the following performance variance could be isolated for the cardiac labor costs between years 2 and 1:

(10-6)
$$V_{cc} = CLC_1 - CLC_2$$
$$= (AWR_1 \times AH_1) - (AWR_2 \times AH_2)$$

where: V_{cc} is the difference in total cardiac labor costs (variance) between years 2 and 1.

This total labor variance (V_{cc}) is comprised of a labor rate and a labor efficiency variance.[5] The labor rate variance is computed as:

(10-7)
$$\text{Labor Rate Variance} = AH_2 \times (AWR_1 - AWR_2).$$

The labor efficiency variance is computed as:

(10-8)
$$\text{Labor Efficiency Variance} = AWR_1 \times (AH_1 - AH_2).$$

The sum of the labor rate and efficiency variances is equal to the total labor performance variance. This may be demonstrated as follows.

$$V_{cc} = [AH_2 \times (AWR_1 - AWR_2)] + [AWR_1 \times (AH_1 - AH_2)]$$
$$= (AWR_1 \times AH_1) - (AWR_1 \times AH_2) + (AWR_1 \times AH_2) - (AWR_2 \times AH_2)$$
$$= (AWR_1 \times AH_1) - (AWR_2 \times AH_2)$$

Although a rate and an efficiency variance can be computed under a cost finding system, the cost finding analysis of variance is not capable of providing the same quality of information derived in a standard cost system. Care must be taken to understand the meaning of cost finding activity contrasts so that effective control actions may be formulated. To provide information useful in evaluating the analysis of variance information developed in a cost finding system, performance statistics other than cost must be developed.

Augmenting the Cost Finding System: Development of Noncost Measures of Performance

To balance the organization's decision-making system, performance should be judged with respect to its effect on all of the performance statistics relevant in making managerial decisions. Control based on only one performance statistic may cause resource allocations that are dysfunctional in achieving the institution's mission. Usually, in standard, and sometimes in expected cost systems, other performance measures are not integrated into the organizational evaluation process because standards and expectations are presumed to be associated implicitly with the organization's goals. Therefore, the analysis of an isolated cost variance from the standard is assumed to imply a set of corrective actions which would be both coordinated with the institution's mission and effective in eliminating undesired performance deviations. Of course, this is more of a theoretic assumption than a practical reality.

In a cost finding system, other performance measures must be used to balance the organization's control process so that corrective actions may be coordinated with achievement of the institution's mission. The reason for this is simply that cost finding contrasts are limited to intra-institutional temporal contrasts or interinstitutional contrasts. The analysis of these variances implies nothing about the desirability of particular corrective actions relative to the mission of the organization. Therefore, noncost measures of performance must be used to augment the analysis of the cost finding variances.

The following case study illustrates the assignment of total costs to activities, the development of noncost measures of performance, and the analysis of variance in an emergency medical services unit.[6] The focus of the case discussion is restricted to the technical aspects of developing particular cost assignments and specifying noncost measures of performance. An analysis of the institutional corrective actions elicited from an analysis of performance variations cannot be presented, given the experimental nature of the institutional participation in this study.

EMERGENCY MEDICAL SERVICES COSTING: A CASE STUDY

Currently, few funding or planning agencies require a disaggregated differentiation of service costs. As a consequence, only aggregated emergency medical services (EMS) costs must be reported, as exemplified by the Medicare Cost Report. This aggregated EMS performance information has been criticized as not providing information useful for evaluating a health care delivery system or making institutional decisions. To be useful, such information must be disaggregated to describe the performance of the elements in the system which are under the decision maker's control (see the responsibility accounting discussion in Chapter 7).

The degree of aggregation found in most current EMS reporting makes the task of rationally evaluating the relationship between EMS costs and unit performance most difficult. Disaggregation of EMS cost information is important to effect both a comprehensive description of the institution's EMS delivery system and managerial change. This study focuses on the disaggregation of EMS cost information to effect a comprehensive description of the EMS delivery system, assuming the means to implement change exist within the political structure of the institution.

Aggregation of Service: Ways of Reporting EMS Performance Statistics

To develop a cost finding system, some meaningful level of activity or service aggregation must be selected. The selected aggregation should be more diverse than complete aggregation (i.e., the EMS unit), and more amalgamated than complete disaggregation (i.e., a particular service task). Once this activity level has been selected, cost assignments may be developed (see Figure 10-2).

EMS services may be categorized into service categories and crisis classes. Service categories are distinct treatment patterns requiring specific EMS resources. Crisis classes are those service groupings which manifest patient-oriented service needs.

Although service categories currently are not mandated aggregations of service, these categories may be developed through interviews with the treatment personnel involved in providing EMS service. First, the diagnoses which occur most frequently in the EMS unit must be delineated. Second, the treatment patterns associated with these diagnoses must be specified. Third, those diagnoses which are related to recognized medical specialties should be assigned to the same service category. Finally, based upon the diagnoses included in each grouping, the service categories should be named. In the nine study hospitals, cardiac, dental, gynecology, orthopedics, and primary medical often emerged as service categories (see Appendix 10-A).

Like service categories, crisis classes currently are not mandated aggregations of service. However, the American Medical Association has suggested the use of the following three crisis classes.

Crisis Class I. *Emergency*: Patient requires immediate attention; delay is harmful to patient. Disorder is acute and potentially threatens life or function.

Crisis Class II. *Urgent*: Patient requires medical attention within a few hours. Patient is in danger if unattended. Danger is acute, but not necessarily severe.

Crisis Class III. *Nonurgent*: Patient does not require the resources of an emergency service. Disorder is minor or nonacute.

Service categories and crisis classes are the major groupings within which the following performance measures may be reported.

1. Cost (the primary control focus)
2. Patient waiting time } Performance statistics augmenting the
3. Staff standby time } cost finding system

These three performance measures are suggested to develop a comprehensive evaluation of the management of EMS resources.

Cost Aggregation and Development of Assignment Equations

As suggested in Figure 10-2, after the various activities are identified, the total costs to be assigned must be specified (aggregation). Then, these total costs must be assigned to the various activities to be controlled (disaggregation).

Development of Total Costs: Cost Aggregation

A number of methods may be used to derive total EMS costs. The simplest method is to use the Medicare Cost Report as the first approximation of total costs and then make the necessary cost reclassification entries. These cost adjustments should attempt to correct any questionable allocations. For example, in one of the study hospitals, seven clerks were assigned to the EMS unit. However, the salaries of two of them were included in the administrative and general costs.[7] In this case, the following cost reclassification entry was necessary:

EMS Unit Costs	$15,650	
Administrative and General Costs		$15,650

To reclassify the costs associated with two EMS unit clerks whose salaries were erroneously classified as part of administrative and general costs.

Once the appropriate costs have been identified and adjusted, the total costs must be assigned (disaggregated) to the various service categories. During the study, four major classes of costs were found to be applicable to EMS service categories: direct salaries (medical and other), other direct costs, indirect costs (principally fixed cost allocations), and ancillary costs.[8] These costs were assigned to the various service categories using a methodology that apportioned the costs on an objective basis.

Direct Salaries Assigned to Service Categories: Cost Disaggregation

Of the four cost classes, the allocation of direct salaries to service categories is the most complex, because recording actual service category treatment time is impractical and surrogate measures must be developed. To assign the direct salary costs for physicians, nurses, and other medical personnel (the three personnel treatment components identified in this study), the average treatment time must be approximated for the various service categories.[9] This approximated average treatment time may be used to apportion direct salaries to EMS service categories.

The total treatment time identified with the hth treatment component in the the ith service category (SC_i^h) is the product of (1) the average time that the hth treatment component takes to treat the various diagnoses constituting that service category, and (2) the number of visits in that service category. This may be represented as:

$$SC_i^h = \left[\sum_{j=1}^{n_i^h} \frac{d_j^h}{n_i^h} \right] \times V_i \quad i = 1, \ldots, k \tag{10-9}$$

where: SC_i^h represents the estimated total treatment time identified with the hth treatment component in the ith service category;
d_j^h represents the average treatment time that the individuals constituting the hth treatment component take to treat diagnosis j;
n_i^h represents the number of diagnoses treated by the hth treatment component in the ith service category;
i is an index for the k service categories;
h is an index identifying the various treatment components (e.g., h = physicians (P), nurses (N), or other medical personnel (OM)); and
V_i represents the number of visits in the ith service category.

Hence, the total treatment time (TTT) provided by the hth treatment component in the EMS unit may be estimated as:

$$TTT^h = \sum_{i=1}^{k} SC_i^h. \tag{10-10}$$

Using these estimates, the total salary paid to the hth treatment component may be allocated among the service categories as follows:

$$AS_i^h = S^h \times (SC_i^h/TTT^h) \quad i = 1, \ldots, k \tag{10-11}$$

where: AS_i^h represents the salary allocated to the *i*th service category from the *h*th treatment component;
S^h represents the total salary dollars paid to the *h*th treatment component; and
SC_i^h/TTT^h represents the treatment time allocation percentage used to allocate the *h*th salary component to the *i*th service category.

Once the total salary paid has been allocated to particular service categories, the per visit salary cost for the *h*th treatment component may be computed for each service category. This computation may be represented as follows:

$$PVSC_i^h = AS_i^h / V_i \tag{10-12}$$

where: $PVSC_i^h$ represents the per visit salary cost of the *h*th treatment component in the *i*th service category.

Note that the salary dollars (S^h) represents total time paid, including both productive and unproductive time (vacation, sick, and standby time) for individuals engaged in the delivery of service in the EMS unit. Hence, in equation (10-11) both productive and unproductive direct salary costs are allocated to the various service categories. To separate the cost of unproductive time from the cost of productive time, the total salary and the total time paid must be known. With this information, the cost of unproductive time for the *h*th treatment component ($CUPT^h$) can be computed as:

$$CUPT^h = S^h \times (1 - TTT^h/TP^h) \tag{10-13}$$

where: TP^h represents the total time paid for the *h*th treatment component during the period.

For example, assume that total salaries for physicians and nurses must be apportioned between two service categories, cardiac and orthopedic (see Appendix 10-A). Suppose the estimated treatment times for the physician (P) and nurse (N) treatment components are as shown in Table 10-1. Suppose, too, that the total number of visits in each service category during several days are as follows.

Cardiac Visits (V_1): 39
Orthopedic Visits (V_2): 108

Table 10-1 Estimated Physician and Nurse Treatment Times in the EMS Unit

Service Category	Estimated Average Treatment Time in the EMS Unit	
	Physician	Nurse
Cardiac (SC_1):		
Congestive Heart Failure	15 minutes	10 minutes
Hypertension	5 minutes	40 minutes
Myocardial Infarction	25 minutes	N/A*
Orthopedic (SC_2):		
Dislocations	15 minutes	5 minutes
Spasms/Pain	5 minutes	30 minutes
Fracture	30 minutes	5 minutes

*Assume that nurses are not used in the EMS Unit for individuals diagnosed as myocardial infarction patients.

Then the total treatment time for the two service categories, SC_1^P, SC_1^N (cardiac) and SC_2^P, SC_2^N (orthopedic) would be formulated as follows.

$$SC_1^P = \left[\sum_{j=1}^{n_1^P} \frac{d_j^P}{n_1^P}\right] \times V_1 = \frac{(15 + 5 + 25)}{3} \times 39 = 585 \text{ minutes;}$$

$$SC_1^N = \left[\sum_{j=1}^{n_1^N} \frac{d_j^N}{n_1^N}\right] \times V_1 = \frac{(10 + 40)}{2} \times 39 = 975 \text{ minutes}$$

$$SC_2^P = \left[\sum_{j=1}^{n_2^P} \frac{d_j^P}{n_2^P}\right] \times V_2 = \frac{(15 + 5 + 30)}{3} \times 108 = 1{,}800 \text{ minutes;}$$

$$SC_2^N = \left[\sum_{j=1}^{n_2^N} \frac{d_j^N}{n_2^N}\right] \times V_2 = \frac{(5 + 30 + 5)}{3} \times 108 = 1{,}440 \text{ minutes}$$

In this case, the total treatment time for physicians and nurses may be computed as:

$$\begin{aligned} TTT^P &= \sum_{i=1}^{2} SC_i^P \\ &= 585 + 1{,}800 \\ &= 2{,}385 \text{ minutes;} \end{aligned}$$

$$\begin{aligned} TTT^N &= \sum_{i=1}^{2} SC_i^N \\ &= 975 + 1{,}440 \\ &= 2{,}415 \text{ minutes.} \end{aligned}$$

If the total salary paid to physicians is \$3,849.60, then the physicians' salary dollars would be allocated as follows (see Problem 10-7):

$$\begin{aligned} AS_1^P &= S^P \times (SC_1^P/TTT^P) \\ &= \$3{,}849.60 \times (585/2385) \\ &= \$944.24 \end{aligned}$$

$$\begin{aligned} AS_2^P &= S^P \times (SC_2^P/TTT^P) \\ &= \$3{,}849.60 \times (1800/2385) \\ &= \$2{,}905.36 \end{aligned}$$

The physician cost per visit for the two service categories would be:

$$\begin{aligned} PVSC_1^P &= AS_1^P/V_1 \\ &= \$944.24/39 \\ &= \$24.21 \end{aligned}$$

$$\begin{aligned} PVSC_2^P &= AS_2^P/V_2 \\ &= \$2{,}905.36/108 \\ &= \$26.90 \end{aligned}$$

Finally, if a total of 43.283 hours were paid in the EMS unit during the period, the cost of unproductive time for the physician component would be (see Question 10-7):

$$\begin{aligned} CUPT^P &= S^P \times \left[1 - \frac{TTT^P}{TP^P}\right] \\ &= \$3{,}849.60 \times \left[1 - \frac{2385}{2597}\right] \\ &= \$314.25. \end{aligned}$$

In this example, as in most practical situations, total visits are not disaggregated to reflect the number of visits for each diagnosis in a particular service category because a significant amount of time and expense is associated with the collection of such detailed visit information. Therefore, only total cardiac visits, $V_1 = 39$, and total orthopedic visits, $V_2 = 108$, have been abstracted from the institution's information systems. However, note that a significantly different salary apportionment could occur if detailed visit information were available and the visits were not uniformly distributed.

For example, assume that the information in Table 10-2 has been collected regarding the treatment mix in the example above.
The physician treatment time per service category would be:

$$SC_1{}^P = \frac{(15 \times 1) + (5 \times 31) + (25 \times 7)}{39} \times 39 = 345$$

$$SC_2{}^P = \frac{(15 \times 36) + (5 \times 41) + (30 \times 31)}{108} \times 108 = \underline{1675}$$

$$\underline{\underline{2020}} \text{ minutes.}$$

The physicians' salary dollars allocation would be:

$$AS_1{}^P = \$3{,}849.60 \times \left(\frac{345}{2020}\right)$$
$$= \$657.49$$
$$AS_2{}^P = \$3{,}849.60 \times \left(\frac{1675}{2020}\right)$$
$$= \$3{,}192.11.$$

Table 10-2 Detailed Visit Information for the Cardiac and Orthopedic Service Categories

Cardiac Visits (V_1):	
Congestive Heart Failure	1
Hypertension	31
Myocardial Infarction	7
Total	39
Orthopedic Visits (V_2):	
Dislocations	36
Spasms/Pain	41
Fracture	31
Total	108

Given this information, the per visit physician salary costs would be:

$$\mathrm{PVSC}_1^P = \$16.86$$

$$\mathrm{PVSC}_2^P = \$29.56,$$

while the cost of unproductive time would be:

$$\begin{aligned}\mathrm{CUPT}^P &= \$3{,}849.60 \times \left[1 - \frac{2020}{2597}\right] \\ &= \$855.30.\end{aligned}$$

As this simple illustration demonstrates, the results obtained using the weighted average method can be dramatically different from those obtained using the simple average method. Although the simple average method is less accurate than the weighted average method when utilization differences exist, the simple average method is less costly to implement. Hence, it is not surprising that the nine hospitals that participated in the EMS study indicated that the simple average method was the only practical alternative for cost allocation purposes.

Other Personnel Costs Assigned to Service Categories: Cost Disaggregation

The other direct salaries involved in servicing the EMS unit can be assigned to service categories according to the number of visits in each service category. This basis of assignment is preferable to direct assignment due to the relative immateriality of the dollars to be allocated and the availability of the visit statistics. Hence, the allocation of other direct salaries can be computed as:

$$\text{(10-14)} \qquad \mathrm{OP}_i = \left[\frac{V_i}{\sum_{j=1}^{k} V_j}\right] \times \mathrm{TSPO} \qquad i = 1, \ldots, k$$

where: OP_i represents the cost of the other personnel salaries allocated to the ith service category;
V_i represents the number of visits in the ith service category; and
TSPO represents the total salary paid to the other EMS personnel.

Other Direct and Indirect Costs Assigned to Service Categories: Cost Disaggregation

The other direct and indirect costs may be assigned to service categories based upon the relative proportion of service category visits. The one exception to this rule is building depreciation for each service category. Depreciation is more equitably and simply assigned according to the floor space, measured in units of square footage, in each service category. However, if any of the other direct and indirect costs are used exclusively in the delivery of services in a particular service category, they should be included in that category.

Ancillary Costs Assigned to Service Categories: Cost Disaggregation

The ancillary cost information is abstracted from three sources: Medicare Report C, Medicare Report CI, and a form containing ancillary charge information on an individual diagnosis basis. The Medicare forms are used to develop a ratio of ancillary cost to ancillary charges. This unit cost multiplier is applied to the accumulated ancillary charges for the ith service category to determine the ancillary cost, AC_i, that should be assigned to the ith service category. This computation is represented as:

(10-15) $$AC_i = TAC_i \times (x/y) \qquad i = 1, \ldots, k$$

where: AC_i represents the ancillary cost allocated to the ith service category;
x represents total ancillary costs (Medicare C);
y represents total ancillary charges (Medicare CI); and
TAC_i represents the total charges in the ancillary department for the ith service category.

Time Statistics

As suggested in Figure 10-2, other performance statistics are necessary to interpret the statistics developed in a cost finding system. Two time statistics, patient waiting time and staff standby time, are suggested in this study to establish an evaluative context for the EMS cost statistics. These time statistics, along with the various cost statistics, may be used to evaluate the state of the EMS system.

Patient Waiting Time: A Noncost EMS Performance Statistic

Patient waiting time is measured as the interval between the time the individual enters the EMS system and the time treatment begins. An individual is considered to have entered when a medical record data sheet is completed by an EMS clerk, diagnosing nurse, or physician. The waiting time interval ceases only when treatment begins, because even though a preliminary diagnosis may be made immediately, treatment may not begin for a considerable period of time. Measuring the time interval from admission to diagnosis ordinarily would not give an accurate measure of the amount of time individuals wait in the EMS system.

The time that individuals spend waiting for ancillary services is included in the patient waiting time computation, because the ancillary services are not in the same general area as the EMS unit in most of the study hospitals. Hence, a patient often must go to some remote location for an ancillary workup. These logistical problems usually give rise to waiting time.

Staff Standby Time: A Noncost EMS Performance Statistic

As indicated previously, total salary paid is allocated to various service categories on the basis of total treatment time (Equation (10-11)). Therefore, a portion of each service category cost is the salary cost of having individuals available but not engaged in the delivery of service (standby time), as differentiated from unproductive time (Equation (10-13)). To evaluate the use of treatment staff personnel, standby time should be identified on a per staff basis and reported along with the patient waiting time and the cost statistics. For example, the standby hours per full-time physician per period (SBH^P) may be computed as (see Question 10-7):

$$\text{(10-16)} \qquad SBH^P = (TP^P - (TTT^P + VST^P))/NS^P$$

where: TP^P represents the actual physician hours paid during the period;
TTT^P represents the total treatment time provided by physicians during the period;
VST^P represents the vacation and sick time paid (in hours) to physicians; and
NS^P represents the number of physicians involved in diagnosis and treatment in the EMS unit.

To illustrate the interpretation of these three statistics—service category cost, patient waiting time, and standby time—consider the following example. Assume that the per visit cost of a particular service category for Hospital A and Hospital B are $27.83 and $12.53, respectively. The time statistics for a selected study week in the two hospitals are represented in Table 10-3. In this case, the lower costs per patient reported by Hospital B may occur because the medical staff is overutilized as implied by the relatively long per patient waiting time. The EMS system of Hospital B may be operating at or beyond its capacity. On the other hand, the higher EMS costs of Hospital A may be related to an underutilized staff, as evidenced by the nominal waiting time and relatively high staff standby

Table 10-3 Statistics Used to Augment the Interpretation of Service Category Cost Information

Service Category	Hospital A	Hospital B
Patient waiting time (per patient)	1 minute	38 minutes
Staff standby time (per physician)	12 hours	0

time. Of course, these evaluative inferences must be examined more systematically before corrective actions are taken. The point of this simple example is to indicate the use of the three statistics in developing an investigative focus. The following example further illustrates the analysis of cost finding statistics.

EMS Costing: An Illustration Using Three Service Categories

In this section, the cost finding statistics for the service categories of three hospitals which participated in an EMS cost finding study are presented. The cost and time statistics for the cardiac, medical, and obstetrics/gynecology service categories are considered.

Cost Finding and Time Statistics

Usually before a cost finding system can be implemented, the costs reported by the hospital for the EMS activity must be adjusted to measure total costs. Material adjustments had to be made to the medical costs reported by the study hospitals (see Table 10-4). Once the total actual EMS costs have been approximated, the service category treatment time allocation percentages (SC_i^h/TTT^h) can be computed. The allocation percentages for physician (P), nurse (N), and other medical (OM) treatment components are reported in Table 10-5.

Table 10-4 Total Direct Costs Statistics for Three Study Institutions

Hospital	Total Costs After Adjustment (1)	Total Costs Before Adjustment (2)	Difference (1 − 2)
1	$1,002,705	$571,797	$430,908
2	753,926	600,552	153,374
3	1,144,723	609,243	535,480

Table 10-5 Treatment Time Allocation Percentages

Hospital	Cardiac (SC_1^h)			Medical (SC_2^h)			ObGyn (SC_3^h)		
	P	N	OM	P	N	OM	P	N	OM
1	3.15*	4.25	15.25	31.27	44.46	8.9	2.94	2.14	5.44
2	13.65	11.37	14.23	31.4	26.69	5.54	2.62	3.30	6.29
3	6.19	9.69	16.69	32.73	36.54	8.12	9.92	6.91	7.54

*From equations (10-9) and (10-10), the treatment time allocation percentage may be computed as:

$$\frac{\sum_{j=1}^{n_1^P} (d_j^P / n_1^P) \times V_1}{TTT^P} = \frac{17.66 \text{ (minutes)} \times 1080}{605{,}485 \text{ minutes}} = 3.15\%.$$

Table 10-6 Per Visit Costs for Three Selected Service Categories

	Cardiac				Medical				ObGyn			
Hospital	Direct Salary (P, N, OM)	Other Direct and Indirect Expenses	Ancillary	Total Cost per Visit	Direct Salary	Other Direct and Indirect Expenses	Ancillary	Total Cost per Visit	Direct Salary	Other Direct and Indirect Expenses	Ancillary	Total Cost per Visit
1	$12.56*	$9.81	$26.84	$49.21	$4.68	$9.81	$7.79	$22.39	$4.55	$9.81	$10.95	$25.31
2	14.47	6.34	4.39	25.20	4.59	6.34	6.01	16.94	7.62	6.34	3.93	17.89
3	16.80	6.60	6.27	29.67	4.77	6.58	9.40	20.75	7.06	6.58	5.78	19.42

*The per visit costs (see equation (10-12)) for the direct salary component of the cardiac service of hospital 1 are computed as follows:

$$\left[\frac{S^P \times 3.15\% + S^N \times 4.25\% + S^{OM} \times 15.25\%}{V_1}\right] = \frac{\$9{,}788.00 + \$2{,}365.00 + \$1{,}425.00}{1080} = \frac{\$13{,}578.00}{1080} = \$12.56.$$

The products of these percentages and the salary paid each of the respective treatment components are combined with the other direct and indirect expenses per visit (which are combined for presentation purposes) and ancillary costs per visit to develop per visit total cost (see Table 10-6).

As suggested, these cost statistics should be augmented by other noncost measures of performance. In this case, standby time and waiting time were collected. However, only the waiting time statistics are reported (Table 10-7), because the participating institutions requested that the standby statistics be withheld from publication.

Cost Finding Analysis of Variances: EMS Temporal Contrasts

In a cost finding system such as the one discussed here, two contrasts are possible: (1) contrasts of performance statistics among hospitals, and (2) temporal performance contrasts for the institution. Given the autonomous nature of hospitals and the information required to isolate and analyze cost finding variances, interhospital analysis of variance is not a reasonable alternative. Therefore, temporal cost contrasts have been computed. The following example examines the performance variance for the direct salary component of the cardiac service category for one of the study hospitals over a two-year period.

The per visit direct salary components of the cardiac service category for the first and second years are $12.43 and $12.56, respectively. The temporal performance variance of $.13 ($12.56 − $12.43) certainly does not appear to be significant. Although the management may assume that the variance of $.13 need not be investigated, this is not a valid assumption because the per visit salary component is composed of a number of elements. Analysis of variance can have investigative meaning only when the elements of the performance contrasts are completely disaggregated and the disaggregated elements are contrasted. In this case, the various elements which constitute the computation of the per unit direct salary component, as represented in Table 10-8, must be examined.

Table 10-7 Waiting Time per Patient (minutes) in Three Study Institutions

Hospital	Cardiac	Medical	Ob/Gyn
1	5.6	6.9	2.2
2	3.9	2.0	6.8
3	1.0	11.2	18.6

Table 10-8 Analysis of Salary Component: Cardiac Service

Component	Hospital 1, Year 1	Hospital 1, Year 2
Direct Physician	$ 6,989.00	$ 9,788.00
Nurses	6,346.00	2,365.00
Other Medical	7,878.00	1,425.00
Total Cost	$24,106.00	$13,578.00
Number of Cardiac Visits	1,939	1,080
Per Unit Cost	$12.43	$12.56

Assume that after examining these figures, the administrator decides to investigate the nursing and the other medical components. The decline of $3,981 ($6,346 − $2,365) in direct nursing salaries must be analyzed in terms of the volume of nursing hours and the per hour cost. In the first year, 1,468 nursing hours were used in the EMS department, yielding a wage rate of $4.32 per hour ($6,346/1,468). In the second year, 541 nursing hours were used in the EMS department, yielding a wage rate of $4.37 per hour ($2,365/541). Therefore, this variance is primarily one of efficiency (see Footnote 5).

The other medical direct salary hours for the first and second years were 993 hours and 458 hours, respectively, yielding the following wage rates:

Year 1 = ($7,878/993) = $7.9335347 per hour

Year 2 = ($1,425/458) = $3.1113537 per hour.

Given this information, the total other medical performance variance of $6,453 ($7,878 − $1,425) may be described in terms of the labor rate variance and the labor efficiency variance as follows:

$$\text{Labor Rate Variance} = AH_2 \times (AWR_1 - AWR_2) \quad (10\text{-}7)$$

$$\text{Labor Efficiency Variance} = AWR_1 \times (AH_1 - AH_2) \quad (10\text{-}8)$$

where: $AWR_{1,2}$ are the actual wage rates for the other medical personnel for years 1 and 2;
$AH_{1,2}$ are the service hours of the other medical personnel for years 1 and 2; and
the subscripts 1,2 indicate respective years.

Hence, the labor rate and labor efficiency variances for other medical direct salary hours would be:

$$\text{Labor Rate Variance} = 458 \times (\$7.9335347 - \$3.1113537)$$
$$= \$2,208.56$$

$$\text{Labor Efficiency Variance} = \$7.9335347 \times (993 - 458)$$
$$= \$4,244.44$$

giving a total variance of $6,453.

In this case, these variance results are consistent with the administrator's expectations, because in the second year the EMS unit began referring various cardiac cases to a new cardiac unit. Since these patients formerly were treated by nurses and interns (who are classified as other medical personnel) in the EMS unit, the number of direct nursing hours and direct other medical hours used in the treatment of cardiac patients were reduced in the second year. Furthermore, cardiac patients treated in the EMS unit in the second year were treated primarily by paramedic trainees (other medical personnel), who are paid lower salaries than interns. Hence, the direct other medical wage rate was lower in the second year than in the first.

Appendix 10-A

Diagnosis Classification

Based Upon Interviews with EMS Personnel, Study Hospital #3

Cardiac
- Congestive Heart Failure (CHF)
- Hypertension
- Myocardial Infarction

Major Trauma
- Concussion
- Gun Shot Wounds (GSW)
- Knife Wounds
- Contusions (EYE/ORBIT)

Surgical
- Appendicitis
- Tonsillitis

Orthopedic
- Dislocations
- Spasms/Pain
- Fracture

Obstetric/Gynecologic
- Pregnancy
- Pelvic Inflammation Disease (PID)
- Vaginitis (Inflammation)

Psychiatric
- Suicide Attempt
- Anxiety/Hysteria

Neurological
- Strokes (CVA)
- Seizure Disorder (Convulsions

Medical
- Gastritis
- Gastroenteritis
- Anemia
- Diabetes
- Hyperventillation Problem
- Arthritis
- Headache-Migraine/Tension
- Urinary Tract Infection (UTI)
- Drug Abuse
- Normal Exam-No Significant Findings
- Poisoning Accidental
- Reactions-Allergic, Drug, Chemical, Other
- Dead-on-Arrival (DOA)
- Flu Syndrome

Minor Trauma
- Abcesses
- Bites (Animal-Human-Insect)
- Burns
- Infections/Foreign Body
- Puncture Wounds/Foreign Body

Alcoholic
- Intoxication-Alcoholic "Chemical-Etoh"

Dental
- Dental Clinic
- Accident

NOTES

1. The reasonableness of performance standards included in the tactical budget depends upon how well the performance measures and the tactical plan relate to the mission of the organization. Recall that the tactical budget is presumed to be developed by the chief financial officer or budgeting committee in considering the organization's mission (see Figure 9-1).

2. Note that the following is also true:

$$\text{Direct Labor Performance Variance} = [(\text{SWR} - \text{AWR}) \times \text{SH}] + [(\text{SH} - \text{AH}) \times \text{AWR}]$$

$$= (\text{SWR} \times \text{SH}) - (\text{AWR} \times \text{AH}).$$

3. To illustrate this calculation, consider the following example. Assume that 1,200 units are completed during the period. Further assume that 400 units, 70 percent complete as to material, labor, and overhead, were in process at the beginning of the period. If 200 units, 30 percent complete as to material, labor, and overhead, are in process at the end of the period, the equivalent units of production may be computed as follows.

1. The number of units completed during the period:	1,200
2. Less the number of equivalent units in process at the beginning of the period (400 × .70):	280
Equivalent units completed during the period	920
3. Plus the number of equivalent units in process at the end of the period (200 × .30):	60
Equivalent units of production	980

4. The interview has been paraphrased from the consultant's interview notes.

5. Note that in a cost finding system the term "efficiency" variance may be a misnomer, because instead of being compared with standard performance, performance is compared with that in another period or another institution where the number of service units rendered may be different from the number used to generate the cost finding statistics.

6. This case is abstracted from a report to HEW (HSM 110-71-256 Health Resources Administration). Nine hospitals participated in the study.

7. At the time of this study, inpatient services had a higher reimbursement rate than outpatient services. Hence, the cost allocation was biased in favor of inpatient services.

8. During the early phases of the study, costs were classified as direct variable, indirect variable, direct fixed, and indirect fixed. After various classification efforts, the following four cost assignment groupings were formulated: direct salaries (DVC), other direct costs (DVC, DFC), indirect costs (IVC, IFC), and ancillary costs (DVC). The grouping simplified the allocation system and was preferred by the participating institutions.

9. This treatment time information may be difficult to gather, requiring either engineering studies of the time and motion variety or the elicitation of various treatment times from the appropriate EMS staff. In this study, the latter method was elected. The treatment time information was gathered in three institutions with little or no complication. The various estimates were all reasonably close.

Questions and Problems

Question 10-1. Discuss the relationship between tactical budgeting systems and variance analysis in a cost finding system.

Question 10-2. Evaluate and discuss the following statement: If standard measures of performance exist, the organization may use cost finding information to develop a standard cost accounting system.

Question 10-3. Prepare a diagram which details the relationships among the budgeting process, the development of expected performance measures, and the control of operations.

Question 10-4. Assume you are the manager of a service laboratory. Develop a comprehensive set of cost allocation equations such as those developed in the EMS case study, and indicate what performance variances you would analyze.

Question 10-5. The difference between performance standards and expectations may be useful in developing insights regarding long-range policy changes which may be required to achieve the mission of the institution. Assuming that the contrast {standards vs. expectations} is used to provide such planning information, suggest how the contrast {standard vs. actual} may be used to generate useful operational and long-range planning information.

Question 10-6. Assume you are a consultant investigating the inability of the hospital's budgeting system to provide information useful in controlling hospital resources. During an interview with a physician who is a responsible department head, the following comment is made: "So you want to know how I use the budgeting variance reports (they are generated monthly and are about 30 pages). Well, I bring them home for my kids to take to school for art class. The backs of the reports make great finger painting paper."

Required:

a. What are at least four possible reasons for the comments made by the department head?
b. Suggest a means of correction for each reason.
c. How would you evaluate the cost and benefit of each corrective action taken in (b)?

Question 10-7. Consider Equations (10-13) and (10-16). Is it possible for the $CUPT^h$ or SBH^h to be negative? Interpret a negative $CUPT^h$ or a negative SBH^h.

Problem 10-1. You are the administrator of a large progressive prepaid group. For a number of years, you have been studying the control possibilities afforded by an expected cost system. You have concentrated on the labor component of activity, since this component represents 81 percent of your organization's controllable cost. You intend to put several departments on the expected cost system on July 1, 19X1. During March, you collect the following information regarding the general medical clinic:

GMC Expected Costing Information

	Total	Physician	Nurse
1. Actual Hours Worked	1,350	337.5	1,012.5
2. Actual Payroll	$9,639.00	$4,455.00	$5,184.00
3. Expected Salary per Hour	—	$12.00	$5.50
4. Number of Patients	3,570	—	—
5. Expected Service Hours per Patient	—	.1	.5

Required:

a. Compute and analyze the variance for the physician and the nursing components of the GMC.
b. Write a letter to the head of nursing explaining the meaning of the variances.
c. After receiving the letter, the head of nursing attempts to verify your figures, but is unable to do so. The figures developed by the head of nursing are as follows.

Efficiency Variance

$$\$5.12\ [1012.5 - 1785] = \$3{,}955.2$$

Price Variance

$$1785\ [\$5.12 - \$5.50] = \underline{678.3}$$

$$\underline{\underline{\$4{,}633.5\ A < E}}$$

Why are these figures different from those developed in (a)?

Problem 10-2. The following information is provided by Dawkins Memorial Hospital.

Department A

	19X1	19X2
Total patient waiting time (hours)	1,344	2,562
Total patient visits	20,160	21,960
Total payroll	$219,700.80	$221,005.16
Total hours paid	26,280	21,436
Vacation time and other nonproductive time (hours)	3,232	3,258

Treatment Time Statistics (constant over years 1 and 2)

	Average Treatment Time (minutes)	
Service Category I	19X1	19X2
Diagnosis A	23	23
Diagnosis B	8	8
Diagnosis C	19	19
Number of visits	1,931	1,824
Service Category II		
Diagnosis D	11	11
Diagnosis E	27	27
Number of visits	797	1,041
Other Service Categories		
Diagnosis F-n	47	47
Number of visits	17,432	19,095

Required:

a. Compute the salary cost allocated between service categories I and II *and* the other service categories for 19X1 and 19X2.
b. Compute the cost allocations to service categories I and II for 19X1 and 19X2.
c. Compute the per patient waiting time for years 19X1 and 19X2.
d. Compute the cost of staff slack time. What assumption must you make to complete this computation?

Problem 10-3. You are the medical director of a large prepaid group practice, which maintains a laboratory. During the year, technicians worked 4,916 hours in the laboratory, creating a total wage expense of \$23,411.18. After careful consideration, you ascertain that the average time required to complete a laboratory procedure is 12 minutes. During the year 19,617 laboratory procedures were performed. Part-time technicians are hired periodically during the year in an attempt to minimize paying overtime. If no overtime is paid, the wage rate is expected to be \$4.35 per hour.

Required:

a. Given this information, analyze the labor performance variance.
b. Comment on the possible use of this information.
c. Is the use of variance analysis for monitoring laboratory performance proper? Defend your answer.

Problem 10-4. Under what conditions would the EUS be approximately equal to the number of whole units completed during the period? When the EUS equals the whole units completed during the period and output measures exist, could a standard or expected cost system be used to generate meaningful control information? Defend your answer.

Problem 10-5. The medical director of a large teaching hospital is attempting to develop a cost accounting system. The director asks you to explain why budget contrasts are developed monthly. After considerable thought, you are unable to defend a monthly period for the generation of variance information. You are then asked how one ascertains the timing of variance information for various activities monitored by a standard or expected cost accounting system. Write a memo explaining how you would ascertain the appropriate timing for generating performance variance information.

Problem 10-6. Equation (10-11), $AS_i^h = S^h \times [SC_i^h/TTT^h]$ indicates how the total salary of the hth treatment component (S^h) is to be allocated to the ith service category. Develop an equation which would indicate how the total salary of the hth treatment component would be allocated (a) on a crisis class basis, and (b) on a crisis class basis within a service category.

Problem 10-7. Given the information provided on page 366, assume the nursing salaries paid are \$1,795.00, which represents 2,133 minutes of service. Use this information to develop AS_1^N and AS_2^N. Also compute and interpret the cost of unproductive time for the nursing component.

Chapter 11

Capital Budgeting: Selection of Strategic Decision Alternatives

"Up ahead, the road divided into three and, as if in reply to Milo's question, an enormous road sign, pointing in all three directions, stated clearly:

DIGITOPOLIS

5 Miles
1,600 Rods
8,800 Yards
26,400 Feet
316,800 Inches
633,600 Half Inches

AND THEN SOME

'Let's travel by miles,' advised the Humbug; 'it's shorter.'

'Let's travel by half inches,' suggested Milo; 'it's quicker.'

'But which road should we take?' asked Tock. 'It must make a difference.'

As they argued, a most peculiar little figure stepped nimbly from behind the sign and approached them, talking all the while. 'Yes, indeed; indeed it does; certainly; my, yes; it does make a difference; undoubtedly.'

When he reached the car, the figure doffed his cap and recited in a loud clear voice:

'My angles are many.
My sides are not few.
I'm the Dodecahedron.
Who are you?'

'What's a Dodecahedron?' inquired Milo, who was barely able to pronounce the strange word.

'See for yourself,' he said, turning around slowly. 'A Dodecahedron is a mathematical shape with twelve faces.'

'Perhaps you can help us decide which road to take,' said Milo.

'By all means,' he replied happily. 'There's nothing to it. If a

small car carrying three people at thirty miles an hour for ten minutes along a road five miles long at 11:35 in the morning starts at the same time as three people who have been traveling in a little automobile at twenty miles an hour for fifteen minutes on another road exactly twice as long as one half the distance of the other, while a dog, a bug, and a boy travel an equal distance in the same time or the same distance in an equal time along a third road in mid-October, then which one arrives first and which is the best way to go?'

'Seventeen!' shouted the Humbug, scribbling furiously on a piece of paper.

'Well, I'm not sure, but ——' Milo stammered after several minutes of frantic figuring.

'You'll have to do better than that,' scolded the Dodecahedron, 'or you'll never know how far you've gone or whether or not you've ever gotten there.'

'I'm not very good at problems,' admitted Milo.

'What a shame,' sighed the Dodecahedron. 'They're so very useful. Why, did you know that if a beaver two feet long with a tail a foot and half long can build a dam twelve feet high and six feet wide in two days, all you would need to build Boulder Dam is a beaver sixty-eight feet long with a fifty-one-foot tail?'

'Where would you find a beaver that big?' grumbled the Humbug as his pencil point snapped.

'I'm sure I don't know,' he replied, 'but if you did, you'd certainly know what to do with him.'

'That's absurd,' objected Milo, whose head was spinning from all the numbers and questions.

'That may be true,' he acknowledged, 'but it's completely accurate, and as long as the answer is right, who cares if the question is wrong? If you want sense, you'll have to make it yourself.'

'All three roads arrive at the same place at the same time,' interrupted Tock, who had patiently been doing the first problem.

'Correct!' shouted the Dodecahedron. 'And I'll take you there myself. Now you can see how important problems are. If you hadn't done this one properly, you might have gone the wrong way.'

'I can't see where I made my mistake,' said the Humbug, frantically rechecking his figures.

'But if all the roads arrive at the same place at the same time, then aren't they all the right way?' asked Milo.

> *'Certainly not!' he shouted, glaring from his most upset face. 'They're all the* wrong *way. Just because you have a choice, it doesn't mean that any of them has to be right.' "*
>
> Norton Juster
> *The Phantom Tollbooth**

As noted in Chapter 9, management should ascertain the quantitative effects of specific long-range planning alternatives on the achievement of the mission of the organization. Without a sense of the interrelationship between the various capital alternatives and their expected effects on the mission of the organization, the strategic decision process is not likely to be effective. In this chapter, a normative model, called the relevance model (Lusk, 1974), is used to develop insights regarding the type of information required for an effective long-range planning process. This normative relevance model has a simple operational analogue, the eigenvalue prioritization model (Saaty, 1977). In the second part of the chapter, this prioritization approach is examined.[1]

THE RELEVANCE MODELING APPROACH

A simple organizational scenario is outlined to facilitate the discussion of the relevance model. The basic organizational model in this scenario is an institution in which (1) demands for funds to support capital investment activities exceed the supply of funds, and (2) investment decisions must be made considering general and program activities. The mission of the institution is a generalized welfare specification detailed enough to allow the measurement and evaluation of the interrelationship between the mission and the activities of the institution.

Three basic levels of activity exist within the institution: general, program, and investment activities. The general activities are the major institutional functions which result from programs (e.g., medical research), and they support or enable the mission of the institution to be realized. The program activities are groupings of specific technologies and their related staffs, which support the various general activities in the institution. For example, a hospital may have a clinical scholars program which in part supports the general activity of medical research. The investment

---

activities are specific capital projects and investment alternatives proposed by various institutional personnel. Each activity level is an integral part of the institution's operations, and, therefore, must be evaluated in the capital budgeting process.

To evaluate each level of activity, a set of qualitative or quantitative criteria must be developed by management. For example, "improving patient welfare" may be an evaluation criterion useful in evaluating various general activities. In the following discussion of the relevance model, these evaluation criteria shall be noted as EC_k^i, where i indicates the pertinent activity category and k represents a particular evaluation criterion.

Relevance Model Requirements

In addition to the information provided by the scenario, the relevance model requires the specification of a planning, programing, budgeting (PPB) hierarchy of activities. The evaluation criteria (EC_k^i) applicable to these basic institutional activities must be weighted according to their impact in achieving the mission of the organization. Further, the specific activities within each basic activity category (general, program, or investment) must be weighted with respect to the evaluation criteria for the pertinent category. The relevance model combines all this information to yield a set of priority weights which reflect each investment's relative contribution to achievement of the institutional mission. However, the derivation of the various weights is a very complex task. A matrix approach simplifies the derivation of the relative criterion weights and of the activity weights for specific criteria. This matrix is called the relevance matrix.

Relevance Matrix

The relevance matrix is a numerical construct consisting of a series of rows and columns that aid in evaluating the relative contribution of a number of specific alternative activities to the mission of the organization. A relevance matrix must be constructed for each basic activity category. The evaluation criteria for the category under consideration form the first column of the matrix. In the second column, each criterion is weighted with respect to its impact on the mission of the organization, so that the sum of the weights equals one. In the third and subsequent columns, each specific activity in the category is weighted with respect to its impact on each criterion, so that the sum of the activity weights on each equals one. The criterion weights (column 2) are noted as CW_k^i. The activity weights (columns 3, 4, . . .) are noted as AW_{kj}^i, where i indicates a particular activity category, k indicates a particular evaluation criterion, and j indicates the specific activity. Hence, for an activity category, i, with m criteria and n specific alternative activities,

$$\sum_{k=1}^{m} CW_k^i = 1 \text{ and } \sum_{j=1}^{n} AW_{kj}^i = 1.$$

For example, assume that the general activities category (G) has two evaluation criteria, EC_1^G and EC_2^G. If the group of individuals responsible for evaluating the criteria[2] believe that EC_1^G is four times as important as EC_2^G in achieving the organization's mission, then the following criterion weights will be assigned to EC_1^G and EC_2^G, respectively: $CW_1^G = .8$ and $CW_2^G = .2$. As required, the sum of these criterion weights

$$\sum_{k=1}^{2} CW_k^G$$

equals one. Furthermore, if the institution engages in four general activities, each must be judged with respect to the general activities criteria. Assume that general activities 1 and 2 are considered to be of equal importance with respect to EC_1^G. In addition, assume that general activities 3 and 4 are of equal importance with respect to EC_1^G. If the group responsible for assigning the activity weights judges that general activities 1 and 2 will each have four times the impact on EC_1^G of either general activity 3 or general activity 4, then the following weights will be assigned to the respective general activities: $AW_{11}^G = .4$, $AW_{12}^G = .4$, $AW_{13}^G = .1$, and $AW_{14}^G = .1$. Again, the sum of the weights ($\sum_{j=1}^{4} AW_{1j}^G$) equals one. To complete the matrix for the general activities category, this same procedure would be used to weight the four general activities with respect to EC_2^G.

Once the relevance matrix has been constructed, a specific activity's contribution to the mission of the organization can be computed as the vector product (see Appendix 11-B) of the criterion weights and the activity weights. These vector products indicate the relative impact of the specific activities on the mission of the organization, and may be included as the final row in the relevance matrix. Each vector product, called the relevance weight, is noted as RW_j^i, where i and j indicate activity categories and specific activities, respectively. The sum of these vector products also equals one (i.e., for activity category i with n specific alternative activities, $\sum_{j=1}^{n} RW_j^i = 1$).

The relevance matrix that would be constructed for a program activity category (P) which has three criteria and three programs is shown in Figure 11-1. The contribution of the third specific program activity to the mission of the organization is computed as $RW_3^P = (CW_1^P \times AW_{13}^P) + (CW_2^P \times AW_{23}^P) + (CW_3^P \times AW_{33}^P)$. This vector computation must be completed for each specific activity in each activity category. The sets of relevance weights for the specific activities over all activity categories are used to determine the relevance value for each alternative investment activity. For computational convenience, these relevance weights are placed in a relevance lattice.

Relevance Lattice

The relevance lattice is a network representing the organization's PPB relationships. Its nodes are horizontally stratified by activity category and vertically stratified by the general, program, and investment activity interrelationships.[3] The first step in calculating the relevance value for a particular investment activity (RV_j, where j represents the particular investment activity) is to find the product of (1) the relevance weight for that investment activity and (2) the related relevance weights at the other activity levels. Once this product has been computed for all investment activities,

Figure 11-1 Program Activity Relevance Matrix

Program Activity Category: P

Evaluation Criteria		Program Activity 1	Program Activity 2	Program Activity 3	
Name	Weight				
EC_1^P	CW_1^P	AW_{11}^P	AW_{12}^P	AW_{13}^P	$\sum_{j=1}^{3} AW_{1j}^P = 1.0$
EC_2^P	CW_2^P	AW_{21}^P	AW_{22}^P	AW_{23}^P	$\sum_{j=1}^{3} AW_{2j}^P = 1.0$
EC_3^P	CW_3^P	AW_{31}^P	AW_{32}^P	AW_{33}^P	$\sum_{j=1}^{3} AW_{3j}^P = 1.0$
	$\sum_{i=1}^{3} CW_i^P = 1.0$	RW_1^P	RW_2^P	RW_3^P	$\sum_{j=1}^{3} RW_j^P = 1.0$

each product is divided by the sum of the products to find the relevance value of each investment activity. Hence, for an organization with n alternative investment activities, $\sum_{j=1}^{n} RV_j = 1$. The concepts of the relevance lattice may be more clearly elucidated by the following example.

Assume that a particular institution has two activity categories, general (G) and investment (I). If the institution engages in three general activities, each supported by one investment activity, then two relevance matrices, yielding six relevance weights, would have to be constructed. The relevance lattice for these six relevance weights is shown in Figure 11-2. In this simple case, the relevance value for each investment activity would be computed as:

$$\text{Investment Activity 1: } RV_1 = (RW_1^G \times RW_1^I)/A$$
$$\text{Investment Activity 2: } RV_2 = (RW_2^G \times RW_2^I)/A$$
$$\text{Investment Activity 3: } RV_3 = (RW_3^G \times RW_3^I)/A$$

where: $A = \sum_{j=1}^{3} RW_j^G \times RW_j^I$.

Figure 11-2 Simple Relevance Lattice

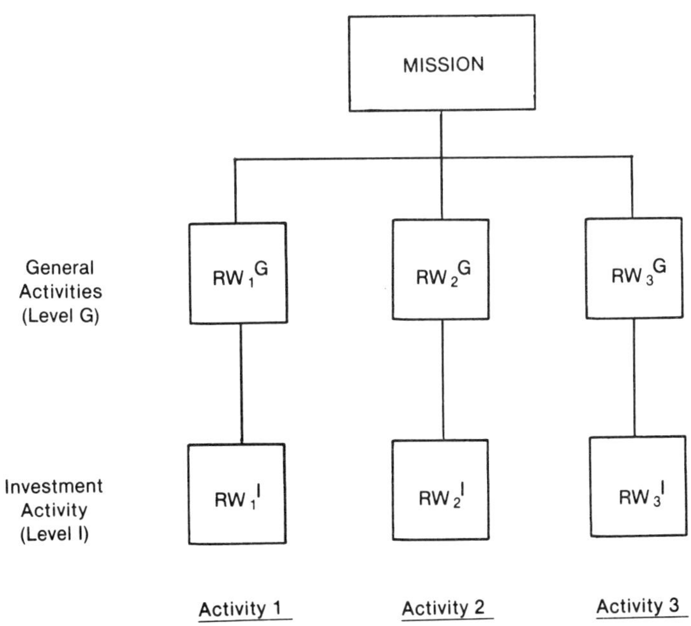

Relevance Model Information Flows

The relevance model requires judgment information from the managers of the organization. This information is transformed by the relevance model into a numerical value useful in planning the organization's investment activities. Figure 11-3 details the relevance model information flows from the development of the mission of the organization through the final investment decision. All of the elements of the model are encompassed by these information flows.

As shown in Figure 11-3, the system's scenario is used to develop the mission of the organization (also see Chapter 9). Given the mission, the general activities that characterize institutional functions can be formulated. Then, the various institutional programs can be placed among these general activities according to the support that each program activity gives to each general activity, remembering that some program activities may support more than one general activity (Appendix 11-A). As investment opportunities are proposed, they may be placed among the program activities according to the support they provide to each. In some cases, the proposed investment activity will require the formulation of a new program activity. In any case, the mission and the general, program, and investment activities form the PPB hierarchy of activities, the first informational input to the relevance model.

To evaluate the proposed investment activities, evaluation criteria that are pertinent to the various activity categories must be developed. In addition, the relative importance of these criteria must be quantified. Different evaluation criteria are pertinent to different activity categories, and criteria within each activity category are weighted relative to each other, without regard for the criteria of other activity categories. These criteria and their weights form the second informational input to the relevance model.

Once the evaluation criteria have been developed for each activity category, the specific activities can be evaluated using these criteria. The procedure for quantifying these judgments has been outlined previously. These activity weights, in conjunction with the criterion weights, form the elements of the relevance matrix. Hence, the quantified evaluation of the specific activities forms the third and final input to the relevance model.

Also, as shown in Figure 11-3, a separate relevance matrix is prepared for each activity category. The information in each of these matrices can be developed to produce one relevance weight for each specific activity. Hence, a set of relevance weights—at least one from each activity category—will be used to evaluate each investment activity. This set of relevance weights can be converted into one relevance value by placing the relevance weights in the relevance lattice and performing the proper calculations (see

Figure 11-3 Relevance System Information Flows

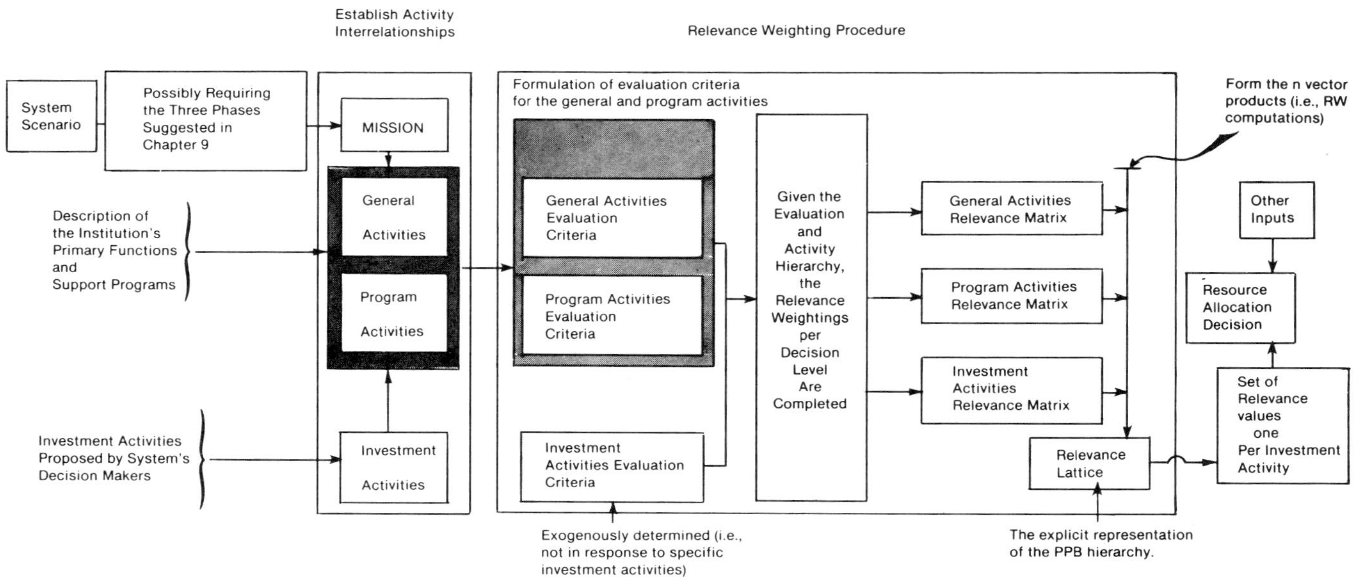

Appendix 11-A). The relevance values are the quantitative transformation of the input information. These values are used along with other information to develop the organization's investment plan.

The information flows of Figure 11-3 are illustrated in detail in the following example, which also illustrates the matrix computations and the use of the relevance lattice.

Relevance Setting: A Hospital Illustration

In this example, the hospital under consideration is assumed to have as its mission To Utilize Scarce Hospital Resources to Best Deal with Local Health Problems. The hospital supports teaching, research, and health care delivery activities. For expositional simplicity, each of these general activities is supported by only one program activity. An intern/extern training program supports the teaching activity. A program to develop general research competence, rather than categorical program research such as cardiovascular research, supports the research activity. Finally, a program to extend medical care into the community supports the health care delivery system.

Three investment activities, one to support each program, have been proposed by various individuals in the hospital: (1) invest in new medical classroom equipment, (2) acquire an electronic analog/digital computer system, and (3) start a health maintenance organization (HMO). To develop priority weights for these investment alternatives, the hospital will use the relevance model. Hence, in addition to the information already provided, evaluation criteria must be specified. Then, the relative value of each of these criteria and the impact of the specific activities within each category on each criterion can be quantified for the relevance matrix.

Activities Evaluation: Relevance Matrices

Four evaluation criteria have been developed by management to evaluate the general activities:[4]

- EC_1^G: provide for patient welfare,
- EC_2^G: contribute to the status of the hospital,
- EC_3^G: establish a fund-generating potential, and
- EC_4^G: provide resource control effectiveness.

The group responsible for evaluating these criteria has decided that EC_1^G is twice as important as EC_3^G, which is twice as important as EC_2^G. This group also judged that while EC_4^G is not as important as EC_1^G, it is more important than EC_3^G. Hence, the following weights should be assigned to the respective criteria:

	Criterion Weight
EC_1^G (provide for patient welfare):	$CW_1^G = .4$
EC_2^G (status of the hospital):	$CW_2^G = .1$
EC_3^G (fund generation potential):	$CW_3^G = .2$
EC_4^G (resource control potential):	$CW_4^G = .3$

Note that the sum of these weights equals one as required.

This same ranking procedure, ascertaining the ordering and magnitude of weights, is used to determine the relevance weighting for each general activity with respect to each general activities category criterion. For example, assume those responsible for weighting the general activities feel that health care delivery has four times the impact of teaching and research combined, which have been judged as equally important in providing for patient welfare (EC_1^G). Therefore, the following weights should be assigned to the general activities of teaching, research, and health care delivery.

		Teaching	Research	Health Care Delivery
EC_1^G	.4	.1	.1	.8

The general activities category matrix of Figure 11-4 can be prepared once all of the general activities have been weighted with respect to all of the general activities category criteria. Note that the vector products, yielding the relevance weights, are represented in the last row of the general activities relevance matrix. These vector products have been computed as follows.

Teaching	*Research*	*Health Care Delivery*
$.4 \times .1 = .04$	$.4 \times .1 = .04$	$.4 \times .8 = .32$
$.1 \times .1 = .01$	$.1 \times .1 = .01$	$.1 \times .8 = .08$
$.2 \times .3 = .06$	$.2 \times .6 = .12$	$.2 \times .1 = .02$
$.3 \times .7 = .21$	$.3 \times .2 = .06$	$.3 \times .1 = .03$
$RW_1^G = .32$	$RW_2^G = .23$	$RW_3^G = .45$

Note that the sum of the relevance weights also equals one.

Figure 11-4 Relevance Matrix—General Activities Category: *G*

		General Activities		
Evaluation Criteria	Criteria Weights	Teaching	Research	Health Care Delivery
EC_1^G: Provide for Patient Welfare	.4	.1	.1	.8
EC_2^G: Status of the Hospital	.1	.1	.1	.8
EC_3^G: Fund Generation Potential	.2	.3	.6	.1
EC_4^G: Resource Control Potential	.3	.7	.2	.1
Entry on Relevance Lattice: General Level		.32	.23	.45

Preparing the program activities category relevance matrix requires a similar procedure. First, the program activities category criteria must be defined. Then, these criteria must be weighted. Finally, the specific program activities must be weighted with respect to these criteria. In this case, the hospital uses the following evaluation criteria to assess program activities:

- EC_1^P: program achievement within one year with existing personnel;
- EC_2^P: continuity of fund flow (state, federal or philanthropic); and
- EC_3^P: provide an environment attractive to eminently qualified physicians.

The group responsible for evaluating these criteria has weighted the respective criteria as follows:

- EC_1^P: $CW_1^P = .5$
- EC_2^P: $CW_2^P = .3$
- EC_3^P: $CW_3^P = .2$

Again, these weightings sum to one. After each of the program activities has been weighted with respect to each of the criteria, the program activities category relevance matrix of Figure 11-5 is complete. The relevance weights again have been included in the matrix. The derivation of these relevance weights is as follows.

Physician Training	*Research*	*Extended Care*
$.5 \times .1 = .05$	$.5 \times .1 = .05$	$.5 \times .8 = .40$
$.3 \times .1 = .03$	$.3 \times .2 = .06$	$.3 \times .7 = .21$
$.2 \times .2 = .04$	$.2 \times .7 = .14$	$.2 \times .1 = .02$
$RW_1^P = .12$	$RW_2^P = .25$	$RW_3^P = .63$

A relevance matrix also must be prepared for the investment activities category. The investment activities criteria and the corresponding weights in this case are:

- EC_1^I: yearly economic return (revenue over direct cost), $CW_1^I = .1$;
- EC_2^I: potential to increase hospital utilization, $CW_2^I = .6$; and
- EC_3^I: ability to validate the proposed investment benefits prior to fund commitment, $CW_3^I = .3$.

Now each of the proposed investment activities can be evaluated with respect to the investment activities criteria, and the matrix in Figure 11-6 can be prepared. The relevance weights in this matrix have been computed as follows.

Classroom Equipment	*Computer System*	*HMO*
$.1 \times .1 = .01$	$.1 \times .2 = .02$	$.1 \times .7 = .07$
$.6 \times .4 = .24$	$.6 \times .5 = .30$	$.6 \times .1 = .06$
$.3 \times .3 = .09$	$.3 \times .2 = .06$	$.3 \times .5 = .15$
$RW_1^I = .34$	$RW_2^I = .38$	$RW_3^I = .28$

Figure 11-5 Relevance Matrix—Activities Category: *P*

		Program Activities		
Evaluation Criteria	Criteria Weights	Intern/ Extern Training	Develop Research Competence	Extend Care into the Community
EC_1^P: Program Achievement Within One Year	.5	.1	.1	.8
EC_2^P: Continuity of Fund Flow	.3	.1	.2	.7
EC_3^P: Attractive Physician Environment	.2	.2	.7	.1
Entry on Relevance Lattice: Program Level		.12	.25	.63

Figure 11-6 Relevance Matrix—Investment Activities Category: I

		Investment Activities		
Evaluation Criteria	Criteria Weights	Investing in new Medical Classroom Equipment	Acquisition of Computer System	Starting a Health Maintenance Organization (HMO)
EC_1^I: Yearly Economic Returns (Revenue over Direct Cost)	.1	.1	.2	.7
EC_2^I: Increase Hospital Utilization	.6	.4	.5	.1
EC_3^I: Ability to Validate the Proposed Benefits Prior to Fund Commitment	.3	.3	.2	.5
Entry on the Relevance Lattice: Investment Level		.34	.38	.28

Investment Evaluation: Relevance Values

Most institutions have no systematic means of choosing among proposed investment activities. However, if management had established only investment activity criteria, the highest priority would be given to the electronic computer system. At the investment activities level, this investment is the most desirable of the three proposed investments. Unfortunately, its impact on the organizational mission is uncertain.

By using the relevance lattice of Figure 11-7, the three investment activities can be evaluated according to their relative contribution to the mission of the hospital. The relevance value for each of the three investments can be computed from this relevance lattice (see Table 11-1). An examination of these relevance values shows that the HMO would make a greater contribution to the mission of the hospital than either of the other two investment alternatives. Note that while this investment is the least important at the investment activity level, it has the greatest relevance value when considering all of the activity levels.

Evaluation of Relevance Model Output

As indicated in Figure 11-3, the relevance values are a set of priority weights that can be used to allocate capital resources. However, the use-

Figure 11-7 Relevance Lattice*

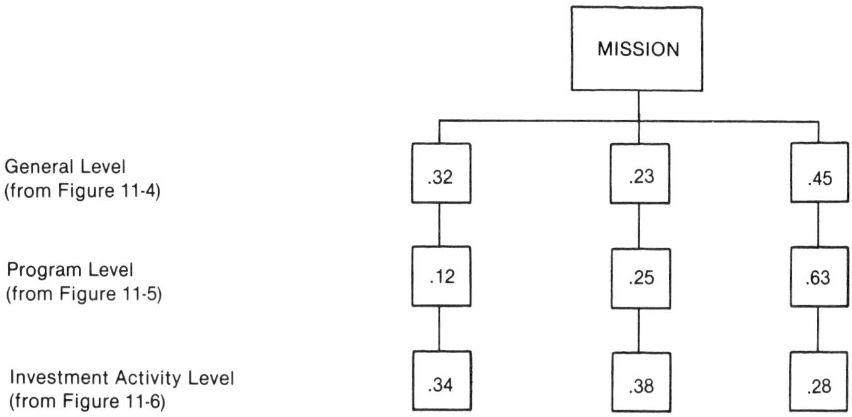

Table 11-1 Computation of Relevance Values

Investment Alternatives	Investment Level (RW_j^I)	Program Level (RW_j^P)	General Level (RW_j^G)	$\frac{(RW_j^I \times RW_j^P \times RW_j^G)}{A} = RV_j$
Classroom Equipment	.34	.12	.32	1.31/11.44 = .12
Computer System	.38	.25	.23	2.19/11.44 = .19
HMO	.28	.63	.45	7.94/11.44 = .69

fulness of the priority weights derived from the relevance model depends upon the accuracy of the hierarchical specifications and the validity of the various criteria and criterion weights. If the criteria, criterion weights, or hierarchical specifications are inaccurate, the relevance values could lead to, or reinforce, misallocations of resources.

The relevance model may not be applicable in a health care setting if operational peculiarities of the health care industry prohibit the accurate measurement of criterion and activity weights or the accurate specification of the hierarchical relationships. Developing criterion weights for the organization's activity categories has inherent problems because the relationship between a particular criterion and the mission of the organization becomes rather arbitrary as one moves down the PPB hierarchy. This rela-

*This PPB hierarchy was assumed for this example to simplify the analysis. In practice, this straightforward ordering is seldom found.

tive remoteness of criterion weights is one major problem in implementing the relevance model. However, even if the criterion and activity weights are accurate, they must be placed in the relevance lattice before the relevance values can be computed. Since the relevance lattice is merely a graphical representation of the formal statement of the PPB hierarchy, the accuracy of the hierarchical specifications will directly affect the relevance values. Unfortunately, in most cases, specifying the PPB hierarchy with any degree of confidence is very difficult. Hence, although the relevance model is important in developing normative insights to the requirements of a priority weighting model, it may be very difficult to implement.

PRIORITIZATION MODEL REQUIREMENTS

A prioritization model, such as the relevance model, requires a systematic analysis of decision alternatives so that a priority weight may be developed for each decision alternative. This type of systematic analysis requires (1) the explicit enumeration of a set of decision alternatives so that comparisons may be made between alternatives, (2) the development of a set of criteria so that each alternative can be judged with respect to the other alternatives on each criterion, and (3) the evaluation of each criterion with respect to its relative importance in achieving the organization's mission. Unfortunately, most of the existing models which develop priority weights for decision alternatives require the use of criteria that can be measured objectively.[5] Since this degree of problem specification is beyond the measurement abilities of most health care institutions, these models are not appropriate for most health care applications. However, the eigenvalue prioritization model uses judgmental as well as objective evaluation criteria, and is therefore well suited to most health care alternative selection problems.

THE EIGENVALUE PRIORITIZATION MODEL

To develop managerially relevant information regarding alternative selection in complex decision situations, Saaty (1977) has developed a prioritization model which accepts as inputs (1) pairwise judgments regarding the impact of the various decision alternatives on each evaluation criterion, and (2) pairwise judgments regarding the relative importance of each criterion to the mission of the organization. These judgments are recorded in judgment matrices. The judgment matrices are constructed so that if n decision alternatives are judged with respect to m evaluation criteria, m judgment matrices each of size $n \times n$ and one criteria judgment matrix of size $m \times m$ will be constructed. The judgmental information represented in these matrices is abstracted by computing the *eigenvector* associated with the maximal *eigenvalue* of each matrix.[6] The eigenvector of a particular $n \times n$ judgment matrix represents the judgmental information of the matrix in an $n \times 1$ vector of weights analogous to the activity weights of the relevance model. Similarly, the eigenvector of an $m \times m$ criteria judgment matrix produces a set of m weights analogous to the criterion weights of the relevance model. These $m + 1$ eigenvectors are, after adjustment, used to develop the priority weights for the decision alternatives analogous to the relevance values of the relevance model.

Requirements of the Eigenvalue Prioritization Model

The elements required to operationalize the eigenvalue prioritization model are (1) a delineated set of decision alternatives, noted as $\{a_i, i{:}1, \ldots, n\}$; (2) a set of criteria used to describe the decision alternatives $\{C_j, j{:}1, \ldots, m\}$; and (3) a judgmental measurement scale which has only the numeric descriptors, $\{1,2,3,4,5,6,7,8,9\}$. Once the decision alternatives and the evaluation criteria have been specified, pairwise comparisons may be made among the n alternatives on each criterion. If the evaluation criteria are well conceived relative to the decision alternatives, then an individual is expected to be able to make pairwise alternative comparisons and render a judgment regarding the intensity of the difference between alternatives. The numeric descriptors of the judgmental measurement scale are used to quantify this intensity, as shown in Table 11-2. This measurement scale is also used to quantify the intensity of the differential impact of each criterion on the mission of the organization when pairwise comparisons are made among the criteria.

Table 11-2 Description of Weights Assigned to Alternative a_x When Compared to Alternative a_y*

1:	if alternative a_x and alternative a_y are equally preferred on a particular criterion.
3:	if a_x is weakly preferred to a_y on a particular criterion.
5:	if a_x is strongly preferred to a_y on a particular criterion.
7:	if a_x is demonstrably preferred to a_y on a particular criterion.
9:	if a_x is absolutely preferred to a_y on a particular criterion.

*The measurement scale values 2, 4, 6 and 8 may be used if the primary descriptors are not sufficiently representative of the individual's judgment of the intensity quantified by $\{1,3,5,7,9\}$.

Development of Judgment Matrices

The results of the pairwise decision alternative comparisons are recorded in a judgment matrix of the form:

$$\|A\|_j = a^j{}_{hi}$$

where: h and i indicate that the hth alternative is being evaluated against the ith alternative, $h = 1, \ldots, n,$ and $i = 1, \ldots, n$;
j denotes a particular criterion, $1 \leq j \leq m$; and
each integer value in $\|A\|_j$ (subsequently noted as A_j) is selected from the measurement scale represented in Table 11-2.

A_j is constructed so that element $a^j{}_{hi}$ is in the hth row and the ith column. The properties of A_j are such that (1) if $h = i$, then $a^j{}_{hi} = 1$, and (2) for all $a^j{}_{hi}$, $a^j{}_{hi} = 1/a^j{}_{ih}$.[7]

The judgments rendered and recorded in A_j represent the perceived interrelationships among the n alternatives. For most health care alternative selection problems, the nature of the criteria will require that judgmental matrices be developed. However, in some cases, measurable or objective bases of evaluation exist, such as payback and return on investment. When objective measures exist, judgments do not have to be quantified on the {1,3,5,7,9} scale. Instead, the objective measures may be used to develop an $n \times n$ ratio matrix.

Development of Ratio Matrices

In a ratio matrix R_j, each entry is a ratio of the value of the row decision alternative and the column decision alternative. Hence, matrix element $r^j{}_{hi}$ would be the ratio of the value of the hth decision alternative to the value of the ith decision alternative for the jth criteria. For example, if three investments have a rate of return of 8, 2, and 4 percent, respectively, the 3 × 3 ratio matrix would be as follows.

$$R_j = \begin{bmatrix} \frac{.08}{.08} & \frac{.08}{.02} & \frac{.08}{.04} \\ \frac{.02}{.08} & \frac{.02}{.02} & \frac{.02}{.04} \\ \frac{.04}{.08} & \frac{.04}{.02} & \frac{.04}{.04} \end{bmatrix} = \begin{bmatrix} 1 & 4 & 2 \\ 1/4 & 1 & 1/2 \\ 1/2 & 2 & 1 \end{bmatrix}$$

Note that this ratio matrix has the same properties as the judgment matrix, A_j (i.e., $r^j{}_{hi} = 1$ when $h = i$, and $r^j{}_{hi} = 1/r^j{}_{ih}$).

Abstracting the Eigenvector Associated with the Maximal Eigenvalue

Once the judgment and ratio matrices have been developed, a set of weights that sum to one and reflect the relative impact of each decision alternative on a particular criterion can be abstracted from each matrix. This is accomplished by computing the eigenvector associated with the maximal eigenvalue for a particular judgment or ratio matrix. The computed eigenvector is an $n \times 1$ vector that contains the set of judgmental weights.

An iterative procedure is used to generate this normalized (i.e., sums to one) maximal eigenvector[8] for the jth judgment (or ratio) matrix as follows.[9]

Algorithm (1)

$$\underset{n\times 1}{\bar{d}_1} = [\underset{n\times n}{A_j} \cdot \underset{n\times 1}{\bar{e}}]\cdot[\underset{1\times n}{\bar{e}^T} \cdot \underset{n\times n}{A_j} \cdot \underset{n\times 1}{\bar{e}}]^{-1}$$

$$\bar{d}_2 = [A_j \cdot \bar{d}_1]\cdot[\bar{e}^T \cdot A_j \cdot \bar{d}_1]^{-1}$$

$$\vdots \qquad \vdots$$

$$\bar{V}_j \equiv \bar{d}_q = [A_j \cdot \bar{d}_{q-1}]\cdot[\bar{e}^T \cdot A_j \cdot \bar{d}_{q-1}]^{-1}$$

where: $\bar{d}_i$ represents the approximation of the maximal eigenvector after the ith iteration;

$\bar{e}$ represents a unit column vector of size $n \times 1$;

$\bar{e}^T$ represents the transpose of the unit column vector (see Appendix 11-B); and

$\bar{V}_j$ represents the computed normalized maximal eigenvector for the jth judgment or ratio matrix.

The iterative procedure of algorithm (1) stops when $\bar{d}_q \approx \bar{d}_{q+1}$. At this point, the normalized maximal eigenvector, $\bar{V}_j$, is set equal to $\bar{d}_{q+1}$.

Judgmental Consistency: A Quantification of the Effectiveness of the Judgment Process

The relative consistency of the pairwise judgments within each matrix also can be measured. A matrix is consistent if a proportionate relationship exists among the decision alternative preference judgments. For example, if decision alternative g is weakly preferred to decision alternative h (i.e., $a_{gh} = 3$), while decision alternative h is weakly preferred to decision alternative i (i.e., $a_{hi} = 3$), then consistency exists if alternative g is absolutely preferred to alternative i (i.e., $a_{gi} = 9$). In other words, a matrix is consistent if its elements are transitive (i.e., $a_{gh} \times a_{hi} = a_{gi}$).

Transitivity is assumed in most mathematical studies of decision making. However, in practice, preference relationships between alternatives may not be transitive. For example, alternative A may be preferred to alternative B, while alternative B is preferred to alternative C, and alternative C is preferred to alternative A. Transitivity is not, however, a precondition for rational behavior, since rational people may have judgments which are not transitive. In any case, where nontransitive or inconsistent behavior is evidenced in the eigenvalue prioritization model, a measure of relative inconsistency is important.

Relative Inconsistency

Eigenvalues can be used to approximate relative inconsistency in a particular matrix. The eigenvalues of a matrix are the real or complex roots of the equation derived from the determinant of the matrix. The largest root, or maximal eigenvalue, for a particular matrix is called λ_{max}. The difference between λ_{max} for a particular matrix and λ_{max} for a consistent matrix of the same size indicates the degree of inconsistency of the particular matrix. Comparing this difference with a measure of the greatest inconsistency that could occur for a matrix of similar size yields an approximation of the relative inconsistency of a judgment matrix.

To perform the prescribed calculations, λ_{max} must be defined for a consistent, a moderately inconsistent, and a completely inconsistent matrix. A consistent matrix has only one real nonzero root, which is equal to the trace of the matrix, $TR(A_j)$—i.e., the sum of the elements in the main diagonal of the matrix. Hence, $\lambda_{max} = TR(A_j) = n$, if A_j is consistent. However, if A_j is inconsistent, λ_{max} will be greater than $TR(A_j)$. Therefore, $\lambda_{max} > n$, if A_j is inconsistent. In addition, if the measurement scale used to make the matrix entries has α as an upper limit, the magnitude of λ_{max} for any matrix of a particular size will have an upper limit. The upper limit for λ_{max}, called λ_{sup}, is the largest root of the following matrix.

$$\underset{n\times n}{\|B\|} = \begin{bmatrix} 1 & \alpha & 1/\alpha & \alpha & 1/\alpha & \cdots \\ 1/\alpha & 1 & \alpha & 1/\alpha & \alpha & \cdots \\ \alpha & 1/\alpha & 1 & \alpha & 1/\alpha & \cdots \\ 1/\alpha & \alpha & 1/\alpha & 1 & \alpha & \cdots \\ \vdots & \vdots & \vdots & \vdots & \vdots & \end{bmatrix}$$

Of course, the size of this matrix in any specific case depends upon the size of the matrix being analyzed for inconsistency.

Given these eigenvalues, the degree of relative inconsistency of a matrix can be measured as:

$$\theta_j^i = \frac{\lambda \max - n}{\lambda \sup - n}$$

where: θ_j^i denotes the relative judgmental inconsistency represented in a particular judgment matrix developed by individual i considering criterion j.

This relative inconsistency is expressed as a percentage because the range of θ_j^i is [0, 1]. Recall that if the judgment matrix is consistent, then $\lambda_{max} = n$ and $\theta_j^i = 0$, while if the matrix is completely inconsistent, $\lambda_{max} = \lambda_{sup}$ and $\theta_j^i = 1$. Since the measure of relative inconsistency, θ_j^i, is expressed as a percentage, the *relative consistency* of any matrix developed by individual i for the jth criterion can be calculated as $1 - \theta_j^i$.

This measure of relative consistency can be used to evaluate the quality of the judgment process and to adjust the judgmental weights as represented in the maximal eigenvector. Eigenvectors developed from inconsistent matrices should not be given as much credibility as eigenvectors developed from consistent matrices. Multiplying each eigenvector by the relative consistency, $1 - \theta_j^i$, of the matrix from which it was abstracted will adjust the eigenvector to reflect the credibility of the judgmental weights. Hence, the set of adjusted judgmental weights is calculated as:

$$\bar{w}_j = \bar{V}_j[1 - \theta_j^i].$$

Therefore, judgments which are completely inconsistent, i.e., $\lambda_{max} = \lambda_{sup}$, will be factored out of the evaluation process, judgments which are relatively inconsistent will be deemphasized, and judgments which are consistent, i.e., $\lambda_{max} = n$, will be unaltered in developing priority weights.

Computing the Set of Priority Weights

The m consistency adjusted maximal eigenvectors form the columns of an $n \times m$ matrix that represents the judgmental weights assigned to the decision alternatives for each of the m evaluation criterion.[10] This matrix is noted as:

$$\underset{n \times m}{\|P\|} = [\bar{w}_1 \bar{w}_2 \bar{w}_3 \cdots \bar{w}_m].$$

To produce the set of priority weights for the n decision alternatives, P must be multiplied by the maximal eigenvector of the criteria judgment matrix.

The criteria judgment matrix, C, is an $m \times m$ matrix. The pairwise evaluations represented in this matrix are made by using the same measurement scale used to develop the alternatives judgment matrices. The maximal eigenvector, $\bar{V}_c$, of C is an $m \times 1$ vector that represents the relative importance of each evaluation criterion to achievement of the institutional mission.

Given the decision alternative evaluation matrix, P, and the maximal eigenvector, $\bar{V}_c$, representing the relative importance of the m criteria, the priority weights for the n decision alternatives may be computed as follows.

$$\frac{P \cdot \bar{V}_c}{\bar{e}^T \cdot P \cdot \bar{V}_c} = \underset{n \times 1}{\bar{i}^*}$$

The elements of $\bar{i}^*$ represent the relative priorities of the n investment alternatives.[11] The relative importance of each of the n decision alternatives in the priority vector $\bar{i}^*$, has been derived considering the relative importance of each of the n decision alternatives on each of the m criteria and the relative importance of the criteria in facilitating the achievement of the organizational mission. The following example illustrates the derivation of the priority weights in the eigenvalue prioritization model.

An Illustrative Example: A Hospital

Assume that a hospital has three investment alternatives, a_1, a_2, and a_3. Further assume that management intends to evaluate these three alternatives on three criteria: C_1, the internal rate of return (IRR); C_2, improving the status of the hospital; and C_3, increasing the census of the hospital. Given this information, the first step in the eigenvalue prioritization model is to develop the alternative ratio or judgment matrices for each of the three criteria.

Development of the Ratio and Judgment Matrices

The IRR, C_1, can be computed from the institution's accounting data. Hence, a ratio matrix can be developed for this criterion. Assuming that the IRR (stated in percentage terms) for the three investments is .137, .421, and .097 for a_1, a_2, and a_3, respectively, the ratio matrix for the first criterion would be as follows.

$$R_1 = \begin{bmatrix} \frac{.137}{.137} & \frac{.137}{.421} & \frac{.137}{.097} \\ \\ \frac{.421}{.137} & \frac{.421}{.421} & \frac{.421}{.097} \\ \\ \frac{.097}{.137} & \frac{.097}{.421} & \frac{.097}{.097} \end{bmatrix} = \begin{matrix} 1 & .325 & 1.412 \\ \\ 3.08 & 1 & 4.34 \\ \\ 7.08 & .230 & 1 \end{matrix}$$

The extent to which an investment will improve the status of the hospital, C_2, cannot be determined explicitly. Hence, a judgment matrix must be developed for C_2. Assume the following preference relationships exist among the three investment alternatives on C_2: a_3 is weakly preferred to a_1; a_1 is weakly preferred to a_2; and a_3 is absolutely preferred to a_2. Therefore, the following values selected from the measurement scale (Table 11-2) will be assigned to the nine pairwise comparisons.

a_3 judged against a_1, noted as $a^2{}_{31}$, is valued at 3
a_1 judged against a_2, noted as $a^2{}_{12}$, is valued at 3
a_3 judged against a_2, noted as $a^2{}_{32}$, is valued at 9
a_1 judged against a_3, noted as $a^2{}_{13}$, is valued at 1/3 (i.e., $1/a^2{}_{31}$)
a_2 judged against a_1, noted as $a^2{}_{21}$, is valued at 1/3 (i.e., $1/a^2{}_{12}$)
a_2 judged against a_3, noted as $a^2{}_{23}$, is valued at 1/9 (i.e., $1/a^2{}_{32}$)
a_1 judged against a_1, noted as $a^2{}_{11}$, is valued at 1
a_2 judged against a_2, noted as $a^2{}_{22}$, is valued at 1
a_3 judged against a_3, noted as $a^2{}_{33}$, is valued at 1

These quantified judgments are recorded in a judgment matrix as follows.

$$A_2 = \begin{matrix} & a_1 & a_2 & a_3 \\ a_1 & a^2{}_{11} & a^2{}_{12} & a^2{}_{13} \\ a_2 & a^2{}_{21} & a^2{}_{22} & a^2{}_{23} \\ a_3 & a^2{}_{31} & a^2{}_{32} & a^2{}_{33} \end{matrix} = \begin{bmatrix} 1 & 3 & 1/3 \\ 1/3 & 1 & 1/9 \\ 3 & 9 & 1 \end{bmatrix}$$

Since objective measures do not exist for the third criterion, increasing the census of the hospital, a judgment matrix must also be developed for C_3. Assume that pairwise judgments are made among the alternatives with respect to C_3 and recorded in matrix A_3.

$$
A_3 = \begin{array}{c} a_1 \\ a_2 \\ a_3 \end{array}
\overset{\begin{array}{ccc} a_1 & a_2 & a_3 \end{array}}{\begin{bmatrix} 1 & 1/7 & 3 \\ 7 & 1 & 1/7 \\ 1/3 & 7 & 1 \end{bmatrix}}
$$

The development of these ratio and judgment matrices is the first step in the eigenvalue prioritization model. The next step involves abstracting the eigenvector associated with the maximal eigenvalue of each ratio or judgment matrix. These three maximal eigenvectors form the columns of the 3 × 3 alternatives evaluation matrix P.

Abstraction of Maximal Eigenvectors

Algorithm (1) is used to abstract the eigenvectors associated with these three matrices. The derivation of the maximal eigenvector for matrix A_2 is illustrated as follows.

Iteration 1

$$
\bar{d}_1 = \begin{bmatrix} 1 & 3 & 1/3 \\ 1/3 & 1 & 1/9 \\ 3 & 9 & 1 \end{bmatrix} \cdot \begin{bmatrix} 1 \\ 1 \\ 1 \end{bmatrix} \div \left([1, 1, 1] \cdot \begin{bmatrix} 1 & 3 & 1/3 \\ 1/3 & 1 & 1/9 \\ 3 & 9 & 1 \end{bmatrix} \cdot \begin{bmatrix} 1 \\ 1 \\ 1 \end{bmatrix} \right)
$$

$$
= \begin{bmatrix} 39/9 \\ 13/9 \\ 117/9 \end{bmatrix} \div (169/9)
$$

$$
= \begin{bmatrix} 39/169 \\ 13/169 \\ 117/169 \end{bmatrix} = \begin{bmatrix} .231 \\ .077 \\ .692 \end{bmatrix}
$$

Iteration 2

$$\bar{d}_2 = \begin{bmatrix} 1 & 3 & 1/3 \\ 1/3 & 1 & 1/9 \\ 3 & 9 & 1 \end{bmatrix} \cdot \begin{bmatrix} 39/169 \\ 13/169 \\ 117/169 \end{bmatrix} \div \left([1, 1, 1] \cdot \begin{bmatrix} 1 & 3 & 1/3 \\ 1/3 & 1 & 1/9 \\ 3 & 9 & 1 \end{bmatrix} \cdot \begin{bmatrix} 39/169 \\ 13/169 \\ 117/169 \end{bmatrix} \right)$$

$$= \begin{bmatrix} 117/169 \\ 39/169 \\ 351/169 \end{bmatrix} \div (507/169)$$

$$= \begin{bmatrix} 117/507 \\ 39/507 \\ 351/507 \end{bmatrix} = \begin{bmatrix} .231 \\ .077 \\ .692 \end{bmatrix}$$

In this case, the maximal eigenvector is abstracted in two iterations. Since $\bar{d}_2 = \bar{d}_1$, the maximal eigenvector for A_2 is $\bar{V}_2 = [39/169 \quad 13/169 \quad 117/169]^T$. This same procedure is used to derive the maximal eigenvectors for the other two matrices.

After algorithm (1) has been applied to all three matrices, the maximal eigenvectors for the respective matrices are:

$$R_1\!: \ \bar{V}_1 = [.21 \quad .64 \quad .15]^T$$
$$A_2\!: \ \bar{V}_2 = [.23 \quad .08 \quad .69]^T$$
$$A_3\!: \ \bar{V}_3 = [.24 \quad .33 \quad .43]^T$$

These eigenvectors best reflect the ratio and judgment information previously represented in the matrices R_1, A_2, and A_3. For example, in matrix A_2, alternative a_3 dominated both a_1 and a_2, while a_1 was preferred to a_2. The weights of $\bar{V}_2$ reflect this relationship. The weight assigned to a_3 is .69, which dominates the weights assigned to both a_1 and a_2. In addition, the weight assigned to a_1, .23, is greater than the weight of a_2, .08. Hence, the maximal eigenvectors reflect the information represented in the matrices from which they were abstracted. However, before these eigenvectors can be used to form the alternatives evaluation matrix, they must be adjusted for consistency.

Derivation of the Consistency Adjustment Information: $1 - \theta_j{}^i$

The eigenvalues of the three matrices may be derived by solving for λ_{max} in the following equation.

$$A_j\bar{V}_j = \lambda_{max} \times \bar{V}_j$$

For example, in matrix R_1, the eigenvalue, λ_{max}, would be derived as follows.

$$R_1 \cdot \bar{V}_1 = \lambda_{max} \times \bar{V}_1$$

$$\underset{3 \times 3}{\begin{bmatrix} 1 & .325 & 1.412 \\ 3.08 & 1 & 4.34 \\ .708 & .230 & 1 \end{bmatrix}} \cdot \underset{3 \times 1}{\begin{bmatrix} .21 \\ .64 \\ .15 \end{bmatrix}} = \lambda_{max} \times \underset{3 \times 1}{\begin{bmatrix} .21 \\ .64 \\ .15 \end{bmatrix}}$$

After performing the necessary multiplication on the left side of this equation, the following algebraic relationship is established.

$$\begin{bmatrix} .63 \\ 1.92 \\ .45 \end{bmatrix} = \lambda_{max} \times \begin{bmatrix} .21 \\ .64 \\ .15 \end{bmatrix}$$

Hence, $\lambda_{max} = 3.0$ for matrix R_1. If these operations are performed for matrices A_2 and A_3, the resultant λ_{max} are 3.0 and 6.5, respectively.

These maximal eigenvalues enable the computation of the consistency adjustment for the three eigenvectors, $\bar{V}_1$, $\bar{V}_2$, and $\bar{V}_3$. However, before this computation can be performed, the maximal eigenvalue for a consistent 3×3 matrix and for a completely inconsistent 3×3 matrix must be derived. The maximal eigenvalue of a consistent 3×3 matrix is equal to the trace of the matrix, or the sum of the numbers in the main diagonal, i.e., 3.0. The maximal eigenvalue of the most inconsistent 3×3 matrix (B):

$$B_{3\times3} = \begin{bmatrix} 1 & 9 & 1/9 \\ 1/9 & 1 & 9 \\ 9 & 1/9 & 1 \end{bmatrix}$$

is $\lambda_{sup} = 10.1$. Hence, the computation of the relative inconsistency, $\theta_j{}^i$, for each of the three matrices, R_1, A_2, and A_3 is:

$$A_j\colon \theta_j{}^i = \frac{\lambda_{max} - n}{\lambda_{sup} - n}$$

$$R_1\colon \theta_1{}^i = \frac{3 - 3}{10.1 - 3}$$

$$= 0$$

$$A_2\colon \theta_2{}^i = \frac{3 - 3}{10.1 - 3}$$

$$= 0$$

$$A_3\colon \theta_3{}^i = \frac{6.5 - 3}{10.1 - 3}$$

$$= \frac{3.5}{7.1}$$

$$= .49.$$

Since each of these values represents the relative inconsistency of A_j as a percentage, the relative consistency of A_j will be $1 - \theta_j{}^i$. Therefore, the maximal eigenvectors for the ratio and judgment matrices would be consistency adjusted as follows.

$$R_j\colon \bar{w}_j = \bar{V}_j \times (1 - \theta_j)$$

$$R_1\colon \bar{w}_1 = \begin{bmatrix} .21 \\ .64 \\ .15 \end{bmatrix} \times (1 - 0) = \begin{bmatrix} .21 \\ .64 \\ .15 \end{bmatrix}$$

$$A_j\colon \bar{w}_j = \bar{V}_j \times (1 - \theta_j{}^i)$$

$$A_2\colon \bar{w}_2 = \begin{bmatrix} .23 \\ .08 \\ .69 \end{bmatrix} \times (1 - 0) = \begin{bmatrix} .23 \\ .08 \\ .69 \end{bmatrix}$$

$$A_3\colon\ \bar{w}_3 = \begin{bmatrix} .24 \\ .33 \\ .43 \end{bmatrix} \times (1 - .49) = \begin{bmatrix} .122 \\ .168 \\ .220 \end{bmatrix}$$

The Alternatives Evaluation Matrix

These consistency adjusted maximal eigenvectors combine to form P, the matrix that represents the judgmental weights assigned to the decision alternatives, as follows.

$$P = \begin{bmatrix} .21 & .23 & .122 \\ .64 & .08 & .168 \\ .15 & .69 & .220 \end{bmatrix}$$

This matrix must be multiplied by the maximal eigenvector of the criteria judgment matrix $\bar{V}_c$ to yield the final set of priority weights for alternatives a_1, a_2, and a_3.

Derivation of the Maximal Eigenvector of the Criteria Judgment Matrix

To derive the set of weights that reflect the relative importance of each criterion in achieving the mission of the hospital, a criteria judgment matrix must be developed. In this case, assume that C_1 is weakly preferred to C_2 and to C_3, while C_2 and C_3 are equally preferred. The resultant criteria judgment matrix will be as follows.

$$\|C\| = \begin{matrix} \\ C_1 \\ C_2 \\ C_3 \end{matrix} \begin{matrix} \begin{matrix} C_1 & C_2 & C_3 \end{matrix} \\ \begin{bmatrix} 1 & 3 & 3 \\ 1/3 & 1 & 1 \\ 1/3 & 1 & 1 \end{bmatrix} \end{matrix}$$

Using algorithm (1), the maximal eigenvector of the criteria judgment matrix is $\bar{V}_c = [.6\ .2\ .2]^T$. The elements in this vector represent the relative importance of each criterion in achieving the institution's mission.

Derivation of Priority Weights for the Decision Alternatives

Once the alternatives evaluation matrix, *P*, and the maximal eigenvector of the criteria judgment matrix, $\bar{V}_c$, are known, the vector of priority weights for the decision alternatives can be derived as follows.

$$\bar{i}^* = \frac{\begin{bmatrix} .21 & .23 & .122 \\ .64 & .08 & .168 \\ .15 & .69 & .220 \end{bmatrix} \cdot \begin{bmatrix} .6 \\ .2 \\ .2 \end{bmatrix}}{[111] \cdot \begin{bmatrix} .21 & .23 & .122 \\ .64 & .08 & .168 \\ .15 & .69 & .220 \end{bmatrix} \cdot \begin{bmatrix} .6 \\ .2 \\ .2 \end{bmatrix}}$$

$$= \begin{bmatrix} .1964 \\ .4336 \\ .2720 \end{bmatrix} \div .902$$

$$= \begin{bmatrix} .218 \\ .481 \\ .301 \end{bmatrix}$$

In this case, the eigenvalue prioritization model indicates that the second investment alternative is considered to be the most important in achieving the organizational mission. This information would be used to guide the investment selection process.

RELEVANCE MODEL AND EIGENVALUE PRIORITIZATION MODEL CONTRAST: A STUDENT EXPOSURE

The perspective of the relevance model is much broader than that of the eigenvalue prioritization model. The relevance model delineates the organizational decision making structure and the respective institutional goals at each organizational level. Various alternative resource allocations or investment opportunities are evaluated within the relevance model with respect to the impact of these alternatives in effecting particular organizational states. The eigenvalue prioritization model, as used here, is a more specialized technique, concerned primarily with the selection of an investment alternative from a set of alternatives. Although each model has different information demands, both may be used to provide priority information regarding the selection of investments.

Model Contrast

To provide a contrast between the results of the relevance model and the results of the eigenvalue prioritization model, a group of five students[12] were given the same scenario information as the group which developed the relevance matrices in the illustration beginning on page 396. These students were asked to make pairwise evaluations among the three investment alternatives:

a_1 = medical classroom equipment
a_2 = electronic analogue/digital computer system
a_3 = health maintenance organization (HMO)

on each of the ten criteria:

C_1: provide for patient welfare
C_2: status of the hospital
C_3: fund generation potential
C_4: resource control potential
C_5: program achievement within one year
C_6: continuity of fund flow
C_7: attractive physician environment
C_8: yearly economic return
C_9: increase hospital utilization
C_{10}: ability to validate proposed benefits prior to fund commitment.

The students also were asked to prepare the 10×10 criteria judgment matrix required in the eigenvalue analysis. The results of this student exposure are given in Table 11-3. Note that in each case, a_3 was given the highest priority weight. This alternative also was preferred in the relevance model.

The eigenvalue investment priority weights developed by these students compare favorably[13] with the weights derived by the students using the

Table 11-3 Investment Alternative Weights Generated with the Eigenvalue Prioritization Model

Individual	a_1	a_2	a_3
A	.06	.25	.69
B	.19	.22	.59
C	.20	.25	.55
D	.15	.35	.50
E	.14	.15	.71
Relevance Weights from Table 11-1	.12	.19	.69

relevance model. However, no significance can be attached to the proximity of the eigenvalue and relevance weights because the student samples in both cases were small. Nonetheless, recognizing that similar information can be generated with the eigenvalue prioritization model and the relevance model is important.

Conclusion

The relevance model is preferred to the simple planning information discussed in Chapter 9 because this model systematically assigns priority weights to a set of decision alternatives, based on a specific set of evaluation criteria which may include the simple planning information. In addition, since the relevance model requires the delineation of the evaluation criteria at various activity levels, management's understanding of organizational goals, activities, and opportunities can be enhanced. Furthermore, the relevance model causes the investment alternatives to be evaluated with respect to a common denominator (i.e., contribution to the mission of the organization). These advantages make the relevance model valuable in aiding the organization's capital evaluation process.

However, the eigenvalue prioritization model generally is more useful than the relevance model because in addition to systematically assigning priority weights to decision alternatives using a specific set of evaluation criteria and evaluating the investment alternatives with respect to the contribution to the mission of the organization, the eigenvalue prioritization model has three other advantages that increase its usefulness, particularly in a health care environment. First, the operational requirements of the eigenvalue prioritization model are not as complex as those of the relevance model. The relevance model requires a significant number of complex intra- and interhierarchical level comparisons (not required by the eigenvalue prioritization model) that can dissipate user enthusiasm even when only a few hierarchical levels exist. Second, the eigenvalue prioritization model is easily programed to receive the required judgment matrices, while the relevance model is difficult to program because an investment may contribute to various decision levels in a variety of ways. Third, the eigenvalue prioritization model has a simple measure of judgment consistency that can aid in determining the confidence that should be placed in the priority vectors developed. The relevance model has no simple measure that would indicate the degree of confidence that should be placed in the relevance values developed for the decision alternatives. Hence, the eigenvalue prioritization model seems ideal for systematizing the long-range planning process. The model provides an easily implemented, yet systematic means of ranking decision alternatives.[14]

Appendix 11-A

Generalized Relevance System Assuming Three Decision Levels

Figure 11A-1 Relevance Matrix—Level G

		General Activities: G				
General Evaluation Criteria	Criteria Weights	GA_1	GA_2	...	GA_m	
EC_1^G	γ_1	x_{11}	x_{12}	...	x_{1m}	$\sum_j^m x_{1j} = 1$
EC_2^G	γ_2	x_{21}	x_{22}	...	x_{2m}	$\sum_j^m x_{1j} = 1$
⋮	⋮	⋮	⋮	⋮	⋮	⋮
EC_n^G	γ_n	x_{n1}	x_{n2}	...	x_{nm}	$\sum_j^m x_{nj} = 1$
	$\sum_{i=1}^n \gamma_i = 1.0$	Φ_1	Φ_2	...	Φ_m	$\sum_j^m \Phi_j = 1$

$$\text{where } \Phi_k = \sum_i^n \gamma_i \times x_{ik}$$

Figure 11A-2 Relevance Matrix—Level P

		Program Activities: P				
Program Evaluation Criteria	Criteria Weights	PA_1	PA_2	$\ldots$	PA_r	
EC_1^P	δ_1	y_{11}	y_{12}	$\ldots$	y_{1r}	$\sum_j^r y_{1j} = 1$
EC_2^P	δ_2	y_{21}	y_{22}	$\ldots$	y_{2r}	$\sum_j^r y_{2j} = 1$
$\vdots$	$\vdots$	$\vdots$	$\vdots$	$\vdots$	$\vdots$	$\vdots$
EC_q^P	δ_q	y_{q1}	y_{q2}	$\ldots$	y_{qr}	$\sum_j^r y_{qj} = 1$
	$\sum_{i=1}^q \delta_i = 1.0$	φ_1	φ_2	$\ldots$	φ_r	$\sum_j^r \varphi_j = 1$

where: $\varphi_k = \sum_i^q \delta_i \times y_{ik}$

Figure 11A-3 Relevance Matrix—Level I

		Investment Activity: I				
Investment Activity Evaluation Criteria	Criteria Weights	a_1	a_2	...	a_t	
EC_1^I	ϵ_1	z_{11}	z_{12}	...	z_{1t}	$\sum_j^t z_{1j} = 1$
EC_2^I	ϵ_2	z_{21}	z_{22}	...	z_{2t}	$\sum_j^t z_{2j} = 1$
⋮	⋮	⋮	⋮	⋮	⋮	⋮
EC_s^I	ϵ_s	z_{s1}	z_{s2}	...	z_{st}	$\sum_j^t z_{sj} = 1$
	$\sum_{i=1}^s \epsilon_i = 1.0$	θ_1	θ_2	...	θ_t	$\sum_j^t \theta_j = 1$

where: $\theta_k = \sum_i^s \epsilon_i \times z_{ik}$

where: EC^G, EC^P and EC^I are the general, program, and investment activity evaluation criteria, respectively;
γ, δ, ϵ are the weights that reflect the contribution of that level's criteria to the mission;
x, y, z are the weights reflecting the way in which an activity relates to an evaluation criteria; and
Φ, φ and θ are the relevance weightings of the activities (general, program, and investment) for the decision levels G, P, I.

In Figure 11A-1, there are $m + r + t$ investment relevance weights. Each relevance weight is placed on the relevance lattice (Figure 11A-4) to compute the relevance values.

Figure 11A-4 PPB Hierarchy

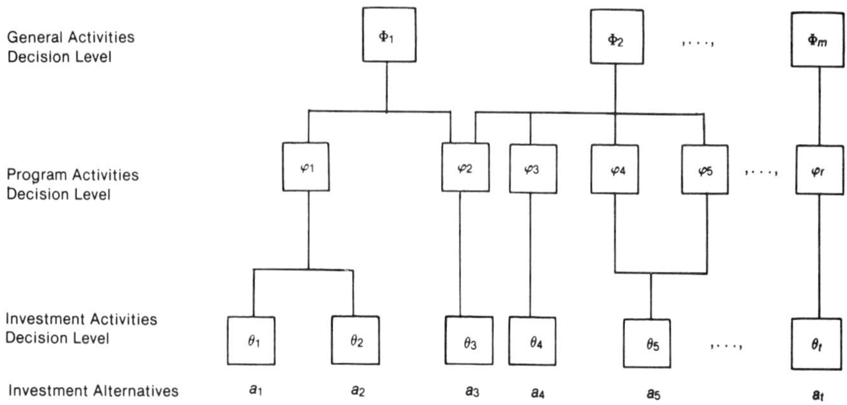

Relevance Values
Investment Activity:

$$RV^1 = (\theta_1 \cdot \varphi_1 \cdot \Phi_1)/A$$
$$RV^2 = (\theta_2 \cdot \varphi_1 \cdot \Phi_1)/A$$
$$RV^3 = (\theta_3 \cdot \varphi_2 \cdot \Phi_1)/A$$
$$RV^4 = (\theta_4 \cdot \varphi_3 \cdot \Phi_2)/A$$
$$RV^5 = (\theta_5(\varphi_4 + \varphi_5))\Phi_2/A$$
$$\vdots$$
$$RV^t = (\theta_t \cdot \varphi_r \cdot \Phi_m)/A$$

where: $A = \sum_{i=1}^{t} f(\theta, \varphi, \Phi).$

Note that investment a_5 contributes to the full support of two different programs, PA_4 and PA_5. In this case, a_5 is weighted by φ_4 and φ_5. If the investment were to make partial contributions, α and β, where $0 < \alpha, \beta \leq 1$, to φ_4 and φ_5, respectively, then the relevance value of a_5 would be computed as $[\alpha\theta_5\varphi_4 + \beta\theta_5\varphi_5]\Phi_2$.

Appendix 11-B

Matrix Operations

Throughout this chapter, various matrix relationships are used to derive planning information. Further discussion of some of these operations may facilitate the reading of the chapter. This appendix examines three matrix operations: (1) scalar multiplication, (2) vector multiplication, and (3) matrix/vector multiplication.

Scalar Multiplication

A vector is a collection of numbers. A *column* vector of *n* elements is represented as shown.

$$\bar{x} = \begin{bmatrix} x_1 \\ x_2 \\ \cdot \\ \cdot \\ \cdot \\ x_n \end{bmatrix}$$

The column vector $\bar{x}$ shall be noted as $\bar{x}_{n \times 1}$, a shorthand method of indicating that vector $\bar{x}$ has n rows and one column of numbers.

A *row* vector of n elements is represented as shown.

$$\bar{x} = [x_1, x_2, \ldots, x_n]$$

In this case, $\bar{x}$ would be noted as $\bar{x}_{(1 \times n)}$ which indicates that $\bar{x}$ has one row and n columns. The only difference between a row and a column vector of size *n* is the way the elements are arranged.

The arrangement of the elements in a vector is important because certain operations are possible if the vectors are arranged in one way, but not possible if they are arranged in another way. When vector arithmetic operations are possible, the vectors are said to be comfortable. Since the only difference between $\bar{x}_{(n\times 1)}$ and $\bar{x}_{(1\times n)}$ is the arrangement of the elements, the two vectors can be algebraically related as

$$\bar{x}^{T}_{(n\times 1)} = \bar{x}_{(1\times n)},$$

which means that $\bar{x}^{T}_{(n\times 1)}$ is the transpose of vector $\bar{x}_{(1\times n)}$ or merely the repositioning of a column vector to make a row vector.

With this background, a scalar may be defined as a single number or a vector of size $\bar{x}_{(1\times 1)}$. Scalars, henceforth noted as k, can multiply a vector of any size. This operation is performed as follows.

$$k \times [x_1, x_2, \ldots, x_n] = [kx_1, kx_2, \ldots, kx_n]$$

For example, the vector generated by multiplying 3 times $\bar{x} = [12, 2, 0, \frac{1}{2}]$ is:

$$3 \times \bar{x} = [36, 6, 0, 3/2].$$

Vector Multiplication

When two vectors are multiplied together, either a scalar or a matrix is produced. In this chapter, vector multiplication which produces a scalar is of particular importance. Therefore, this operation will be examined. The elements in the scalar developed from a vector multiplication are the arithmetic summation of the products of the elements of the vectors being multiplied. For example, consider the following vectors.

$$\bar{x}_{(3\times 1)} = \begin{bmatrix} 4 \\ 5 \\ 3 \end{bmatrix};$$

and

$$\bar{y}_{(1\times 3)} = [2, 4, 1]$$

If these two vectors are multiplied together (i.e., $\bar{y} \cdot \bar{x}$), the following result is obtained.

$$[2, 4, 1] \cdot \begin{bmatrix} 4 \\ 5 \\ 3 \end{bmatrix} = [(2 \times 4) + (4 \times 5) + (1 \times 3)] = 31$$

$$(1 \times 3)\ (3 \times 1)$$

In general, if

$$\bar{x}_{(n\times 1)} = \begin{bmatrix} x_1 \\ x_2 \\ \vdots \\ x_n \end{bmatrix} \text{ and } \bar{y}_{(1\times n)} = [y_1, y_2, \ldots, y_n]$$

the operation $\bar{y}_{(1\times n)} \cdot \bar{x}_{(n\times 1)}$ results in the following scalar:

$$k = [x_1y_1 + x_2y_2 + x_3y_3, \ldots, x_ny_n]$$

Matrix/Vector Multiplication

Size conformability now becomes important in understanding the way that new vectors are formed by multiplying a matrix and a vector. The rule is that the inner subscripts of the matrix and vector being multiplied together must be identical. The multiplication operation forms each new vector element as the sum of a row-column multiplication proceeding from the top row of the matrix. For example, consider $\|A\|$ and $\bar{x}$.

$$\underset{2\times 3}{\|A\|} = \begin{bmatrix} 4 & 3 & 4 \\ 2 & 0 & 1 \end{bmatrix} \qquad \underset{3\times 1}{\bar{x}} = \begin{bmatrix} 4 \\ 5 \\ 3 \end{bmatrix}$$

The new vector will be of size 2 × 1 (two rows, one column) with the following elements.

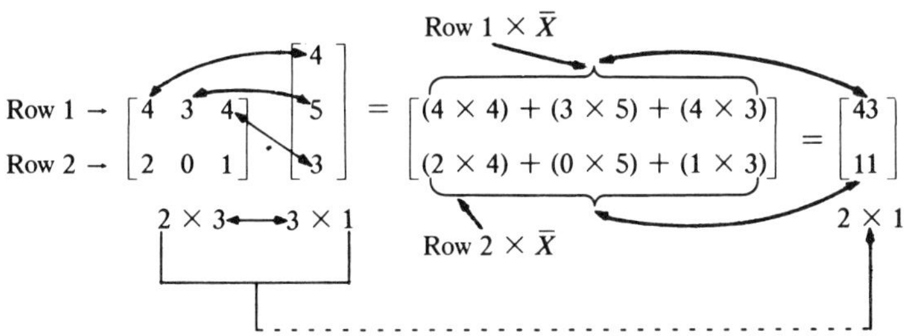

Therefore, each scalar element of the new vector is formed by a vector multiplication of *a* row of the matrix and *the* column vector multiplier. This concept can be generalized for a matrix ($\|A\|$) of size $m \times n$ and a vector $\bar{x}$ of size $n \times 1$ as follows.

$$\underset{m \times n}{\begin{bmatrix} a_{11} & a_{12} & a_{13}, \ldots, a_{1n} \\ a_{21} & a_{22} & a_{23}, \ldots, a_{2n} \\ a_{31} & a_{32} & a_{33}, \ldots, a_{3n} \\ \vdots & & \vdots \\ a_{m1} & a_{m2} & a_{m3}, \ldots, a_{mn} \end{bmatrix}} \cdot \underset{n \times 1}{\begin{bmatrix} x_1 \\ x_2 \\ x_3 \\ \vdots \\ x_n \end{bmatrix}} = \underset{m \times 1}{\begin{bmatrix} \sum_{i=1}^{n} a_{1i}x_i \\ \sum_{i=1}^{n} a_{2i}x_i \\ \vdots \\ \sum_{i=1}^{n} a_{mi}x_i \end{bmatrix}}$$

NOTES

1. The reader is encouraged to reread the capital budgeting section of Chapter 9 before reading this presentation.
2. An important determinant of the quality of evaluative information provided by the relevance model is the constitution of the group of individuals responsible for determining the PPB hierarchical relationships and the various weightings. Care should be taken in selecting the appropriate individuals (see Question 11-7).
3. See Appendix 11-A for a more complete illustration of the relevance lattice.
4. The information provided in this example was developed by a group of second-year MBA students in the Health Care Administration Program at the University of Pennsylvania.
5. Among the models suggested to develop priority weights are multi-dimensional scaling algorithms and network analysis models. Examining these models and their information requirements or their relationship to the priority model to be suggested is beyond the scope of this text.
6. For a lucid discussion of eigenvector analysis, see Hildebrand (1974).
7. These properties are exhibited by the criteria judgment matrix, $\|C\| = c_{jk}$, where j and k indicate that the jth criterion is being evaluated against the kth criterion, $j = 1, \ldots, m$ and $k = 1, \ldots, m$.
8. The eigenvector associated with the maximal eigenvalue shall be referred to as the maximal eigenvector.
9. The basis of this algorithm is the well known iterative procedure for developing the eigenvector associated with the largest eigenvalue. This algorithm often is associated with Vianello or Stodola.
10. The term "consistency adjustment" is used since the maximal eigenvector is multiplied by $1 - \theta_j^i$ which is a measure of consistency. However, the only eigenvectors adjusted (changed) are those developed from inconsistent matrices. The consistency adjustment, as represented here, is an extension of Saaty's model.
11. The denominator is this equation normalizes the final set of priority weights (i.e., makes the weights sum to one).

12. These individuals were health care administration students enrolled in a management control course at the University of Pennsylvania.
13. If the five student weightings are considered as the population, one is unable to show that the relevance weights {.12 .20 .68} belong to a different population at a confidence level of $\alpha \leq .10$.
14. For completeness, note that the eigenvalue prioritization models relies on the eigenvalue transformation of the judgment matrices. While this transformation is order preserving, its precise nature regarding the distribution of judgmental error has not yet been detailed. Further, the measure of inconsistency, θ_j^i, is a surrogate measure for the degree of inconsistency embodied in a particular judgment matrix. The quality of the surrogation depends upon the definition of inconsistency (Lusk (1977)). The implications of these qualifications for the health practitioner are, by and large, inconsequential since the impression of the judgment process precludes the use of the priority weights for anything other than ordinal inference. For example, if $\bar{i}^*$ were the priority vector developed, $\bar{i}^* = [.35, .33, .32]$, no competent analyst would suggest that alternative one dominates the others. Generally, if the priority elements in the maximal vector differ at some reasonable level of α confidence, the imprecisions which may be introduced by the transformation and the surrogation are not substantial enough to alter the statistical inferences as to priority dominance.

Vector and Matrix Problems

Problem 11B-1. Compute the following, where $\bar{x} = [x_1, x_2]$:

a. $[4, 8, 3] \cdot \begin{bmatrix} 3 \\ 2 \\ 1 \end{bmatrix}$

b. $\bar{x} \cdot \bar{x}^T$

c. $\left[[4, 8, 3] \cdot \begin{bmatrix} 3 \\ 2 \\ 1 \end{bmatrix} \right] \cdot \bar{x}$

d. $[4, 8, 3] \cdot \bar{x}^T$

Answers

a. 31

b. $[x_1^2 + x_2^2]$

c. $[31x_1, 31x_2]$

d. Not conformable

Problem 11B-2. Compute the following, where $\|A\| = \begin{bmatrix} a_{11} & a_{12} \\ a_{21} & a_{22} \end{bmatrix}$

a. $\begin{bmatrix} 4 & 8 & 3 \\ 3 & 2 & 1 \end{bmatrix} \cdot \begin{bmatrix} 3 \\ 2 \\ 1 \end{bmatrix}$

b. $\|A\| \cdot \|A\|$

c. $\|A\| \cdot \left[\begin{bmatrix} 4 & 8 & 3 \\ 3 & 2 & 1 \end{bmatrix} \cdot \begin{bmatrix} 3 \\ 2 \\ 1 \end{bmatrix} \right]$

d. $\begin{bmatrix} 3 \\ 2 \\ 1 \end{bmatrix} \cdot \|A\|$

Answers

a. $\begin{bmatrix} 31 \\ 14 \end{bmatrix}$

b. $\begin{bmatrix} a_{11}^2 + a_{12}a_{21} & a_{11}a_{12} + a_{12}a_{22} \\ a_{11}a_{21} + a_{22}a_{21} & a_{21}a_{12} + a_{22}^2 \end{bmatrix}$

c. $\begin{bmatrix} 31a_{11} + 14a_{12} \\ 31a_{21} + 14a_{22} \end{bmatrix}$

d. Not conformable

Questions and Problems

Question 11-1. Summarize the steps involved in constructing a relevance matrix and relevance lattice.

Question 11-2. For purposes of developing a relevance lattice, how would you differentiate between general, program, and investment level activities?

Question 11-3. What does it mean when an investment activity has the highest overall relevance value, although it does not have the highest relevance weight on the investment level?

Question 11-4. The program activities evaluation criteria may change when different investment activities are being evaluated. Is this desirable? Defend your answer.

Question 11-5. What is the advantage for either the relevance model or eigenvalue prioritization model of keeping the investment evaluation criteria constant regardless of the set of investment alternatives being analyzed?

Question 11-6. In Figure 11-3, there is a box for "other inputs." What are these other inputs? How should they be used with the results of relevance analysis?

Question 11-7. What criteria would you use to select individuals to conduct (a) a relevance analysis, and (b) an investment analysis using the eigenvalue prioritization model? Discuss any differences in the sets of criteria.

Question 11-8. What information would you gather to evaluate the effectiveness of the relevance and eigenvalue prioritization models over time?

Problem 11-1. Compute the maximal eigenvectors for the following matrices and interpret the entries in each vector.

$$\|A\| = \begin{bmatrix} 1 & 2 \\ 1/2 & 1 \end{bmatrix} \qquad \|B\| = \begin{bmatrix} 1 & 1/5 & 3 \\ 5 & 1 & 1/5 \\ 1/3 & 5 & 1 \end{bmatrix} \qquad \|C\| = \begin{bmatrix} 1 & 1 & 1 \\ 1 & 1 & 1 \\ 1 & 1 & 1 \end{bmatrix}$$

$$\|D\| = \begin{bmatrix} 1 & 1 & 5 \\ 1 & 1 & 7 \\ 1/5 & 1/7 & 1 \end{bmatrix} \qquad \|E\| = \begin{bmatrix} 1 & 3 & 9 \\ 1/3 & 1 & 3 \\ 1/9 & 1/3 & 1 \end{bmatrix}$$

Problem 11-2. Compute the maximal eigenvalue for the five matrices in Problem 11-1.

Problem 11-3. a. Compute the inconsistency measure and the consistency adjustment $(1 - \theta_j^i)$ for the matrices in Problem 11-1.

b. Assume matrices B, D, and E were developed by three individuals in the organization. How would you use the inconsistency information to evaluate their judgments?

Problem 11-4. Carefully consider the following matrix. Without using algorithm (1), compute the eigenvalue and eigenvector for matrix ||F||.

$$\|F\| = \begin{bmatrix} 4/4 & 4/6 & 4/3 & 4/19 \\ 6/4 & 6/6 & 6/3 & 6/19 \\ 3/4 & 3/6 & 3/3 & 3/19 \\ 19/4 & 19/6 & 19/3 & 19/19 \end{bmatrix}$$

Problem 11-5. Assume the hospital administrator had five individuals in the organization evaluate two investment alternatives (a_1, a_2) on six criteria. The prioritization vectors developed by these individuals were:

$$\begin{array}{lcc} & a_1 & a_2 \\ I_1^A: & [.70 & .30]^T \\ I_2^A: & [.80 & .20]^T \\ I_3^P: & [.23 & .77]^T \\ I_4^P: & [.18 & .82]^T \\ I_5^P: & [.40 & .60]^T \end{array}$$

where: the superscript indicates whether the individual was an administrator (A) or a physician (P).

The five individuals also met as a group and generated the following prioritization vector.

$$\begin{array}{lcc} & a_1 & a_2 \\ \text{Group:} & [.45 & .55]^T \end{array}$$

Required:

a. How would you use this information in evaluating the selection of investment alternative a_1 or a_2?

b. What would your answer be if the group prioritization vector was $[.17, .83]^T$?

Problem 11-6. a. Prove that any 2 × 2 judgment matrix is consistent.
b. Prove that any 3 × 3 consistent matrix is a ratio matrix.

Problem 11-7. a. Assume matrices B and D in problem 11-1 were generated by one individual. They reflect this person's judgment regarding three long-range planning alternatives. Further assume that matrix A in problem 11-1 is the criteria judgment matrix. Compute $\bar{i}^*$.
b. Assume that the eigenvectors from matrices B and D are not consistency adjusted. Recompute $\bar{i}^*$ and compare it with the priority alternative weights developed in part (a).

Problem 11-8. a. Assume matrices C, D, and E in problem 11-1 were generated by one individual. They reflect this person's judgment regarding three long-range planning alternatives. Further assume that matrix B in problem 11-1 is the criteria judgment matrix. Compute $\bar{i}^*$.
b. Assume that the eigenvector developed from the criteria matrix B is consistency adjusted. Recompute $\bar{i}^*$ and contrast it with the priority weights developed in part (a). Discuss the implication of your result.

Problem 11-9. You have been engaged by the board of managers of a large chain of extended care nursing homes to assist in the refinement of their long-range planning process. You suggest the use of the eigenvalue prioritization model. After a number of intensive sessions, the following criteria judgment matrix is developed by the board of managers:

$$\begin{array}{c} \\ C_1 \\ C_2 \\ C_3 \\ C_4 \end{array} \begin{array}{c} \begin{array}{cccc} C_1 & C_2 & C_3 & C_4 \end{array} \\ \begin{bmatrix} 1 & .2 & .25 & .2 \\ 5 & 1 & 5 & 3 \\ 4 & .2 & 1 & .3 \\ 5 & .3 & 3 & 1 \end{bmatrix} \end{array}$$

where: C_1 represents the *Pride the Principle Managers Have in the Organization*
C_2 represents the *Maximization of Long-Run Profits*
C_3 represents the *Freedom To Take Managerial Actions Over Time*
C_4 represents the *Rapport with the Regional Hospital Community*

The mission of the organization was specified as: *Provide for Corporate Security*.

The president of the organization wonders if a particular investment alternative or project proposal could be evaluated independently, that is, without reference to how it compares with another investment alternative or project proposal. The president feels this is important because very often only one investment alternative is considered at a particular time.

Required

Suggest a generalized model that uses the information in the criteria matrix to develop a priority weight for a single investment alternative. Discuss how this priority weight may be used in the evaluation of the investment alternative.

Chapter 12

Simulation

Man tries to make for himself in the fashion that suits him best, a simplified and intelligible picture of the world.

A. Einstein

A recurring theme in this text is that the control function of nonprofit institutions is a complex task. To assist in developing relevant control information, a number of techniques and models have been suggested. Unfortunately, discussions of these techniques and models often failed to go beyond specifying information useful for control, because the actual control process is so complex that the normative examination of (1) how control information is used in making decision rule modifications and (2) how these specific modifications are likely to affect the performance of the institution is most difficult. The previous chapters, however, do provide the background needed to study the effects of decision rule modifications on institutional performance. Hence, simulation, the only practical means of analyzing the effects of decision rule modifications on institutional performance, will be examined in this chapter.

THE BASIC SIMULATION MODEL

In most cases, experimentation with an ongoing management process is not desirable. Simulation is a method of analyzing the performance of a system with a model that attempts to abstract and then replicate the structure of real world events. The simulation model is constructed to incorporate the function of the system, rather than merely describe it. The simulation model is designed to (1) accept decision rule modifications which would be impossible to perform on an experimental basis in the institution's management control system, and (2) provide the analyst with insights regarding the effects of those modifications on specific institutional control variables.

Many different types of simulation exist. The most useful in ascertaining the effects of a decision rule modification on institutional performance is the symbolic simulation, which represents the organization's resource conversion process as mathematical or statistical functions. These mathematical or statistical representations are used to determine the effects of decision rule modifications.

In a health care context, the four principal elements of a symbolic simulation are:[1]

Inputs, which enter the health care process. Examples of inputs are the number of emergency medical services (EMS) patients, the number of requests for laboratory procedures, etc. Normally, inputs occur at varying time intervals.

Process, which is the interaction of institutional personnel and technology to convert input to output. The EMS process may be described by the manner in which the medical and administrative personnel use the institution's resources to deliver service to EMS patients.

Decision Rules, which are managerial policy statements used to determine the nature of particular process interactions. For example, a decision rule may specify how many physicians are to be available to deliver service in the EMS unit during various periods of the week.

Output, which is the result of processing inputs. Generally, the output of the institution cannot be measured accurately (e.g., the degree of patient welfare). However, numerous process statistics, such as physician hours, procedure costs, or inpatient days for specific treatments, usualy can be used to infer changes in the system's output (see the cost finding system, Chapter 10).

Dynamic Stochastic Simulations

Symbolic simulations may differ with respect to time and measurement orientation (see Figure 12-1). To simulate most decision problems realistically, *dynamic stochastic* simulations are required. These simulations provide information about events that occur over time where accurate measures of input processing over time do not exist, but where reasonable estimates of input processing over time can be developed.

Figure 12-1 Simulation Categorization

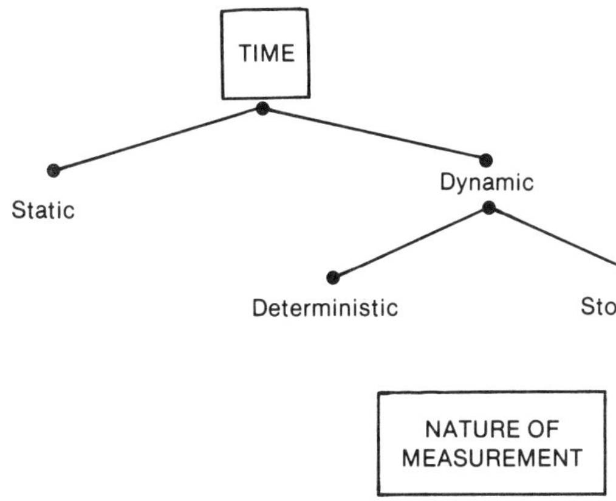

Since the results of *stochastic processes* are not known with certainty, only expectations can be developed regarding the realization of a stochastic process. For example, assume that the number of error-free laboratory procedures is generated from a stochastic process. In any given period, the actual number of error-free laboratory procedures cannot be predicted precisely. However, by using the mean value of error-free laboratory procedures as the expectation, variance information (σ^2) can be used to develop confidence intervals regarding the probability that the actual number of error-free procedures will fall into some interval about the expectation.

The results of *dynamic processes,* on the other hand, change as a function of time. For example, the arrival rate of EMS patients may differ dramatically by day of the week. In this case, the process generating EMS patient arrivals is dynamic. If the number of patient arrivals is not known with certainty, the EMS process is also stochastic.

Monte Carlo Technique

Stochastic processes complicate the simulation process because management cannot be sure which values will result from the stochastic process. To deal with this uncertainty, the stochastic process may be characterized by a probability density function. Once the appropriate density functions are developed, random draws are selected from each of the density functions. Then these randomly selected draws are used in the simulation process. To represent the stochastic variation, a number of random draws are made from the density functions. For each random draw, a simulation is conducted. Therefore, given n random draws, n solutions are generated by the simulation. The results of these n solutions usually are represented by a probability density function (see Figure 12-2). This process of (1) formulating probability densities to represent stochastic processes, (2) making random selections from these probability densities, and (3) using these

Figure 12-2 EMS Simulation Used to Ascertain the Approximate Need for Physicians to Staff the EMS Unit

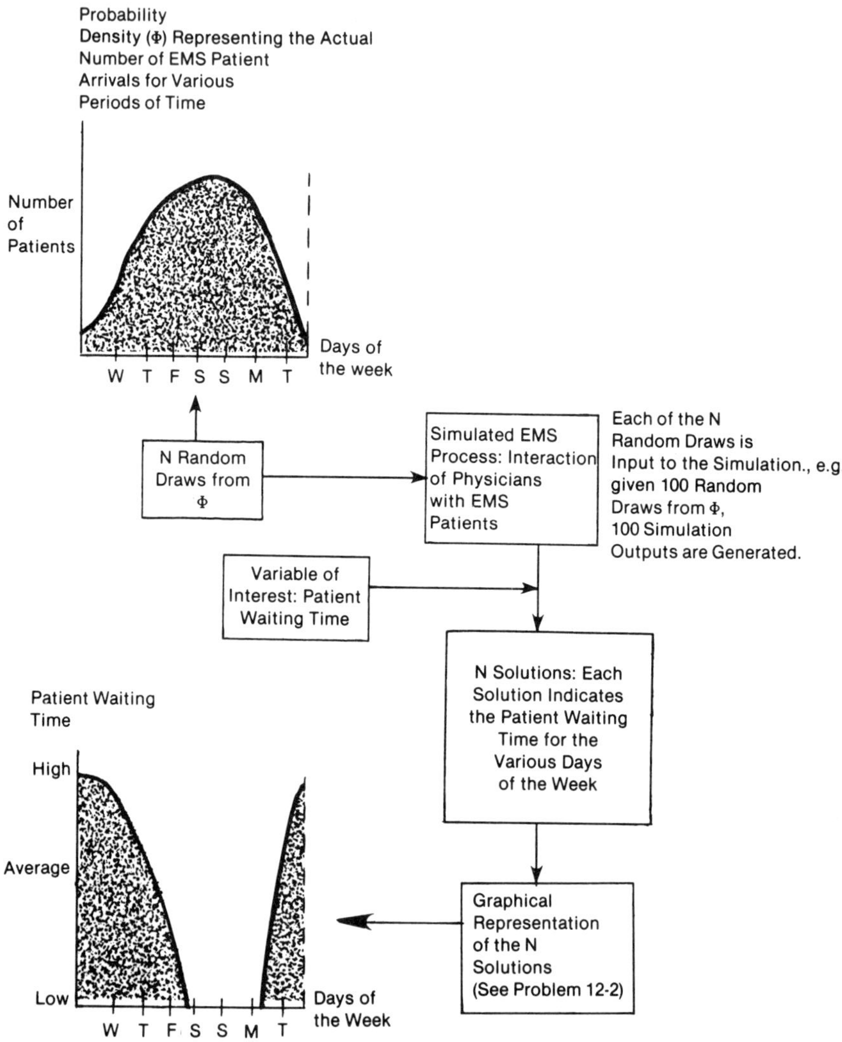

random selections to solve the simulation repeatedly is referred to as the Monte Carlo technique.

To illustrate how stochastic processes are characterized by probability density functions and how random draws are selected from each of the density functions, assume that the physician diagnosis times in the EMS unit are shown in Table 12-1. The probability density function representing how often a patient requires a particular diagnosis time is shown in Figure 12-3. Using the Monte Carlo technique, every individual entering the EMS unit is randomly assigned one of these diagnostic times.

The assignment of diagnosis times to individuals entering the EMS system is accomplished most simply by selecting numbers from a uniform distribution in the interval [0,1]. If, for example, that number falls in the interval [0, .25), the diagnosis time assigned to the individual is assumed to be 12 minutes. Using this rationale, the following Monte Carlo assignment would be developed:

Random Number Interval	*Diagnostic Time Assigned*
[0,.25)	12 minutes
[.25,.50)	15 minutes
[.50,.75)	18 minutes
[.75, $.91\overline{6}$)	21 minutes
[$.91\overline{6}$,1.]	24 minutes

where: the brackets, [,], mean the interval includes the boundary; and
the parenthesis,), means the interval does not include the boundary.

Table 12-1 Physician Diagnosis Times in EMS Unit

Diagnosis Density (see Figure 12-3)	
Diagnosis Time*	Frequency
Less than 12 minutes	3/12
At least 12, but less than 15 minutes	3/12
At least 15, but less than 18 minutes	3/12
At least 18, but less than 21 minutes	2/12
At least 21, but less than or equal to 24 minutes	1/12

*Determined from a time study of diagnosis times during a selected period.

Figure 12-3 Diagnosis Time Density and Corresponding Random Number Interval

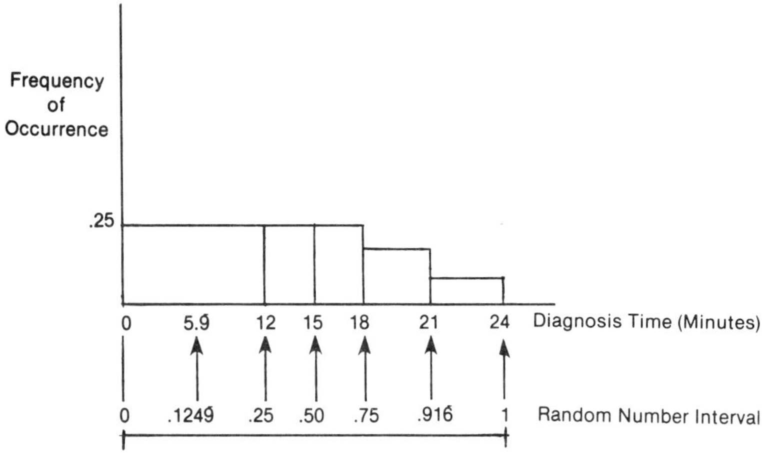

Hence, each individual would be assigned a diagnosis time of 12, 15, 18, 21, or 24 minutes.

Another means of assigning diagnosis times to individuals is to draw from the diagnosis density function represented in Figure 12-3. This is accomplished by relating the number selected in the [0,1] interval to the number of minutes that corresponds to that number. For example, if two random numbers, $.124\bar{9}$ and .75, are drawn, the number of minutes associated with each would be 5.9 and 18 minutes, respectively (see Figure 12-3). Using this assignment rule, any diagnosis time represented in the diagnosis density function may be assigned.

Hence, once a stochastic process has been characterized by a probability density function, a number of methods can be used to make random selections from that density function. In the first selection method described above, only five specific times are assumed to characterize the entire interval. The second selection method, on the other hand, assumes a continuous interval. Regardless of the selection method used, however, the selected physician diagnosis time is used in conjunction with the other facts of the problem to generate the simulation.

ILLUSTRATIVE SIMULATION EXAMPLE

The administration of Memorial Hospital is interested in developing a decision rule which the physician in charge of the EMS unit may use to determine how many physicians are required for duty during a two-day period (see Question 12-7). The EMS diagnostic services are conducted in four examination carrels in which individuals are examined privately. Physicians to staff these carrels are available on-call from other service areas of the hospital. However, during the two-day time period, the demand for physician diagnostic expertise fluctuates significantly, so that satisfactorily balancing the use of physicians and patient waiting time is a difficult task.

Since management is unwilling to experiment with the EMS system to determine the consequences of various staffing decision rules on (1) physician time spent in the EMS unit and (2) patient waiting time, the information in Tables 12-2 and 12-3 has been gathered over some representative time period so that a number of decision rules can be evaluated using a simulation (see Problem 12-5). The diagnosis times in Table 12-2 are averages for all physicians, and the interarrival time intervals in Table 12-3 are the average times between individual arrivals at the diagnostic carrels. For purposes of the simulation, patients are assigned to the shortest queue, and queue switching is permitted.

Table 12-2 Physician Diagnosis Information

Physician Diagnosis Time Density	Percentage of the Time (Density A)
[0, 12) minutes	3/12
[12, 15) minutes	3/12
[15, 18) minutes	3/12
[18, 21) minutes	2/12
[21, 24] minutes	1/12

Table 12-3 Patient Interarrival Information

Patient Interarrival Density	**First 1/2 of Day 1; Last 1/2 of Day 2** (Density B)	**Last 1/2 of Day 1; First 1/2 of Day 2** (Density C)
One patient per:		
[0, 6) minutes	3/12	8/12
[6, 12) minutes	6/12	2/12
[12, 18) minutes	2/12	1/12
[18, 24] minutes	1/12	1/12

Management's current policy is to have two diagnostic carrels open and staffed by physicians at all times. Based upon an EMS call schedule, other physicians may be used to staff the other two carrels. Once a decision is made to open or close a carrel, 60 minutes are required to convert the carrel from one status to the other. When a carrel is opened, it is staffed by a physician and available to receive a patient.

The management problem is to determine how many physicians are needed and how they will be assigned to various carrels. Two variables are of interest and will be used to evaluate the various staffing decision rules.

Variable 1.—The Average Waiting Time in Long Lines. A long line is assumed to exist if three individuals are waiting and a fourth person joins that queue. The amount of time spent until the queue reaches three or less is recorded as time spent waiting in long lines.

Variable 2.—The Amount of Time Physicians Spend in the EMS Unit.

To develop decision-relevant information regarding this management problem, various technical aspects of this simulation problem, such as carrel status switching, decision rule specification, testing decision rules, validating the simulation, and selecting a decision rule to be implemented, must be considered.

Carrel Status Switching

In the EMS example, a carrel can be in any one of the following five states:

1. CL—closed.
2. BO—60-minute, nonproductive setting-up period which requires a physician.
3. OP—open for diagnostic services.
4. WC—the decision has been made to close the carrel, but individuals are waiting for service. Those in line when the decision to close is made will be served, but no new individuals will be accepted.
5. BC—60-minute, nonproductive closing-down period which requires a physician.

Since carrels 1 and 2 are open at the start and must remain open throughout the two-day period, their status will always be "OP." Carrels 3 and 4, which are closed at the start, can go through the following sequence of status switches:

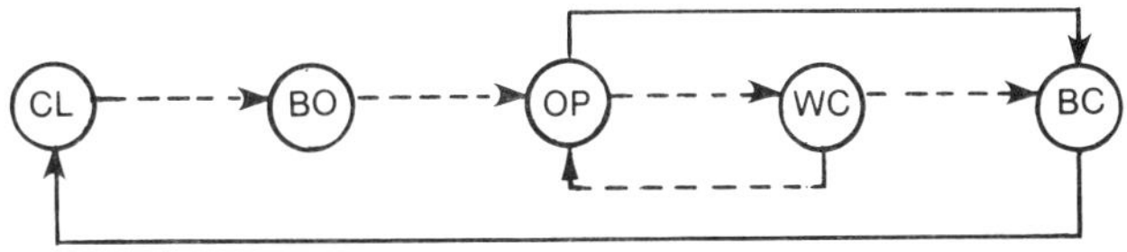

Most of the above status changes should be clear. Whether a carrel goes from "OP" directly to "BC," or has to pass through the intermediate "WC" state depends on whether or not individuals are at the carrel when the decision is made to close it. The switch from "WC" back to "OP" is an option which allows for the unlikely but possible case in which a decision is made to close a carrel at which one or more individuals are waiting, but before their service can be completed, a number of arrivals makes reopening the carrel desirable. The simulation program makes these status switches in a time-oriented, rather than event-oriented, mode. [2]

Decision Rule Specification

The purpose of the EMS study and, therefore, of the simulation program is to find a decision rule which represents a satisfactory balance between the use of physician time and the average amount of waiting time in long lines. In general, average waiting time in long lines can be reduced by keeping more carrels open for longer periods of time, but this requires more physician time.

A decision rule can be either time or status reactive. A *time reactive* decision rule opens and closes carrels on the basis of time. For example, in view of the increased arrival rate during the middle 24-hour period, one decision rule might be to open the third carrel at the beginning of the last half of the first day (which requires switching it from "CL" to "BO" one hour before it is to be used), and to begin closing it one hour before the end of the first half of the second day. A *status-oriented* decision rule, on the other hand, opens and closes carrels based on the current number of individuals in particular lines. For example, one status-oriented decision rule might begin to open a new carrel when the queue lengths at all currently open carrels are eight people or greater, and begin to close a carrel when the queue lengths at all currently open carrels are five people or fewer.

The function of a time or status reactive decision rule is to determine when a carrel should be opened and when one should be closed. Specifically, either type of decision rule must perform the following status switches.[3]

1. From "CL" to "BO";
2. From "OP" to either "WC" or "BC"; and
3. Optionally from "WC" back to "OP."

Sample Decision Rules

The following are examples of decision rules which will be used in the simulation to provide management with data regarding the staffing of the EMS service carrels.

Decision Rule 1:
The simplest decision rule is to do nothing at all, which means never opening carrels 3 and 4. This time-oriented decision rule requires no instructions and minimizes total physician-minutes, presumably at the cost of maximizing average waiting time spent in long lines.

Decision Rule 2:
A more complex, time-oriented decision rule is to (1) open the third carrel as soon as possible and keep it open throughout the two-day period, and (2) open the fourth carrel during the peak arrival period. Recall that to have the fourth carrel open at time t_k, it must be switched into the "BO" status at time t_{k-1} due to the 60-minute delay.

Decision Rule 3:
One possible status-oriented decision rule would be to open a new carrel if the average number of individuals at any currently open carrel is greater than five, and to leave it open until the end of that 12-hour period.

Decision Rule 4:
Another status-oriented decision rule is to open a new carrel when each of the currently open carrels has a queue length of three or more, and to close a carrel when each of the currently open carrels has a queue length of one or less.

Decision Rule 5:
An example of a time-oriented decision rule is to open carrel 3 as soon as possible and keep it open while carrel 4 remains closed throughout the two-day period.

Decision Rule 6:
Another time-oriented decision rule is to open carrel 3 at time t_k (i.e., switch it into state "BO" at t_k), and begin to close it at time t_h, where t_k represents the beginning of the second half of the first day and t_h represents the end of the first half of the second day. Carrel 4 remains closed.

Testing Decision Rules: Monte Carlo Selection

These six decision rules may be used by management to process the simulated arrivals for the two-day period. For a particular simulation, random draws are made from density B (Table 12-3), which represents the interarrival rates for the first half of the first day and the second half of the second day, and density C (Table 12-3), which represents the interarrival rates for the second half of the first day and the first half of the second day. Specific individual arrivals are assigned diagnosis times based upon random selections made from density A (Table 12-2).

For example, at the beginning of the first simulation for decision rule 4, the first individual arrived after 3.24 minutes. This individual was assigned a diagnosis time of 11.42 minutes and was sent to diagnostic carrel 1. The next individual arrived 12.92 minutes after the first individual, was assigned a diagnosis time of 18.02 minutes, and was sent to the unoccupied diagnostic carrel 1. The third individual arrived 0.31 minutes after the second, was assigned a diagnosis time of 6.11 minutes, and was sent to diagnostic carrel 2 because carrel 1 was occupied. These random selections continued for the two-day period.

At the end of the simulation, the total time spent in long lines must be divided by the number of individuals who were in long lines during the two-day period. This value equals the average waiting time spent in long lines. The total amount of time spent by physicians in staffing the diagnostic carrels must be recorded and reported as total physician time. These two statistics from the first simulation for decision rule 4 were:

Variable 1—Average waiting time in long lines: 103 minutes, and
Variable 2—Total physician time: 10,711 minutes.

Using only one simulation for the two-day period as the basis for judging the effect of a decision rule on the variables of interest is unwise. Therefore, multiple simulations must be conducted for each decision rule. One hundred simulations were conducted for decision rule 4, the results of which are represented by the two histograms in Charts 12-1 and 12-2:

Variable 1—Average waiting time in long lines: Chart 12-1. A histogram showing the distribution of average waiting time spent in long lines for each of the 100 simulations, and

Variable 2—Total physician minutes: Chart 12-2. A histogram showing the distribution of total physician-minutes for each of the 100 simulations.

The data represented in Charts 12-1 and 12-2 provide information regarding the effect of a particular decision rule on the average number of minutes individuals spent in long lines, and on the time physicians spent in the EMS unit.

Chart 12-1 Distribution of Average Waiting Time in Long Lines for 100 Simulations: Decision Rule 4*

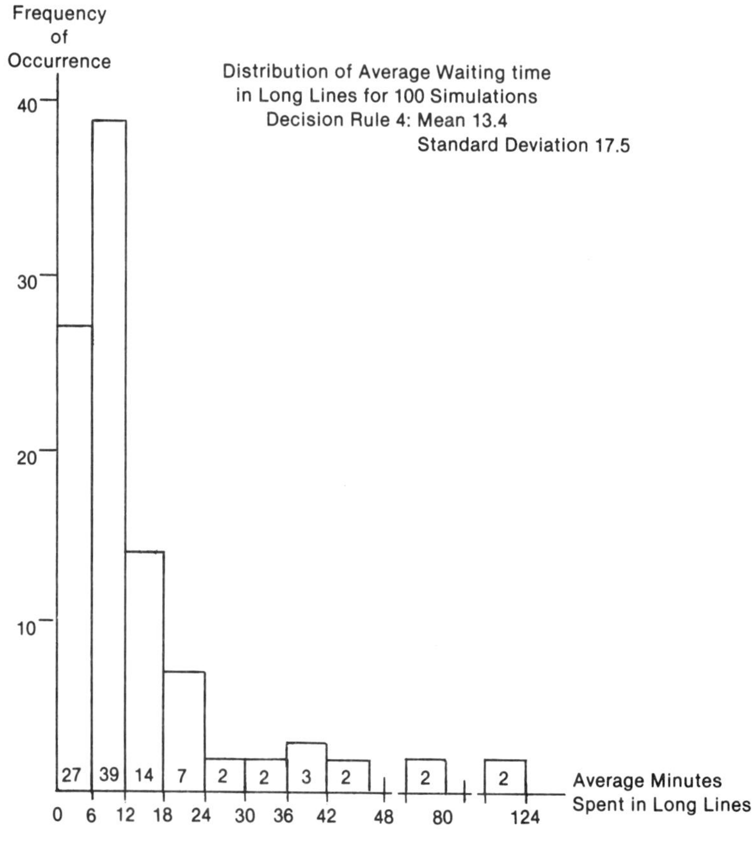

*To represent the results of the 100 simulations in a histogram, intervals of six minutes were constructed. For example, in 27 simulations the average waiting time in long lines was six minutes or less.

To facilitate decision rule comparisons, the information in Charts 12-1 and 12-2 should be summarized statistically and presented in an axis space as a probability ellipse, as shown in Figure 12-4 (see Problem 12-3). This ellipse, which is centered at the means of the two variables, results from plotting the points from the joint distribution of the total physician minutes and the average waiting time which may be expected to occur 95 percent of the time (see Appendix 12-A). The shape and orientation of the ellipse depends upon

Chart 12-2 Distribution of Total Physician Diagnosis Minutes for 100 Simulations: Decision Rule 4*

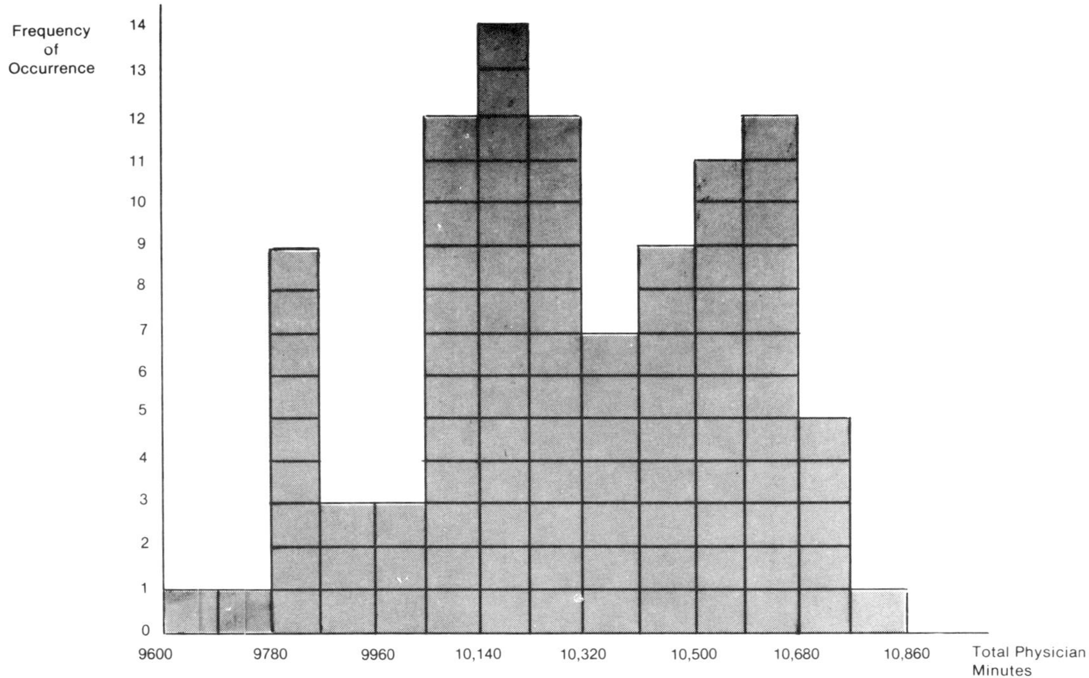

*To present these results in a histogram, intervals of 90 minutes were constructed. For example, in one simulation, total physician minutes was in the interval [9600–9690].

Figure 12-4 Graphical Representation of the Probability Ellipse Covering 95 Percent of the Joint Distribution of Total Physician Minutes and Average Patient Waiting Time

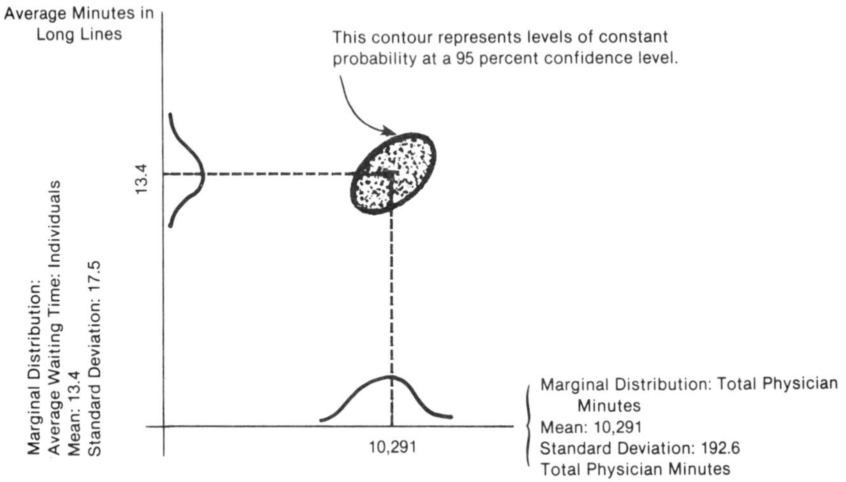

the variances and the association between the two variables. The probability density and ellipse results developed from the simulation for the six decision rules tested are presented in Figure 12-5.

Validating the Results of the Simulation

Before management acts to select a particular decision rule from among the six decision rules represented in Figure 12-5, the results of the simulation must be validated. Since the implementation of a particular decision rule usually requires a substantial organizational resource commitment, management should consider only those decision rules which represent valid modifications of the system. A decision rule may be considered invalid for two reasons: (1) it is incompatible with the system being simulated, or (2) it is compatible, but the assumptions made in constructing and programing the simulation would cause invalid inferences to result from analyzing the simulation results according to that decision rule. To reject a decision rule for either reason, the following three validation procedures are necessary: (1) professional judgment must be secured to ascertain the simulation's reasonability; (2) repeated simulations and comparisons of the results must be done under various and varying assumptions (sensitivity analysis); and (3) statistical tests must be used to judge the comparability of simulated and

Figure 12-5 Probability Densities and Ellipses Representing a 95 Percent Confidence Interval for the Average Minutes in Long Lines Versus Total Physician Minutes for Six Decision Rules

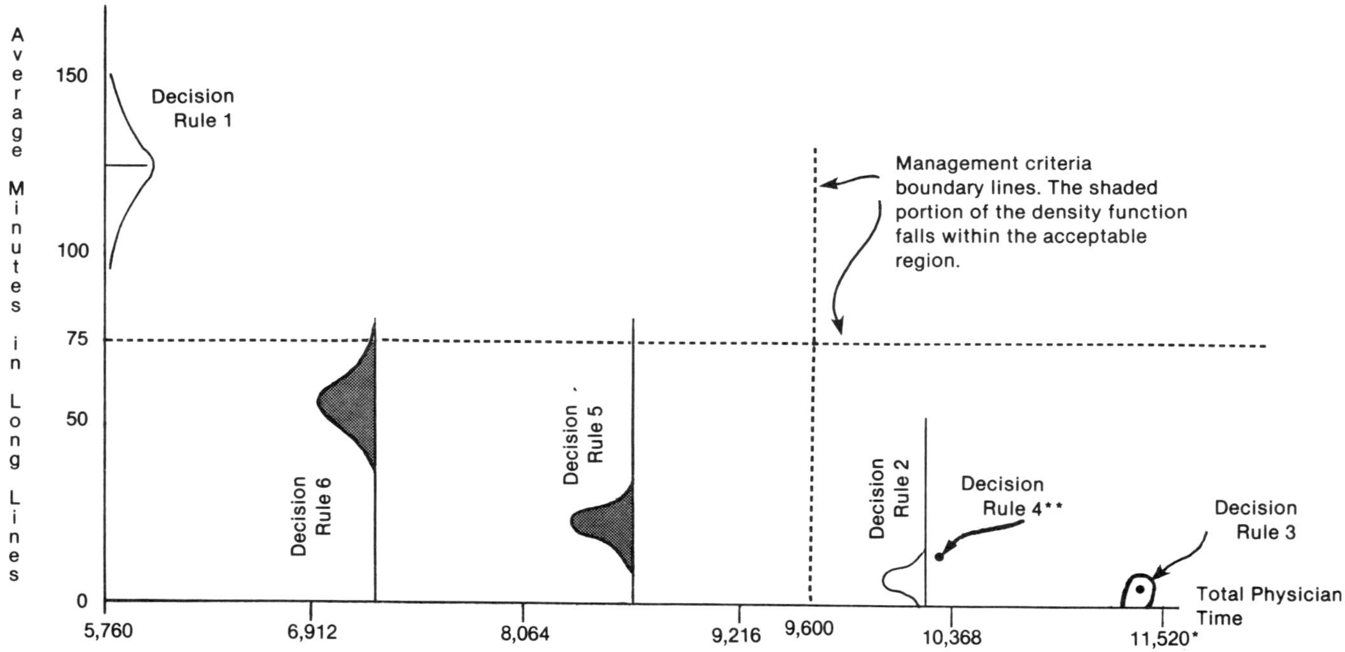

*Total Physican Time Cannot Exceed 11,520 minutes
**See Figure 12-4

historical data. These procedures are important in rationalizing management's proposed actions, and should be used to ascertain which decision rules will be further analyzed by management to select and implement a particular decision rule.

Professional Judgment

By subjecting the simulation model to the scrutiny of other professionals who are familiar with the process and the results which should be generated, a sense of the reasonability of the simulation may be ascertained. This is critical because important qualitative relationships usually exist which cannot be incorporated in the simulation, but which may affect the successful implementation of a particular decision rule. Hence, professional judgment can be an important factor in isolating decision rules which are unreasonable in light of the many factors which cannot be integrated into the analysis mathematically or statistically.

Sensitivity Analysis

Simulations of complex systems often incorporate numerous decisions rules and various assumptions which are used in conjunction with the decision rules to process simulated inputs. Ascertaining how sensitive the results of the simulation are to varying the assumptions underlying the decision rules is important because if the results of a simulation differ significantly depending upon the assumptions used, the analyst must determine if the various assumptions are reasonable given the problem simulated. If a particular assumption is incompatible with the known behavior of the system being simulated, the simulated results developed using that assumption must be excluded from the analysis. If, on the other hand, assumptions generate approximately the same results and these assumptions are reasonable given the system simulated, the analyst may select the assumption most easily accomplished when the decision rule selected is implemented.

For example, the results of the simulations represented in Figure 12-5 are generated assuming that individuals would be assigned to the carrel with the shortest queue and that queue switching would occur. An important validating question might be: What would the results have been if individuals were not permitted to switch from one queue to another? To ascertain the effect of queue switching, this assumption was changed so that no switching was permitted. The results of these two simulations, compared in Figure 12-6, indicate that queue switching does not affect the results of the simulations materially. Therefore, queue switching is a relatively insensitive assumption and if any decision rule is selected for implementation, no particular queue switching policy need be enforced as long as individuals are always assigned to the carrel with the shortest queue.[4]

Figure 12-6 Comparison of Queue Switching with No Queue Switching for the Six Decision Rules

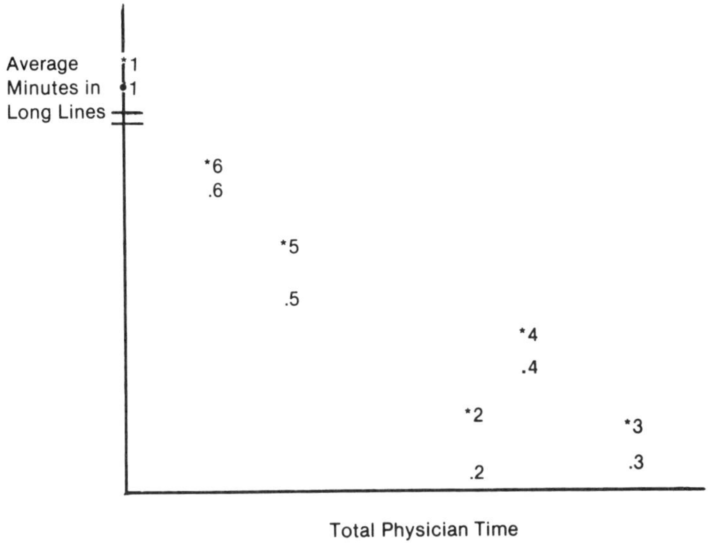

where: · Represents the average results of 100 simulations with queue switching permitted; and
* Represents the average results of 100 simulations with queue switching not permitted.

Statistical Testing

When empirical distributions of the outputs of the simulation exist, the simulation results can be tested statistically against these empirical distributions. These statistical results may lend insights regarding the congruity of the actual process interactions and the simulated ones. After stating the relevant hypotheses (i.e., the simulated phenomenon is not distributed differently from the empirical phenomenon) either parametric or nonparametric statistical testing may be used to ascertain the similarity of the simulated and the empirical distribution. Statistically significant differences between the two may cast doubt on the validity of a particular decision rule or processing assumption.

Selecting a Decision Rule to Be Implemented

After the results of the simulation are validated to the satisfaction of management, the decision rules which generated valid simulated results must be analyzed further to ascertain which decision rules will be selected and implemented. The two stages in selecting a particular decision rule are as follows.

Figure 12-7 General Process of Decision Rule Selection Using a Simulation

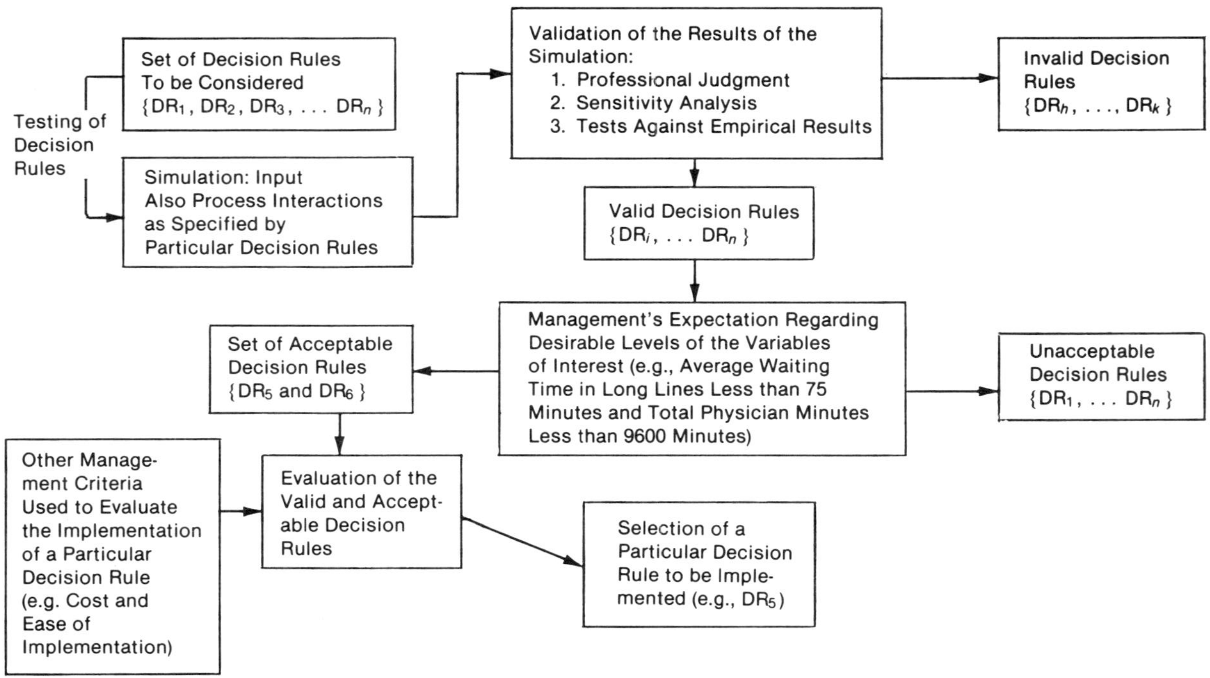

(1) Management must ascertain which of the valid decision rules satisfy specific requirements regarding the variables of interest. For example, assume that management decides that any decision rule which keeps the average waiting time under 75 minutes and the total physician service time under 9,600 minutes would be acceptable. Using these specific limits, management criteria boundary lines may be drawn and the set of acceptable decision rules ascertained visually (Figure 12-5). In this case, the only acceptable decision rules are decision rules 5 and 6, since they alone fall in the acceptable region.[5]

(2) The set of valid and acceptable decision rules must be evaluated in terms of other management criteria. For example, assume that management evaluates proposed systems changes in terms of cost and ease of implementation. If decision rule 5 is both less costly and simpler to implement, it would be selected. This general process of selecting a particular decision rule is represented in Figure 12-7 (see Question 12-6).

Conclusion

Simulation is a technique useful in analyzing the performance of a system with an abstract model. The principal advantages of simulating decision systems are (1) wide applicability (i.e., most health care decision problems can be simulated;) and (2) sytems learning (i.e., in setting up the model, one frequently learns a great deal about the system being simulated). The one principal disadvantage of simulation is that it often is used in place of careful managerial analysis. Simulation should be used only when no other form of managerial analysis is capable of developing decision-relevant information.

NOTES

1. In this chapter, specific examples are used to provide a frame of reference for the many definitional elements required to discuss simulation comprehensively. The frame of reference chosen is an EMS simulation, and consequently, most of the definitional illustrations are drawn from an EMS context.
2. In general, all Monte Carlo simulations can be divided into two groups: those which are time-oriented and those which are event-oriented. In a *time-oriented simulation*, as the hands of an imaginary clock are incremented by one unit of time, the following values are reduced by one time unit:

   a. Time until service is completed at each staffed carrel,
   b. Time until a carrel is to be closed,
   c. Time until a carrel is to be opened, and
   d. Time until the next arrival.

If any of these values are reduced to zero, then an event has occurred and must be processed. If all of the above values remain positive, then no event needs to be processed, the clock again is incremented by another time unit, and the above values again are reduced and compared to zero.

In an *event-oriented simulation,* the event which will occur next is processed. The "time until" of that event is reduced from the "time until" of all unprocessed events. The advantage of this method is that all time periods in which no events occur are eliminated. The disadvantage is that this method is more difficult to understand conceptually and to program. If the characteristics of the system being simulated are such that one or more events occur in most of the time periods (70 percent in the EMS case), then the advantage of the event-oriented method becomes less significant.

3. The user need not be concerned with the following status switches, because they should be performed automatically by the program regardless of the decision rule being used:

   a. From "BO" to "OP";
   b. From "WC" to "BC"; and
   c. From "BC" to "CL."

4. In the example used to illustrate the use of the simulation in this chapter, the decision rules themselves include no assumptions regarding systems behavior. The behavioral assumptions, i.e., queue switching or no queue switching, were programed for all the decision rules. This programing style of keeping the decision rules free from behavioral assumptions where possible allows management to invalidate sets of decision rules based upon erroneous assumptions, rather than have to analyze each decision rule as it is affected by the particular processing assumption. In most cases, this simplifies the validation process dramatically.
5. Note that a small portion of decision rule 6 density function falls outside the acceptable region. However, since the portion of the density function which falls outside the acceptable region represents the probability of decision rule 6 falling in the unacceptable region, it may be ignored in this case (see Question 12-8).

Appendix 12-A

The Probability Ellipse: Its Use in Evaluating Decision Rule Modifications

To clarify Figure 12-5, some discussion of the information represented by a probability ellipse is appropriate. Consider the simulation for decision rule 4, which results in the following statistics for the two variables of interest:

Variable 1: Average waiting time in long lines—Mean: 13.4 minutes; Standard Deviation: 17.5 minutes.

Variable 2: Total physician minutes spent in the EMS Unit—Mean: 10,291 minutes; Standard Deviation: 192.6 minutes.

Assume that no significant correlation exists between these two variables and that management has established the following criteria: (1) A decision rule is acceptable only if the total physician minutes are less than 9,600 minutes, and (2) the average waiting time is less than 75 minutes. Given these criteria specifications and the simulation statistics, management may ask: should decision rule 4 be considered acceptable?

To evaluate this question, management would have to specify some level of confidence so that a statistical inference can be developed regarding the likelihood that variable 1 will be less than 75 minutes *and* variable 2 will be less than 9,600 minutes. Assume that the level of confidence chosen is 95 percent. This means that management will accept decision rule 4 if variable 1 is less than 75 minutes, and variable 2 is less than 9,600 minutes 95 percent of the time. In this case, the likelihood that variable 1 will be less than 75 minutes can be formulated as follows (assuming the 100 simulation observations are population realizations which are normally distributed):

$$(12\text{-}1A) \qquad \frac{13.4 - X}{17.5} = -1.645$$

where: X represents the value of the critical variable (if $X \geq 75$, then decision rule 4 would be rejected; if $X < 75$, decision rule 4 could not be rejected); and 1.645 is the z value representing an approximate 95 percent likelihood of occurrence.

Solving equation (12-1A), the value of X is determined to be 42.19. Therefore, insofar as variable 1 is concerned, decision rule 4 is acceptable because management can be at least 95 percent certain that the average waiting time in long lines will be less than 75 minutes.

However, variable 2 also must be tested before decision rule 4 is accepted. In this case, the likelihood that variable 2 will be less than 9,600 minutes may be formulated as follows (making the same assumptions):

$$(12\text{-}2A) \qquad \frac{9600 - X}{192.6} = -1.645$$

where: X is the value of the critical variable. If $X \geq 9600$, then decision rule 4 would be rejected; if $X < 9600$, decision rule 4 could not be rejected.

Solving equation (12-2A), the value of X is determined to be 9,916.83. Therefore, insofar as variable 2 is concerned, decision rule 4 is not acceptable and must be rejected. Since management requires both variables to be in the acceptable region, decision rule 4 must be rejected as an acceptable decision rule.

A simple and computationally convenient way of representing not only the probability distributions derived from the simulation, but also the association (which may be measured as product moment correlation, f) between the variables, is to plot an ellipse of the joint probability distribution of both variables. Management may choose some level of confidence—90 or 95 percent would seem reasonable for most problems—and sketch the ellipse in the two-dimensional space formed by variables 1 and 2. Management may then draw criteria lines to see if the ellipse is within the acceptable region defined by the criteria lines. For example, in Figure 12-1A, decision rule X would be considered acceptable, whereas decision rule Y would be rejected.

Visually ascertaining the acceptability of particular decision rules depends on the ability to plot them (see Appendix B). In a one, two, and sometimes a

Figure 12-1A Ellipses for Decision Rule X and Decision Rule Y Which Represent 90 Percent Confidence Level

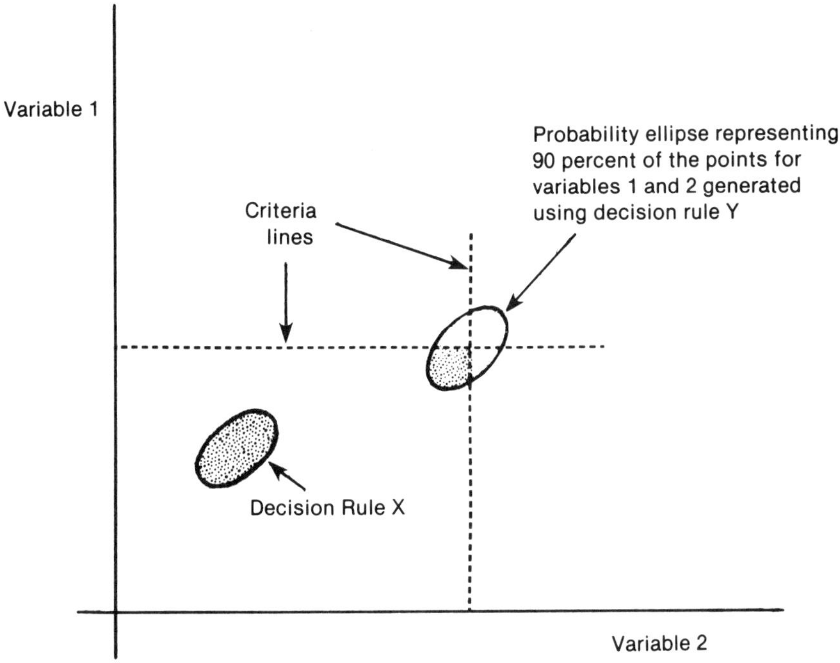

Note: The convex set formed by the criteria lines represents the acceptable region. The portions of the ellipses within the acceptable region are shaded.

---

three dimensional space, plotting is a possibility. However, when the number of variables of interest is four or more, mathematical analysis must be used. In this case, the dimensionality of the axis space would equal the number of variables, and the convex set would be formed by partitioning the space with linear equations. The ellipse would then be oriented in that space and analyzed. This is an arduous but not an overwhelming task given the availability of computationally compatible computer algorithms.

Questions and Problems

Question 12-1. What is the rationale for using simulation? What is a dynamic simulation? What are the advantages of using a dynamic simulation as opposed to a static one?

Question 12-2. Explain how random number generation is used in a Monte Carlo simulation. Why is it used?

Question 12-3. What are time-oriented and event-oriented simulations?

Question 12-4. What is a status-oriented decision rule? A dynamic one? Can static simulations have dynamic decision rules? Can dynamic simulations have static decision rules?

Question 12-5. What are some important cost/benefit considerations regarding the validation of a simulation?

Question 12-6. Figure 12-7 represents the process used to select a particular decision rule; it does not represent a process for implementing a particular decision rule. Expand Figure 12-7 to incorporate implementation information. Make sure your solution recognizes information provided by the sensitivity analysis.

Question 12-7. The introduction to this chapter suggests that (1) simulation may be used to analyze the effect of decision rule modifications on performance, and (2) the proposed set of decision rule modifications result from management's analysis of control information (see Figure 9-1 or 9-2). Indicate what types of control information may have led management to undertake investigation of the EMS system and to propose various decision rule modifications discussed in the chapter.

Question 12-8. Assume that half of the density function representing decision rule 6 fell outside the acceptable region. Would you consider decision rule 6 to be acceptable? Why?

Problem 12-1. In chapter 4, a heuristic was suggested to provide information regarding the maintenance of safety stock. Recast this safety stock heuristic as a simulation. Explicitly state four different decision rules you would test. How would you validate this simulation?

Problem 12-2. Examine Figure 12-2. What changes in the physician staffing rule are indicated by the graphical output of the simulation?

Problem 12-3. In plotting the probability ellipse for the EMS example (Figure 12-4), the principal axis (the longest one) has a positive slope. What does this mean? Does the orientation of the principal axis conform to your intuition? Defend your answer.

Problem 12-4. Develop a simulation for the selection of capital investments using the IRD and the VA_{IRD} as discussed in Chapter 9.

Problem 12-5. The emergency room is usually open 24 hours each day. Therefore, three eight-hour shifts must be used to provide emergency medical services. Redesign the simulation to reflect varying treatment time by shift. State all of the assumptions made and rationalize each.

Problem 12-6. The institution which served as a model for the simulation reported in the text had a relatively high patient arrival rate for a 24-hour period. Other institutions may experience increased activity for periods of shorter duration. Assume that in a 48-hour period there are four periods of six hours each when the patient arrival rate is relatively high compared to the patient arrival rate during the other 24 hours. How would this fact be programmed for purposes of simulation? Is it possible that Table 12-3 could serve as the patient arrival probability density format?

Chapter 13

Behavioral Considerations

When you believe in things you don't understand, you suffer.
S. Wonder

Various behavioral aspects of the institutional decision framework affect the implementation, operation, and evolution of control models, techniques, and systems. Although a myriad of complex behavioral issues affect institutional control, coalition analysis (i.e., the identification and analysis of individual groupings which affect the organization's decision and control process) is most useful in understanding the possible effects of control actions.

BUDGETARY CONTROL: ITS SEMANTIC DIMENSION

One control system that might benefit from coalition analysis is the budgetary control system because, when institutional performance deviates from expectations or standards, the budgetary control system brings various organizational coalitions together to investigate the reasons underlying the performance deviations. The effective functioning of the organization's budgetary control system depends upon the following three aspects of performance measurement:

- *Denotative*—Data: the performance data generated by the organization's information system;
- *Connotative*—Semantic: the perception of the importance of the variance contrasts; and
- *Evaluative*—Feedback and Reward-Penalty: the institutional reaction to the variance information generated by the control system.

Therefore, the coalitions must consider each of these aspects to isolate and evaluate the principle reasons for the performance deviations. Once this has been accomplished, the organization's resource conversion process can be modified appropriately.

In most organizational settings, the denotative dimension of budgetary control is highly structured, representing the measurable performance statistics. For example, a cost control system measures actual performance, contrasts actual with budgeted performance, and reports any significant deviations. These variance contrasts represent one of the denotative outputs of the budgetary control system.

The effectiveness of the evaluative dimension in motivating corrective action depends upon management's perception of the variance contrasts, i.e., the connotative dimension. For example, if cost variances are unfavorable but management does not perceive cost as an important control dimension, corrective actions are not likely to be initiated. Therefore, some indication of the connotative predisposition of the various decision coalitions is necessary to structure the evaluative dimension of the institution's control system effectively.

When the organization's control procedures fail to effect the desired performance, adjustments in either the denotative, connotative, or evaluative dimension may be selected to deal with the control problem. The usual reorientation response is to correct the denotative dimension by altering the type of information currently measured. If this reorientation response fails to eliminate the performance deviations, the institution may resort to rationalizing an alteration in the evaluative dimension. Although these tactics may eliminate the performance deviations, they do so only by redefining the problem in a way that eliminates the need for corrective actions.

To modify the institution's resource conversion process effectively, all three aspects of performance measurement should be considered. The evaluative and denotative aspects of performance evaluation have been examined in previous chapters. The connotative aspects of performance measurement will be examined here through a technique that aids in developing insights to the semantic disposition of the coalitions involved in the organization's control system.

The Semantic Differential

The pioneering research into the use of the semantic differential as a measurement construct was conducted by C. E. Osgood et al. (1957). The basis of the semantic differential is the unique encoding (the selective and consistent connotative responses evoked by objects) performed by individuals. According to the investigators,

> It is apparent that if we are to use linguistic encoding as an index of meaning, we need (a) a carefully devised sample of alternative verbal responses which can be standardized across subjects, (b) these alternatives to be elicited from subjects rather than emitted so that encoding fluency is eliminated as a variable, and (c) these alternatives to be representative of the major ways in which meanings vary.

To formalize this encoding, Osgood and his associates suggest representing semantic responses (the connotative dimensions) in a dimensionally unspecified Euclidian space.[1] Each dimensional extreme of the space is represented by a set of bipolar adjectives. In theory, the semantic space should be defined by a minimum spanning set of bipolar adjectives (axes in the semantic space). Unfortunately, a precise definition of the spanning set cannot be deduced.

Through a factor analysis, however, a series of bipolar adjectives have been suggested to define the semantic space. The factor analysis groups the bipolar adjectives along three dimensions—evaluative, potency, and activity. The minimum spanning set for the semantic space usually is considered to be included in these three dimensions because bipolar adjectives in the evaluative dimension explain 68.5 percent of the common variation, while the bipolar adjectives in the potency and activity dimensions explain an additional 28.1 percent of the common variation.

Semantic Interaction: A Measure

To measure the semantic disposition of the interacting organizational coalitions, the systems analyst must (1) determine which dimensions best characterize the concepts useful in defining the coalition's interrelationships, (2) select bipolar adjectives[2] which most appropriately define the coalition's semantic disposition, and (3) have the respondents indicate on a scale of one to seven how each concept is related to each set of bipolar adjectives.

For example, if the semantic response for concept Q is to be measured on all three dimensions (evaluative, potency, activity), the following scoring grid may be used:

Concept Q

good	:	:	:	:	:	:	bad
awful	:	:	:	:	:	:	nice
weak	:	:	:	:	:	:	strong
sharp	:	:	:	:	:	:	dull
dirty	:	:	:	:	:	:	clean
large	:	:	:	:	:	:	small
passive	:	:	:	:	:	:	active
fast	:	:	:	:	:	:	slow
valuable	:	:	:	:	:	:	worthless
heavy	:	:	:	:	:	:	light

In this case, the adjectives relate to the factor dimensions as follows.

Evaluative Dimension	Potency Dimension	Activity Dimension
good—bad	weak—strong	sharp—dull
dirty—clean	large—small	passive—active
awful—nice	heavy—light	fast—slow
valuable—worthless		

If a coalition member responding to concept Q feels that the concept is good as opposed to bad, a check (✓) should be placed in the far left interval on the bipolar good-bad scale, indicating a score of seven. If, on the other hand, a coalition member feels that concept Q is bad as opposed to good, a check should be placed in the extreme right interval, indicating a value of one. Furthermore, if the respondent has a neutral feeling about the "goodness or badness" of concept Q, a check should be placed in the mid-interval on that scale, indicating a score of four.

The score assigned to each response does not depend on whether the check is toward the right or toward the left of the mid-interval. Instead, each bipolar adjective set contains an adjective describing a desirable attitude and another describing an undesirable attitude. Scores of seven are associated with the desirable adjectives, and scores of one are associated with the undesirable ones. Furthermore, to avoid biasing the solicited responses, the desirable adjectives in some bipolar sets are placed on the right of the scoring grid, while the desirable adjectives in other bipolar sets are placed on the left of it.

Each respondent should use the scoring grid to show the relationship between each concept and each bipolar adjective set. Once this scoring procedure has been completed, the arithmetic means of the assigned scores can be used to indicate each respondent's semantic score for each concept. For example, assume that respondent A scores concept Q as follows.

Concept Q

good	✓							bad
awful					✓			nice
weak						✓		strong
sharp				✓				dull
dirty					✓			clean
large				✓				small
passive			✓					active
fast		✓						slow
valuable	✓							worthless
heavy			✓					light

The arithmetic means or the semantic score for concept Q, as rated by respondent A, would be:

$$(7 + 5 + 6 + 4 + 5 + 4 + 3 + 6 + 7 + 3)/10 = 5.0.$$

Similarly, the semantic score would be computed for the ratings assigned by each respondent to each concept. Therefore, given four concepts and three respondents, 12 semantic scores describing the aggregate connotative disposition to the specific concepts tested would be generated.

Since the semantic scores quantify the attitudes of individuals in various coalitions, these scores can be used to ascertain if statistically significant differences exist among the attitudes of organizational coalitions. If connotative differences do exist, they can be used to develop insights regarding the possible reaction of the coalitions to control information (see Figure 13-1). Hence, the effectiveness of the semantic differential depends on the variance in the responses elicited from the members of the various coalitions. However, the variance in the elicited responses depends on the bipolar adjectives selected to define the semantic space.

Definition of the Semantic Space in a Specific Context

To select a set of bipolar adjectives for specific connotative problems, a thesaurus factor analysis can be conducted. The evaluative, potency, and

Figure 13-1 Use of the Semantic Differential to Develop Control Information from Identified Organizational Coalitions

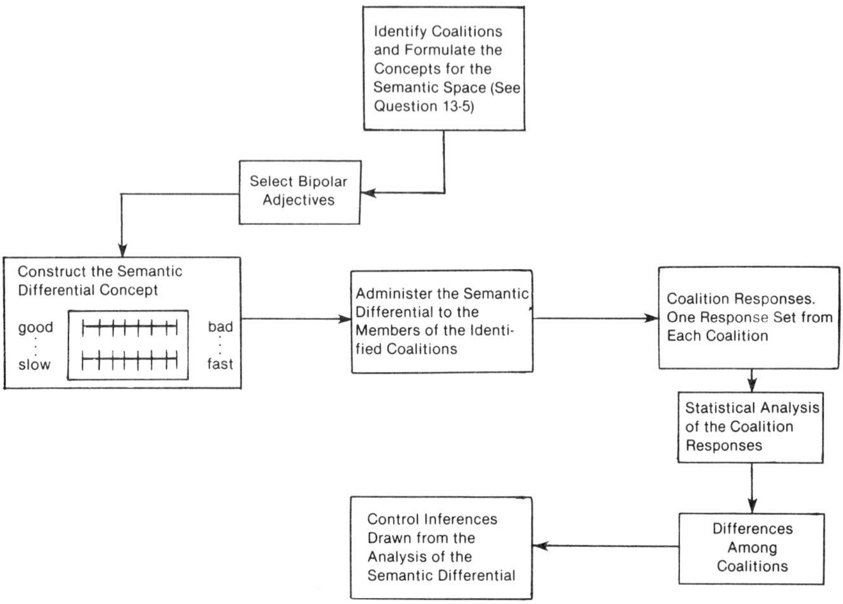

activity factors generated by this analysis may be used to determine the bipolar adjectives. This approach, in essence, replicates Osgood's thesaurus study for a particular problem.

An alternative to this expensive replication would be to select the required number of bipolar adjectives based upon the magnitude of the factor loadings reported in Osgood's study. The problem with selecting bipolar adjectives in this manner is that in different research settings the semantic impact evoked by these bipolar adjectives may bear no relationship to the magnitude of Osgood's factor loadings. For example, a set of bipolar adjectives may have generated a low factor loading, owing to the nature of the concepts and the respondent group used in the thesaurus study. However, for a different group of concepts and respondents, that bipolar adjective set may evoke a significant semantic response. Hence, by selecting adjectives based solely upon Osgood's study, a high preponderance of midinterval (neutral) responses may be evidenced, indicating an inapplicable pairing of concepts and adjectives. Recognizing these problems, an alternative bipolar adjective selection methodology is suggested (see Lusk (1973)).

Variance Ordering: A Bipolar Selection Rationale

The following six steps are useful in researching semantic response problems:

1. Select from Osgood's thesaurus study a set of bipolar adjectives for each factor dimension (evaluative, potency, activity) applicable to the study.
2. Select a representative sample of individuals from the group whose semantic responses are to be sampled in the primary study.
3. Prepare the pretest concept-adjective test blocks which distributes the concepts and bipolar adjectives randomly within concepts.
4. After administering the pretest material, compute the variance from the midpoint of each bipolar adjective for the concepts across individuals.
5. Order the bipolar adjectives based upon their response variance computed in the preceding step.
6. Select the required number of bipolar adjectives from the variance rank-ordered bipolar adjectives. (Adjectives with larger variances will be preferred over those with smaller variances.)

The rationale for these pretest procedures is that when bipolar adjectives are used, the midpoint yields no information since it represents the neutral point. Therefore, by rank ordering the variance of bipolar adjectives, those which evoke the greatest semantic response can be isolated. The following example further illustrates the usefulness of this bipolar adjective selection technique and also illustrates the semantic differential concepts in a practical setting.

AN ILLUSTRATIVE EXAMPLE: HOSPITAL RESOURCE CONTROL

Assume that the administrator of a large urban hospital is interested in investigating why the operational budgeting system does not seem to be generating information useful in either evaluating performance or controlling operations. To solve this hypothetical problem, interviews were conducted with medical and administrative personnel at several hospitals. During these interviews, the connotative dimensions of budgetary control appeared to involve the following four concepts (see Question 13-4).

C_1 = Health Care Delivery
C_2 = Cost Consciousness
C_3 = Economic Management
C_4 = Patient Welfare

If the *control potential* of a hospital budgeting system depends upon the connotative interrelationships between the medical and administrative coalitions relative to these control concepts, budgetary controls will be effective only if both groups have sufficiently differentiated control dispositions to manifest a diverse vesting of interests. However, if both groups have similar control dispositions, then institutional evaluation must be structured to redistribute the decision sensitivities among the coalitions and restore an effective managerial balance between the medical and administrative coalitions. Therefore, the following hypotheses should be tested to measure the connotative dimension of the budgetary control system.

H_1: The medical and administration coalitions represent different connotative dispositions.

H_2: Of the four control concepts, none will dominate the total semantic space (i.e., the space constituted of members of both coalitions).

One would expect H_1 and H_2 to be true for an institution which has an effective budgeting system, because in a managerially balanced system, no concepts should dominate the total semantic space and the various coalitions should have a differentiated control perspective. However, if one concept dominates both coalitions to the extent that it obscures consideration of other concepts, institutional control may be difficult to effect along the dominated dimension.

To test H_1 and H_2, an actual sample of individuals, representing the medical and administrative groups in this case, was chosen.

Medical Group:

32 medical students, interns, residents, physicians, and medical researchers.

Administrative Group:

32 administrative personnel from six hospitals and health care administration students.

In a study of a particular institution, however, all the personnel used to develop the semantic space should be drawn from within the institution. To facilitate the discussion, assume the groups are respresentative of an institution.

Test Results

The semantic differential was administered to these 64 individuals. Each individual was given the four concepts (C_1, C_2, C_3, C_4) to score on ten evaluative bipolar adjectives selected using the maximization of variance criteria. A statistical analysis of the results indicated that both groups scored the four semantic concepts similarly (see Table 13-1). Therefore, these two coalitions could not be differentiated from each other based upon their responses to the four concepts.

The statistical difference between the medical concepts (C_1 and C_4) and the administrative concepts (C_2 and C_3) for both groups, however, was significant at an $\alpha < .001$ level of confidence. Based upon this information, both hypotheses may be rejected because given the individuals selected to score the semantic differential, no statistically significant difference appears to exist between their connotative view of the four concepts. Further, both groups view the medically related concepts (C_1, C_4) as being more important (in a connotative sense) than the cost-related control concepts (C_2, C_3).

The basic conclusion to be drawn from these results would be that the control rationale inherent in the budgetary cost control system may exist at cross-purposes with the priorities established by the medical personnel and adopted by the administrators. These results imply that the institution must establish or reestablish, by whatever means are institutionally available, a diverse coalition vesting of interests. The balancing of the institution's control system is a first priority. Until both groups understand the importance of supporting a control environment which permits a diverse vesting of coalition interests, budgetary cost control is unlikely.

In the context of the problem of budgetary cost control, the semantic differential is a valuable methodology for focusing attention on the reasons precipitating the problem. For example, the information provided by the semantic differential is useful in measuring coalition behavioral dispositions. In addition, the semantic differential may aid in the identification of coalitions and the understanding of various coalition role interactions, which are critically important to the systematic development, implementation, and evolution of control systems. However, merely identifying coalitions and measuring their behavioral propensities fails to provide

Table 13-1 Mean Semantic Differential Scores

Concepts	Group I (Medical)	Group II (Administrative)
C_1: Health Care Delivery	5.21	5.41
C_2: Cost Consciousness	2.76	3.20
C_3: Economic Management	2.49	2.85
C_4: Patient Welfare	5.50	5.54

information regarding the nature of effective corrective actions. This information often may be generated by the analysis of job descriptions.

COALITION VARIANCE ANALYSIS: ANALYSIS OF JOB DESCRIPTIONS

To formulate corrective actions, given the results of a behavioral analysis, management must determine for what activities the coalition members believe the organization is holding them responsible (note this as *expected* responsibility), and for what activities the coalition members believe themselves to be responsible (note this as *actual* responsibility). In the interest of developing a balanced decision system, it is important to be able to judge how a particular coalition should act and react to varying organizational situations. The variance between what the coalition is doing and what it reasonably can be expected to do is of considerable managerial interest (e.g., recall the previous medical/administrative example in which the administrative group was presumed to be concerned with cost and management issues, but proved to be more concerned with the medical concepts).

Analysis of the job descriptions of the coalition members provides an objective basis for developing expected coalition actions and reactions on specific organizational issues. The importance of the analysis of job descriptions cannot be overemphasized. It is the only objective way to develop insights regarding the appropriateness of possible corrective actions where systems imbalances are isolated by the semantic differential (or other behavioral analyses). This behavioral analysis of variance is not technically analogous to the analysis of performance variances, but it is, nonetheless, an important aspect of the development or maintenance of a balanced decision system.

For example, consider the results of the semantic differential exercise discussed previously. One of the failures of the institution's budgeting system may be the lack of polarization of the medical and administrative staff. However, should the medical or the administrative group be admonished? The only way to rationalize and plan a corrective action is to analyze the job descriptions of the members of both coalitions to ascertain if their actions are consistent with organizational expectations.

Description of Hospital Administrator's Position

Consider, as an illustration, the job description of the hospital administrator of a major institution. The formal document describing the functions and responsibilities of the administrator may be constructed as follows:

Position Title: Hospital Administrator

Primary Function. The administrator is responsible for all day-to-day activities of the hospital and for obtaining results in keeping with the policies and objectives established by the executive director of hospitals. The administrator directs the activities of the associate administrator, assistant administrators, medical director, and any other department, project, or function reporting directly to the administrator. The administrator maintains liaison with the professional staff and assists the executive director of hospitals and the dean of the school of medicine in improving and enlarging the professional staff. The administrator assists the executive director in developing long-range plans and programs for the hospital, and is responsible for meeting required standards for licensure and hospital accreditation. The administrator has profit and loss accountability.

Authority. The administrator is authorized to employ and terminate employment of personnel on the authorized hospital personnel budget. The administrator may purchase supplies and incur other obligations within the approved hospital operating and capital budgets, and may negotiate for physicians' services for the hospital.

Accountability.

- To recommend and meet budget objectives for the hospital.
- To support activities leading to operational improvements and cost reductions.
- To implement accounting controls in all sections of the hospital.
- To implement systems changes designed to improve patient care and/or effectiveness of hospital operations.
- To employ and maintain a stable employee work force which meets the standards of quality patient care.
- To develop coordination, cooperation, and understanding among professional staff, administration, and other hospital personnel.
- To support joint programs and cooperative activities between the hospitals.
- To implement programs which enhance medical staff support of the hospitals.
- To report regularly progress in meeting the goals of the hospital to the executive director of hospitals.

Education. A Master's Degree in health care administration or business administration preferred. Equivalent experience in a responsible position will be evaluated in lieu of a degree.

Training and Experience. A minimum of five year's experience as the administrator or associate administrator of a major hospital, preferably a teaching institution, or strong experience with hospitals in a health care related position is required.

Job Knowledge and Professional Experience. The administrator should have complete knowledge of all aspects of modern hospital administration with a strong professional background in organization and leadership skills. The administrator should have current knowledge of federal, state, local, and third party and accreditation regulations which affect hospitals in the health care setting. The administrator should have the personal and leadership ability to maintain strong interpersonal relationships with professional executive personnel.

Variance Analysis

If the semantic differential results are institution-specific, given this hospital administrator job description, a variance appears to exist between the expected responsibility of the administrative coalition (i.e., the duties and responsibilities delineated in the job description) and the actual responsibility of the administrative coalition as inferred from the semantic differential results. The connotative variance analysis does not determine what corrective actions are needed; however, it is suggestive of an investigative focus.

Conclusion

Although the semantic differential may provide information useful in developing an investigative focus when control problems result from a coalition performance imbalance, the costs of developing the information needed by coalition variance analysis must be evaluated against the possible benefits (i.e., the effect of corrective action on institutional performance). These cost/benefit considerations are particularly complex in rationalizing any behavioral analysis. However, notwithstanding the obvious difficulty in objectively ascertaining the benefits of coalition analysis, this cost/benefit information must be ascertained (see Question 13-3).

NOTES

1. The development of the semantic space relies on factor analysis. There are a number of excellent texts on factor analysis; Harman (1976) is recommended.
2. Osgood et al. offer 76 adjectives from the thesaurus study, pp. 47–62.

Questions and Problems

Question 13-1. Why is the analysis of job descriptions important in developing corrective actions based on insights derived from an analysis of the semantic difference among coalitions?

Question 13-2. List at least four criteria which should be used to evaluate the use of the semantic differential in an organization.

Question 13-3. Assume you are a consultant to a large teaching hospital. You have conducted several coalition analyses over the last few years. For the most part, they have provided you with useful information regarding problem definition and solution implementation. You have prepared a proposal which you have delivered to the hospital regarding developing and making operational a planning, programing, budgeting system. As a part of the proposal, you suggest a coalition analysis. However, you do not devote much attention in the proposal to justifying the need for the coalition analysis. At a meeting arranged for you to defend your proposal, you are met with considerable resistance to your entire proposal by the chief of medicine. Your sense of the meeting is that if you are unable to rationalize your proposal to the chief of medicine, no one will support you. The focus of attention is on the coalition analysis. The chief of medicine directs the following statement to you:

> "Look, this is pie-in-the-sky. We don't even know what causes the common cold and you expect us to buy a 'psychological delineation of various decision making coalitions in the institution' so that you can create some utopian budgeting system. You can't be serious. I'm not suggesting that you are trying to fatten your billing, but how much would the study cost be if we amputate this vestigial?"

Required:

How would you respond to this statement?

Question 13-4. Suggest a process for formulating the concepts to be used in the semantic differential.

Question 13-5. How could the semantic differential be used to identify the various coalitions in the institution? Modify Figure 13-1 to represent the identification of coalitions.

Problems 13-1. Assume you have been hired to ascertain the operational feasibility of an intrainstitutional pricing system for the service departments in a large teaching hospital. Assume the price is to be negotiated individually between user and provider departments. The administration hopes that this system will promote resource control in the institution. Design a coalition analysis which will provide insights regarding the operational feasibility of the proposed pricing system.

Problem 13-2. In investigating the design of reports to be used in an information system for a nursing agency, the following semantic differential information was developed.

Individual	Concept A Report Timeliness	Concept B Graphic Presentation	Concept C Report Readability
S_1	6.2	2.1	4.2
S_2	5.8	1.8	5.3
S_3	2.7	4.8	4.8
S_4	3.2	6.1	5.1
S_5	4.7	5.8	5.4
A_1	6.3	2.0	6.0
A_2	5.4	5.4	4.9
A_3	5.9	1.2	5.1
A_4	3.8	6.2	4.8
A_5	6.4	2.2	5.9

Required:

a. Using the semantic scores on concepts A, B, and C, does there seem to be a coalition consisting of supervisors (noted as S_1, S_2, S_3, S_4, S_5) and administrators (noted as A_1, A_2, A_3, A_4, A_5)?
b. What grouping of individuals constitutes two differentiable coalitions?
c. Does the grouping developed in (b) change if only concepts A and B are used? Does this mean the semantic information on concept C is useless?
d. How would the information provided by these three concepts be used in the design of an information system?

Chapter 14

Regionalization

A Prayer for National Health Insurance

I reckon that the sufferings of this present time are not worthy to be compared with the glory which shall be revealed. . . .
Paul, Romans 8:18

The subject of regional control cannot be treated analytically, but must be treated with conjecture, because the political process by which health care change must be effected is complex and no experiential basis exists for predicting confidently the outcome of the National Health Insurance (NHI) issue. Consequently, this chapter focuses on ideas that people close to the NHI problem are vocalizing with some regularity: regionalization, HUB Hospital, rethinking retrospective reimbursement, output definitions, and control of systems technology. Of course, whether or not any substantial thought underlies the elegant political rhetoric remains to be demonstrated. Chances are that the NHI legislation which has been on various administrations "to-do" list will languish on the political back burner because the United States has not experienced a recognized health crisis to develop the momentum needed to formulate and enact such legislation.

The purpose of this chapter is to examine the basic elements of a regionalized system of health care delivery. The regionalization issue is complex with management and control implications for providers, third party payers, and consumers, and a comprehensive presentation of all the aspects of the regionalization model is not possible here. The focus of this chapter, therefore, will be on two elements of a regionalization model—the sociostrategic dimension of regionalization and the elemental conditions necessary to develop a process by which a regionalized delivery system may be effected.

REGIONALIZED CONTROL: A SOCIOSTRATEGIC PLANNING APPROACH

If a health care delivery system's reorientation is to be effective, it must be cast in a sociostrategic framework of anaylsis. A strategic planning approach is necessary because the modification of a health care delivery system involves a major reorganization of the technologies involved. The sociologic aspects must be considered because the success of a reorientation depends upon critical social roles and relationships that must be established, altered, or assumed by the various groups working within the health care delivery system. To effect a sociostrategic systems reorientation, four interrelated elements must be considered: (1) technology, (2) the interaction between providers and regional administration, (3) consumers, and (4) reimbursement.

Technological Reorientation: A Functional Focus

The basic regional delivery configuration often suggested by researchers and politicians is a three-tiered hierarchy interorganization of health care units, which shall be called a medical interorganization (see Figure 14-1). At the periphery of the system and closest to the population is the neighborhood health clinic (NHC), which would serve a population within a defined geographic area.

The NHC would provide health maintenance services and outpatient care. The clinics would be staffed predominantly by nursing and paramedical personnel and would provide services for the majority of patients who do not require specialized care or hospitalization. Each neighborhood clinic would be equipped with only the technology needed for the scope of services which are routinely required in most EMS units in that particular region.

These neighborhood health clinics would be the satellites of a regional hospital which would offer the standard inpatient services and specialized emergency services for the regional population. The regional hospitals generally would serve patients referred from their satellite NHC clinics, but would retain the flexibility of directly accepting both emergency cases and cases that could not be treated at the NHC. The size and number of these regional hospitals would depend upon the total population of the area served. Considerable, rapid, and effective communication between the regional hospitals and the medical center would be required to give the best possible patient care to the community. [1]

At the nucleus of each group of regional hospitals (with their respective satellite clinics) would be the medical center and medical college. The medical center would serve to provide specialized and sophisticated diagnostic and therapeutic facilities (i.e. categorization, see Problem 14-5),

Figure 14-1 Regional Health Care Interorganization

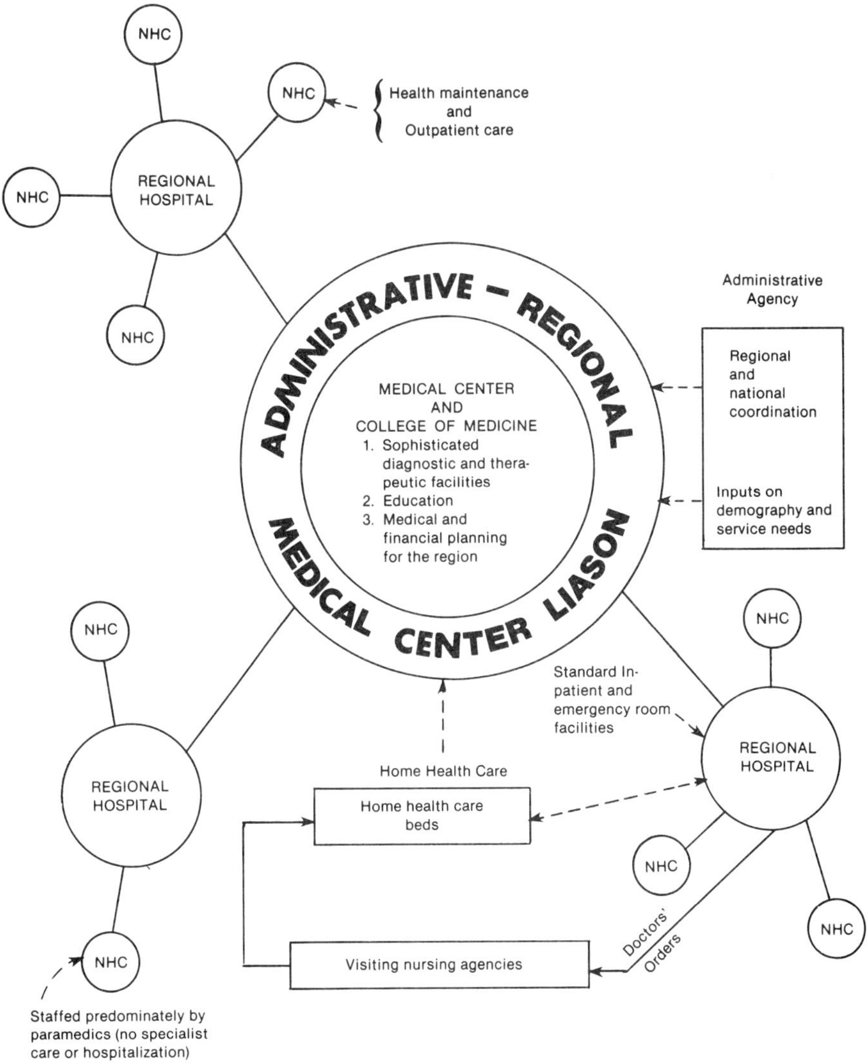

provide training for future physicians and paramedical personnel, and act as the administrative, planning, and control center of the medical interorganization.

Reorganization of the Roles between Health Care Providers and Regional Administration

The reorientation of the systems technology will require an alteration of the roles of those responsible for delivering health care, as well as those responsible for regional administration. The education and training of both providers and administrators must be centralized and updated. In addition, the method of paying providers must be changed, and an incentive system must be devised to encourage cost conscious behavior. A change also must occur in the administration of the various levels of health care delivery, with consumer governance as one possible alternative. Finally, a regional administrative agency must be developed to oversee health care services in the region.

The education and training of providers and administrators must be altered to coincide with the reorientation of the systems technology. The medical center must provide the technology and the environment for the education of allied health personnel. In addition, the pool of qualified personnel must be increased by training individuals and drawing on an already existing population of paramedics. Not only must health technicians, technologists, and physician assistants be trained, but a curriculum and staff to train hospital and medical systems engineers and analysts must be developed. Furthermore, new special skills must be taught so that new technological advancements (e.g., computerized screening and diagnostic techniques) can be utilized most effectively. Finally, special hospital management and administration courses and seminars must be conducted to allow the participants in the health care system to acquire or renew their skills.

Other changes must occur in the method of paying providers and encouraging cost-conscious behavior. Employees in the medical interorganization must be predominantly salaried personnel, a change which should eliminate the relationship between the charges accruing to the patient and the doctor's financial well being. However, other bonus or award arrangements also should be developed and used so that clinics, hospitals, or departments that have reduced costs or have made other significant progress in operational efficiency may be identified and rewarded. These incentives may take the form of direct financial rewards to the individuals involved (administrators, physicians, nurses, etc.), or financial rewards to the institution (e.g., the net revenues which have accrued to a particular department or hospital are retained by it).

In conjunction with this provider reorientation, some individuals suggest that restructuring the hospital's governance is important. One suggested administrative restructuring provides for increased participation on the part of the consumer. Cathcart (1970) suggests that changes in the composition of the board of trustees and in membership policies may be one way of achieving this goal, while consumer participation in policy making committees is another means of achieving better consumer representation. In addition, he suggests that the hospital employees (presumably drawn from the community) can be used effectively in hospital governance. Although Cathcart's consumer governance agreement has a certain "inalienable right" appeal, experiences of many groups with consumer representation generally is mixed, with successful consumer governance interrelationships (such as the one reported by Cathcart) the exception. Therefore, consumer and employee governance representation cannot be recommended categorically.

To coordinate the various regional activities, an administrative agency must be legislatively empowered because this agency must be responsible for determining the appropriateness, adequacy, priority, and location of health care services and facilities. A capital spending fund to modify the medical interorganization should be used under the direction of the administrative agency. The centralization of this aspect of the decision-making process should allow the same agency to coordinate the service and financial priorities of the medical interorganization and thereby enable the managers to eliminate systematically the costs of regional underutilization and nonintegrated planning.

Since the regional agency is presumed to have the responsibility for developing and monitoring the regional health care delivery plan, the administrative agency also should be responsible for evaluating budgets, performing audits, and allocating strategic and tactical funds to the three tiers of the medical interorganization. This is necessary because the medical center probably will not be able to generate sufficient revenue to continue its operations after most of the lucrative services (allergy care, annual physical examinations, immunizations, ordinary surgery, preventative tests, general medical care, maternal and infant care, etc.), formally rendered at the medical center, are transferred to the neighborhood health centers and the regional hospitals. Thus, net revenues collected by the three-tiered providers must accrue to the regional administrative agency and subsequently be allocated to the specific providers in a manner to achieve the regional plan. However, the process by which hospital budgets are evaluated must be dynamic, allowing for the possibility of substituting preventative measures (nursing home care, more accessible health care services, and physician services delivered in the office) for the costly hospital inpatient service alternatives. Therefore, the budget will be a planning document subject to challenging inspection which transcends the mere perpetuation of past utilization.

Consumer Role Reorientation: A Health Maintenance Perspective

If this regionalized system is to work with any degree of success, the consumers of health care services must view health care from a preventative perspective and not merely from a curative one; otherwise, the neighborhood health clinics may not be utilized effectively. The NHC is expected to become a health maintenance organization (HMO), and although the experience of many of the successful HMOs is encouraging, reorienting the consumers' role relative to health maintenance may be difficult.

The most direct way to involve consumers in the health system at the neighborhood health clinic level is through various insurance arrangements. The majority of reimbursement policies presently in use are structured so that the least out-of-pocket expense will be incurred by consumers if they use the hospital inpatient facilities. A series of deductibles makes the use of outpatient facilities and doctors' offices more costly to the consumer and the physician. However, to reverse the adverse utilization effects of these reimbursement policies, the federal or state government could maintain a subsistence preventative medical health care plan for the poor and the infirm, which would be financed through general tax revenues. Further, to limit unnecessary utilization, other consumers (as determined by federal or state standards) could bear a certain proportion of the direct cost of service.

Reimbursement: A Means of Effecting Policy

Reimbursement is fundamental to the growth of the regional system. It provides the basis of economic motivation for the differentiated institutions constituting the regional delivery system. However, the absence of an output definition complicates the effectiveness of the reimbursement pay schedules to motivate productivity, since reimbursement is oriented to units of service delivered which need not be related to productivity. Therefore, to use reimbursement schedules to affect policy, a regional database must be developed so that output surrogates can be formulated and sensibly integrated into an incentive system to provide an allocation of regional resources which facilitates achievement of the region's performance objectives.

Attempting to affect health care policy through reimbursement schedules presumes that the system can be modified in response to various performance criteria considered important in directing the system's resources. A retrospective, full cost reimbursement system is incapable of selective modification. Traditionally, therefore, rather than modifying the reimbursement system, agencies were created to modify the health care institutions directly (i.e., credentialing, certificate of need, HSA, etc.). However, these agencies usually have failed to exert any control because they are not legislatively empowered properly and usually cannot attract sufficient managerial expertise to rationalize their "due process" responsibilities.

An alternative to this system of directly modifying institutions is to modify the reimbursement system. In this case, the reimbursement basis must be changed to prospective and must be based upon allowable costs determined by the regional agency. A prospective budgeting system which is coordinated by the regional agency and reimburses institutions based upon particular performance statistics would enable the regional delivery system to be modified selectively.

The presumption is that prospective reimbursement, used as an economic incentive to achieve regional performance expectations, will vest an interest in achieving economic control. However, regardless of the form of the reimbursement system, quality dysfunctions may arise whenever economic penalty or rewards are sensitive only to cost variations from prospectively determined amounts. (See the EMS case, Chapter 10.) Specifically, the delivery institutions may effect "invisible" reductions in the quality of services to avoid economic penalities, or modify the patient mix to select fewer patients whose care is costly. To check this possibility, performance measures must be developed from the regional database, and effective regional utilization review committees must be created.

CONDITIONS FOR THE DEVELOPMENT OF AN EFFECTIVE REGIONAL HEALTH CARE DELIVERY SYSTEM

As suggested previously, a regional health care interorganization probably will not evolve without a substantial commitment from legislators, providers, third party payers, and consumers. Given this commitment, three systems' conditions must be satisfied to develop an effective regional health delivery system (see Question 14-5). First, a unified accounting and reporting system must be developed for all institutions in the region. This system must be used to develop comparable performance statistics among institutions within regions and among institutions from different regions.[2] Second, a plan must exist to phase the various institutions into the accounting and reporting system. Phasing also must be sensitive to the existing regional bureaucratic structure. In essence, phasing must establish the control protocol among the various agencies concerned with regional delivery. Finally, the administrative agency must be legislatively empowered with authority commensurate to the task. In reviewing a representative number of state proposals, the language confirming regional agency authority is often couched in vague terms which seem certain to inhibit agency effectiveness. However, rather than narrowly spelling out the legislative qualifications, the regional agency should have the ability to plan and monitor the phasing of the elements of the regional medical interorganization and provide for the administrative process necessary to evaluate performance and allocate regional health resources. As noted, these administrative processes may take various forms, from prospective budgeting with rate modification to direct systems control and rate-setting. The critical condition is that only one agency emerge and assume responsibility for the system's effective movement toward the regional performance objectives.

The process of control at the regional level may be developed in much the same way as a control process is developed in an individual institution (see Chapter 10). The agency may develop control information in the region by comparing actual institutional performance to average performance of the other institutions in the region or to regional performance standards if they exist. Then, this information may be used to modify the reimbursement system. However, since individual institutional performance will be compared to other institutions or standards, each institution must be aware of the rules of the competition for resources. The two prevailing regional control philosophies which would affect the allocation of regional resources are performance within standards and outperforming the average.

Performance Within Standards

Under this philosophy, the regional planners are presumed to know the long-range goals for the region as coordinated with national or sectional goals. With this knowledge, the regional planners establish standards of performance which they feel are relevant in effecting regional policy and allocating resources. Then, the performances of all regional institutions are evaluated relative to the standard.

This approach has a number of problems, all of which emanate from the difficult task of accurately setting regional health care output standards. Unfortunately, the health care system is no closer to sensible output performance measures or standards than it was in the mid-1960s. Whether this is due to the political processes or to the measurement problems inherent in the process of regional coordination and control has been vigorously debated. However, no solution appears to be forthcoming.

Outperforming the Average

Under this philosophy of control, institutions which do not compare favorably with the regional averages are allocated fewer regional resources through the reimbursement system. This Darwinian approach to control works for a short period of time; it does, in fact, render the weak incapable of survival. However, after a time, when the only institutions left are the most efficient and effective delivery units, legally changing the reimbursement rules may be difficult. At this point, these surviving institutions may begin to take actions which, in the short run, benefit their position as judged by the competitive statistics, but in the long run are dysfunctional from a regional health care perspective. If a regional system is to be effective, some combination of these two approaches must be used, possibly using the rule of outperforming the average until the desired set of institutions remain, and then effecting standards derived from analyses of their performance as represented in the regional database.

PROPRIETARY HOSPITALS: A FREE ENTERPRISE ALTERNATIVE

Proprietary hospitals should continue to serve the community apart from the medical interorganization. Their existence will insure that any consumer of health care services who is unhappy with the services in the regional system will have an opportunity to exercise the right to select. Also, the proprietary hospitals will provide an employment alternative for those individuals not satisfied with professional opportunities available in the regional system. As Levitan (1970) notes: "The new generation of proprietary hospitals began with the firm conviction that socially responsive, creative capitalism, with reasonable profit as an incentive, can place the operations of the health care system on the same efficient basis as that of other industries."

The services offered by the proprietary hospitals will put them in direct competition with the medical interorganization. If inefficient or ineffective utilization of resources in one system raises costs, the other system probably will benefit from this relative cost difference (see Question 14-8). This competition is healthy and necessary (see Problem 14-2).

SUMMARY

In this final chapter, the emphasis has been on change. The health care delivery systems must be able to change as the environment changes, and the ability of health care institutions to adapt their medical and administrative management systems to the dictates of external forces will, in the final analysis, differentiate successful institutions from those which become part of the fossil record (see Question 14-9).

NOTES

1. Operational models of a regionalized communication network which may be useful in designing an interhospital communication system are the EMS intercounty communication systems developed and sustained under the EMSS Act 1202, 1203, and 1204 DHEW grants.
2. The state of Maryland has developed a comprehensive system of data gathering and reporting which may serve as a model for other states, as well as for the federal government.

Questions and Problems

Question 14-1. What are some difficulties involved in specifying the relationship between regional health care output measures and the cost of activities performed to generate that output?

Question 14-2. What criteria would you use for selecting the location of the medical center and college for a region?

Question 14-3. What are the control advantages of regionalization? What are the control limitations of regionalization?

Question 14-4. At what points in a regional system can you envision consumer participation in the regional decision-making process? Defend your answer.

Question 14-5. What conditions, other than the three discussed in this chapter, are necessary to effect a regional delivery system?

Question 14-6. What are the advantages and disadvantages of an increase in the number of proprietary hospitals from the point of view of the regional administrative agency? From the point of view of the consumer?

Question 14-7. What types of control information would be useful in developing interregional performance variances which could be used in evaluating the administration of the medical center?

Question 14-8. How will conspicuous consumption affect the success of cost competition between proprietary hospitals and the medical interorganization? Does a health maintenance philosophy promote or discourage conspicuous consumption?

Question 14-9. Another perspective is that the medical interorganization should attempt to control its environment rather than react to changes in it. This is often referred to as a preactive perspective. Discuss this perspective.

Problem 14-1. This chapter concentrates on the hospital in the regional health care delivery system because the cost of services delivered in hospitals accounts for a major proportion of consumer expenditure on health care. However, nursing agencies, private group practices, HMOs, and extended care facilities are also important in a regional health care delivery system. Indicate how each of these agencies should be integrated into the regional medical interorganization.

Problem 14-2. One of the most difficult aspects of designing a regional health care delivery system is specifying a reasonable reimbursement price for both the proprietary institutions and the medical interorganization. For example, assume a neighborhood health center treats a fracture. A number of costs may be used to establish the reimbursement price: marginal cost, full cost, or average accounting cost, to mention a few (see Chapter 8). Assume the regional agency fixes the price for a fracture at the average direct variable cost of the nonproprietary institutions in the region. Further assume that the federal and state government contribute substantial funds to the regional system for research, teaching, and administration. Therefore, the pricing of a fracture for the nonproprietary hospitals does not need to generate reimbursement for these subsidized activities.

a. Is the regionally established reimbursement price fair for the proprietary hospital? Should it be?
b. Discuss the reimbursement and control problems which may result from having multiple prices for similar services.
c. Discuss the desirability of having multiple prices for similar services from the consumer's perspective.

Problem 14-3. The services of institutions may be valued at cost or charges. Service costs may be defined as the accumulation of historical costs as they relate to a particular service. Service charges may be defined as the amount at which the institution prices its services. Generally, the two sources of reimbursement are private insurance carriers, which normally pay charges, and the federal government and Blue Cross, which pay costs. Discuss the roles of these two types of third party payers in a regional system where there are proprietary alternatives.

Problem 14-4. The following information was abstracted from *The Medical Directory of Prevailing Charges*, 1977, published by the Health Care Financing Administration.

Average Usual and Customary
Physician Procedure Charges*

	Manhattan	Chicago	Wyoming	Washington, D.C.
Initial complete office visit	$ 44.70	$ 60.00	$ 44.70	$ 51.00
Routine brief office visit	25.00	15.00	8.90	12.80
Radical mastectomy	1,276.00	750.00	510.60	638.00
Colectomy	1,595.00	950.00	522.00	910.00
Appendectomy	500.00	500.00	285.00	319.00
Chest x-ray	25.00	18.00	16.60	15.00
Complete blood count	10.00	9.00	9.25	7.50
Urinalysis	5.00	5.00	3.85	3.80

*Note: Usual and customary charges are established by third party payers profiling the fee schedules of all physicians in a particular area.

Given this information, answer the following questions:

(a) Assuming these figures are accurate, what are some reasons which would account for the various regional differences?

(b) How would this information be used to establish regional price standards?

(c) Assume that you are able to devise an index that accurately uses regional standard of living information to convert the regional usual and customary charge information so that each region may be compared. Assume this conversion factor is .92 for Manhattan and 2.2 for Wyoming. Compute and contrast the normalized usual and customary fees for Manhattan and Wyoming. What regional control information do you have? Assuming the differences you develop are statistically significant, how useful are they in evaluating regional performance differences?

(d) What if the groups selected to prepare the usual and customary charges contain statistically significant different proportions of proprietary and nonproprietary hospitals. Will this effect interregion cost comparisons? If so, how would you adjust for it?

Problem 14-5. In 1971 the state of Illinois received federal money under a presidential initiative to develop a regional emergency medical service system. The spirit of the initiative was to have hospitals in seven geographic regions of the state cooperate (basically within the region) to provide high quality emergency medical services. The demonstration grant specified the following principals in the regional EMS system: the police department, fire department, airport authority, Red Cross (and other related agencies), medical professionals in the region, hospitals, and other agencies responsible for the delivery of health care services.

The demonstration grant was basically addressed to (1) establishing a communication network among the principals, (2) providing for the purchase of mobile EMS units, and (3) providing for the training of emergency medical personnel. Assume that categorization (i.e., certain institutions would be responsible for the treatment of specific EMS cases) is a possibility without a legislative mandate, and that other funding agencies, such as the Robert Wood Johnson Foundation and the Department of Health, Education and Welfare, are interested in funding EMS studies and systems.

Required:

Develop a ten-year strategy to be initiated in 1971 that would be useful in making an institution a medical interorganization.

Problem 14-6. On July 29, 1978, the Carter Administration released through the Office of DHEW the following ten principles which were to form the basis of a national health insurance plan to be operational in 1983:

1. The plan should assure that all Americans have comprehensive health care coverage, including protection against catastrophic medical expenses.
2. Quality health care should be available to all.
3. Americans should have "freedom of choice in the selection of physicians, hospitals and health delivery systems."
4. Unnecessary health-care spending must be reduced with aggressive cost containment and strengthening of the "competitive forces in the health care sector."
5. Additional public and private expenditures should be "substantially offset by savings from greater efficiency."
6. There is to be no additional federal spending until fiscal 1983, and "the plan should be phased in gradually" with consideration given to economic and administrative experience as the plan moves from phase to phase. "The experience of other government pro-

grams, in which expenditure far exceeded initial projections, must not be repeated."

7. The plan would be financed through government funding and contributions from both employers and employees with careful consideration given to the "ability of many consumers to share a moderate portion of the cost of their care."
8. "A significant role" would be reserved for the private insurance industry under government regulation.
9. The plan should promote "ambulatory and preventive services, attracting personnel to underserved rural and urban areas and encouraging the use of prepaid health plans."
10. "The plan should assure consumer representation throughout its operation."

Required:

a. Discuss the definition and measurement problems inherent in each of these ten principles.
b. Many of these ten principles were also suggested in developing a regional medical interorganization. Do these ten principles therefore lead to the development of regional medical interorganizations?
c. How should evidence be gathered to insure that these principles are being satisfied for:
   (i) specific regional interorganizations
   (ii) the coordination of all regional interorganizations

Appendix A

Fundamental Accounting Concepts

In today's economy, goods and services constantly flow between the business sector and the household sector (see Figure A-1). Businesses, including both nonprofit and profit-oriented organizations, receive capital, labor, and entrepreneurial expertise from the household sector in exchange for money. The businesses transform these inputs into goods and services which, in turn, are provided to households in exchange for money. Hence, the economic composition of a business changes over time as goods and services are bought, transformed, and sold. The purpose of accounting is to describe the changing economic composition of the business in monetary terms.

DEFINING THE BUSINESS

A business is an explicitly defined legal entity that is composed of assets, liabilities, and owners' equity. Assets include all items owned by the business that are utilized as the business continues to operate. Generally, assets can be divided into *current assets*, which include cash and other assets that will be sold, consumed, or converted into cash within the ensuing year or the operating period, whichever is longer, and *noncurrent assets*, which will not be sold, consumed, or converted into cash during the ensuing year or operating period. Liabilities include all debts owed by the business. In general, liabilities also are divided into two groups: *current liabilities*, which will be satisfied with current assets within the ensuing year or operating

Figure A-1 Economic Flows Between the Household Sector and the Business Sector

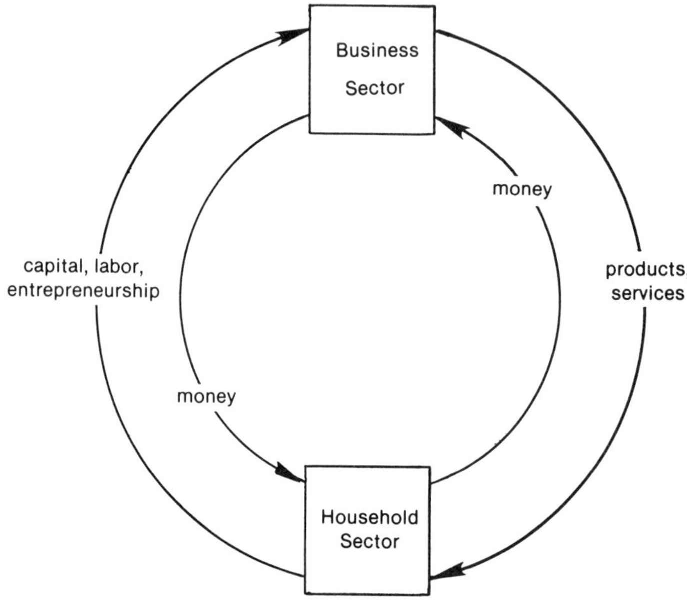

period, whichever is longer, and *noncurrent liabilities*, which will not be satisfied during the ensuing year or operating period. The difference between the value of the assets and the value of the liabilities is called owners' equity. As the economic composition of the business changes, the value of the assets, liabilities, and owners' equity changes. The accounting system delineates the direction and magnitude of these changes in a system of accounts that describes the various types of assets, liabilities and owners' equity associated with the business.

THE DESIGN OF FORMAL ACCOUNTING SYSTEMS

Relatively few of the many economic events that occur affect a particular business, but those that do can be translated into accounting events. As the number of economic events, or transactions, experienced by the business increases, the business's need for a formal accounting system increases.

Five steps are required in a formal accounting system: (1) observation, (2) measurement, (3) recording, (4) record summarization, and (5) statement preparation. The process begins as economic events that affect the business are observed. To translate these economic events into accounting events, the monetary impact of each economic event must be measured. Then, these accounting events, or transactions, can be recorded in the business's formal system of accounts. The information recorded in these accounts is summarized continuously so that the value of the assets, liabilities, and owners' equity can be computed easily. Finally, financial statements are prepared periodically so that interested parties can evaluate the business and plan financing and investing activities.

Transactions Analysis: Observation and Measurement

In order for an economic event to be recorded in a particular business's accounting records, the economic event (1) must be observed by individuals associated with the business, and (2) must be evaluated regarding its monetary effect on the assets, liabilities, or owner's equity of the business. These two activities, observation and measurement, combine to describe the direction and magnitude of the change in the economic composition of the business.

The Fundamental Accounting Equation and the Primary Accounting Condition

As discussed previously, owners' equity is defined as the difference between the value of a business's assets and liabilities. This relationship can be formulated as:

$$\text{Assets} - \text{Liabilities} = \text{Owners' Equity}$$

or,

$$\text{Assets} = \text{Liabilities} + \text{Owners' Equity} \tag{A-1}$$

Equation (A-1) is known as the fundamental accounting equation.

One important insight to the accounting system can be gleaned from the fundamental accounting equation. Since the equation must be true at all times, each transaction that affects the economic composition of the business must leave equation (A-1) true. Hence, each transaction must have at least two parts, an increase in assets and an increase in liabilities or owners' equity, a decrease in assets and a decrease in liabilities or owners' equity, an increase and a decrease in assets, liabilities, or owners' equity, or some other appropriate combination.

To monitor the impact of individual transactions on equation A-1, the double entry accounting system has been devised. Under the double entry accounting system, each transaction affects at least two accounts such that the debits will equal the credits. Debits are accounting entries that are recorded in a left-hand column; credits are entries recorded in a right hand column.[1]

The relationship

$$\text{Debits} = \text{Credits} \tag{A-2}$$

is the primary accounting condition. In order for this condition to exist, a convention must be adopted whereby increases or decreases in particular accounts are recorded as debits or credits. The chosen convention is that credits increase owners' equity. Increases and decreases in all other accounts can be determined accordingly.

For example, since Assets = Liabilities + Owners' Equity, one transaction could increase both assets and owners' equity. By convention, owners' equity increases by a credit. Therefore, assets must increase by debits so that both equations (A-1) and (A-2) can be true. Similarly, a transaction may increase both assets and liabilities. In this case, since assets increase by debits, liabilities must increase by credits. These examples are summarized by the following statement.

> Debits increase accounts to the left of the equal sign in the fundamental accounting equation (equation (A-1)), and credits increase accounts to the right of the equal sign in the fundamental accounting equation.

Conversely, credits will decrease accounts on the left-hand side of equation (A-1) and debits will decrease accounts on the right-hand side.

Cash Basis Accounting vs. Accrual Basis Accounting: The Revenue Principle and the Matching Principle

Many of the economic events that affect a business involve selling its product or service. Since the outflow of the product or service from the business is not always synchronized with the inflow of the cash payment (i.e., credit sales or prepayments may be made), an accounting principle has been established that determines the point at which revenue should be recognized or recorded. This principle is called the revenue principle.

The statement of the revenue principle depends on the business's basis of accounting. Under the cash basis of accounting, revenue is recognized in the period in which the cash associated with a sale is collected, regardless of when the product is delivered or the service is rendered. Under the accrual basis of accounting, on the other hand, revenue is recognized in the period in which a product is delivered or a service is rendered, regardless of when the payment is collected.

Similarly, the time at which expenses are recorded varies between the cash basis and the accrual basis of accounting. Under the cash basis, an expense is recognized in the period in which cash is dispersed for operational inputs, regardless of when these inputs are used. Under the accrual basis, an accounting principle, called the matching principle, has been adopted. This principle states that the expenses associated with the generation of revenue should be recognized in the same period as the associated revenue.

The accrual basis of accounting generally is preferable to the cash basis because the accrual basis produces consistent income streams. Since the accrual basis of accounting matches revenue with the expenses incurred to generate that revenue given that the volume of activity is fairly consistent from period to period, income also will be fairly consistent from period to period. Under the cash basis of accounting, however, a consistent volume of activity will not always produce a consistent income stream because periods in which costly assets are purchased will reflect exceptionally low levels of income, while periods in which no assets are purchased will reflect very high levels of income.

Although a fluctuating income stream may not be inherently bad, evaluating a business that uses cash basis accounting can be quite difficult. For example, the management of a business using the cash basis of accounting may not want to pay the high income taxes associated with the high income of any particular period in which costly assets are not purchased. Therefore, the management may decide to reduce income by acquiring an excessive amount of operational inputs (e.g., inventory) at the end of the period. Unfortunately, this kind of purchasing may not be timely because (1) the costs of the operational inputs may be quite high at the time of the purchase, and (2) by acquiring more operational inputs than are needed, the business will increase the costs associated with storage.[2] In addition, by acquiring large amounts of operational inputs at the end of the period, the business reduces the expenses that could be incurred in the next period. Hence, a high income level in the next period may require even larger end-of-period purchasing. In this case, the business may appear to be well managed, while, in fact, a very poor management policy exists. This tendency toward poor management is the major problem of cash basis accounting. However, businesses that do not own or intend to purchase costly assets can function quite efficiently under a cash basis of accounting.

Throughout the text, the accrual basis of accounting is assumed to be in use. This form of accounting tends to foster effective management and produce accounting information that can be evaluated in a relatively straightforward manner. However, accrual basis accounting alone will not effect efficient management; the proper procedures and controls, as discussed in the text, must be used in conjunction with the accounting information to effect resource control.

Expanding the Fundamental Accounting Equation

Regardless of the basis of accounting used, the results of operations affect the wealth of the owners. Hence, income should increase owners' equity, and losses, or negative income, should decrease owners' equity. This income information could be incorporated in the owners' equity accounts of equation (A-1). However, the accounting system isolates changes in owners' equity that arise from operations, so that the current profitability (revenue less costs) of the business can be evaluated easily. Therefore, equation (A-1) must be expanded to incorporate the income account as follows:

(A-3) Assets = Liabilities + Owners' Equity + Income

Since income is a type of owners' equity account, credits will increase income, and debits will decrease income. This information is useful in interpreting the fundamental accounting equation when expanded to include the two elements of income, revenues and expenses:

(A-4) Assets = Liabilities + Owners' Equity + Revenues − Expenses

Revenues increase income. Therefore, credits will increase revenues. However, expenses decrease income. Hence, debits will increase the magnitude of the expense accounts. Including revenues and expenses in the fundamental accounting equation forms a foundation for the first steps in transactions analysis: observation of economic events that affect the business and isolation of the accounts affected by the observed transactions.

Measuring the Monetary Impact of Transactions

Measuring the monetary impact of transactions begins with the careful observation of economic events. Both the direction and magnitude of any change in the economic composition of a business can be observed. The system of debits and credits can be helpful in ascertaining the direction of the change in any specific account.

As illustrated in Figure A-1, each time goods or services flow to or from the business, a counteracting monetary (cash or credit) flow occurs. These flows provide a consistent basis by which the magnitude of all economic changes can be valued. Hence, the magnitude of change in any asset, liability, owners' equity, revenue, or expense account is determined by the monetary flows that are associated with that change. In some cases, however, particularly when previously purchased operational inputs are used to generate revenue, isolating the monetary flows associated with a particular transaction may be difficult. For example, a hospital may generate revenues of $45 by rendering a service that uses supplies from the inventory. Clearly, the change in the revenue account would be a $45 increase. However, the change in the expense account and the change in the asset account (inventory) seems to be undetermined. In these cases, the cost principle must be used to evaluate the effect of the transaction.

The cost principle states that an asset should be valued at an amount equal to the costs incurred to acquire that asset. Hence, when an asset is used, the asset accounts should decrease by the amount at which the asset used was recorded. In the example above, assume that the supplies originally were purchased for $30. Since this is the value at which the supplies were recorded, assets should decrease by $30 when the supplies are used and, hence, the expense associated with the generation of the $45 of revenue should be $30. The following example further illustrates this concept, as well as the other fundamentals of transactions analysis.

Example

Assume that the following economic events are observed by the Robert Hughes HMO during the first week of January, 19X0:

- Jan. 1, The owners contribute $100,000 in cash to start the HMO.
- Jan. 2, Equipment is purchased; a $20,000 check (#101) is given to Jackson Equipment Co., the seller, and $40,000 is due in ten days.
- Jan. 3, Supplies are purchased for $10,000 cash.
- Jan. 4, Services are rendered to patients; $1,000 is collected in cash; $2,000 is to be billed to various patients. Supplies purchased for $600 are used in rendering these services.
- Jan. 5, Check #102 for $20,000 is sent to Jackson Equipment Co.
- Jan. 6, Checks amounting to $1,600 are received from patients.
- Jan. 7, Wages of $1,200 are paid to employees (Checks #1001–1006).

Each of these economic events is judged to affect the Robert Hughes HMO. The monetary impact of these transactions on specific accounts can be summarized as follows.

Jan. 1,	Dr: Assets (Cash)	$100,000
	Cr: Owners' Equity	100,000
Jan. 2,	Dr: Assets (Equipment)	60,000
	Cr: Assets (Cash)	20,000
	Cr: Liabilities (Accounts Payable)	40,000
Jan. 3,	Dr: Assets (Supplies)	10,000
	Cr: Assets (Cash)	10,000
Jan. 4,	Dr: Assets (Cash)	1,000
	Dr: Assets (Patient Accounts Receivable)	2,000
	Cr: Revenues	3,000
	Dr: Expenses	600
	Cr: Assets (Supplies)	600
Jan. 5,	Dr: Liabilities (Accounts Payable)	20,000
	Cr: Assets (Cash)	20,000
Jan. 6,	Dr: Assets (Cash)	1,600
	Cr: Assets (Patient Accounts Receivable)	1,600
Jan. 7,	Dr: Expenses	1,200
	Cr: Assets (Cash)	1,200

Note that in each case the debits equal the credits. In addition, the assets equal the sum of the liabilities, owners' equity, and revenues less the expenses, as shown below.

	Assets	=	Liabilities	+	Owners' Equity	+	Revenue	−	Expenses
Jan. 1,	+ $100,000	=	$ 0	+	$100,000	+	$ 0	−	$ 0
Jan. 2,	+ 60,000 − 20,000	=	+ 40,000	+	0	+	0	−	0
Jan. 3,	+ 10,000 − 10,000	=	0	+	0	+	0	−	0
Jan. 4,	+ 1,000 + 2,000	=	0	+	0	+	3,000	−	0
	− 600	=	0	+	0	+	0	−	600
Jan. 5,	− 20,000	=	− 20,000	+	0	+	0	−	0
Jan. 6,	+ 1,600 − 1,600	=	0	+	0	+	0	−	0
Jan. 7,	− 1,200	=	0	+	0	+	0	−	1,200
Total,	$121,200	=	$20,000	+	$100,000	+	$3,000	−	$1,800

Hence, at the end of one week, the Robert Hughes HMO has $121,200 in assets, $20,000 in liabilities, $100,000 in owners' equity, $3,000 in revenues, and $1,800 in expenses.

The method by which these transactions are recorded accurately reflects the economic impact of each transaction on the assets, liabilities, owners' equity, revenues, and expenses of the HMO. Nevertheless, information losses occur. For example, the purchase of supplies for cash on January 3, 19X0, appears to have no economic impact on the HMO, since assets increase and decrease by $10,000. However, the actual economic composition of the HMO has changed: supplies valued at $10,000 have been acquired and cash of $10,000 has been relinquished. To avoid this kind of information loss, a more refined method of recording transactions has been developed.

Recording and Summarizing Accounting Information

The actual composition of a business's accounting records depends on the type and size of the business and on the number and complexity of the transactions affecting it. However, most businesses have a general journal and a general ledger which may be complemented or supplemented by any number of special journals or subsidiary ledgers.

The General Journal

The general journal is known as the book of original entry because it is the book in which the raw data of transactions analysis are first recorded. The date of the transaction, the affected accounts, and the magnitude and direction of the change in those accounts must be recorded in the general journal. To provide more complete information regarding the changing economic composition of the business, the account delineations in the general journal are more specific than the general titles of assets, liabilities, owners' equity, revenues, or expenses. For example, if the asset cash increases by $100,000, a specific account called Cash, instead of the general account called Assets, is debited for $100,000. In addition, the general journal contains separate columns for recording debit entries and credit entries. These separate columns enable immediate distinction between debited amounts and credited amounts and also simplify the procedure of checking to see that the debits equal the credits. Since the debit column always precedes the credit column (i.e., the debit column is to the left of the credit column), a convention has been adopted whereby the debited accounts are listed first and the credited accounts are listed second and indented to the right. This standardized format produces uniformity in the general journal, thereby simplifying the presentation of transactions.

Although the information already discussed is sufficient to record changes in the economic composition of the business, the general journal also contains information that can aid in auditing the business. For example, a description of the transaction follows each journal entry. This description should associate the transaction with source documents, such as checks and invoices. In addition, a column called "folio" is included to aid in the audit process. The folio number indicates where each part of each transaction is recorded in the general ledger. This column is completed as the amounts recorded in the general journal are posted to the general ledger (see the discussion of the general ledger below). An example of the general journal is shown in Figure A-2. The entries shown reflect the transactions of the Robert Hughes HMO in the example above.

Special Journals

Sometimes the number of transactions in a specific account becomes so large that recording the transactions associated with that account in the general journal becomes inefficient. In this case, a special journal is created to record the transactions that affect the specific account. For example, most of the transactions of the Robert Hughes HMO affect the cash account. Two special journals, one for cash receipts and one for cash disbursements, could be created to cope with these kinds of transactions.[3] The cash receipts journal for the Robert Hughes HMO is shown in Figure A-3. Accounts, like Accounts Receivable and Service Revenue, that routinely would be associated with cash transactions, are listed in separate columns. Periodically, the columns in this journal are totalled and posted in the general ledger. At the time of posting, the folio column is completed for the miscellaneous accounts, and the general ledger reference for the specific account columns is listed under the column total.

The General Ledger

The general ledger summarizes the information recorded in the journals so that the balance in each account is always known. Hence, each account is located in a different part of the general ledger. The location of each account is noted by an account number. These account numbers correspond to the numbers that were included in the folio columns of the journals.

In addition to the usual debit and credit information, the general ledger contains a column that indicates the current balance in the account. An example of the cash account page in the Robert Hughes HMO general ledger is shown in Figure A-4. The folio column in this case is a cross-reference to the page in the general journal on which the information was first recorded.

Subsidiary Ledgers

Subsidiary ledgers are needed when the transactions within one account become complex. For example, if services are rendered on credit to a number of patients, an accounts receivable subsidiary ledger is needed to record the amount of money owed by each patient. This ledger includes the date and

Figure A-2 Sample Page in the Robert Hughes HMO General Journal

Date	Account	Folio	Debit	Credit
Jan. 1	Cash	101	$100,000.00	
	Contributed Capital	301		$100,000.00
	To record the contribution of $100,000 by the owners.			
2	Equipment	104	60,000.00	
	Cash	101		20,000.00
	Accounts Payable	201		40,000.00
	To record the purchase of equipment from Jackson Equipment Co. for $60,000; $20,000 paid with check #101, $40,000 is due in 10 days.			
3	Supplies Inventory	103	10,000.00	
	Cash	101		10,000.00
	To record the purchase of supplies for $10,000 cash.			
4	Cash	101	1,000.00	
	Patient Accounts Receivable	102	2,000.00	
	Service Revenue	401		3,000.00
	To record services rendered to patients; $1,000 paid in cash, $2,000 due from patients.			
4	Supplies Expense	501	600.00	
	Supplies Inventory	103		600.00
	To record the use of $600 of supplies in rendering services to patients.			
5	Accounts Payable	201	20,000.00	
	Cash	101		20,000.00
	To record a $20,000 payment by check #102 to Jackson Equipment Co.			
6	Cash	101	1,600.00	
	Patient Accounts Receivable	102		1,600.00
	To record the collection of $1,600 due from patients.			
7	Wage Expense	502	1,200.00	
	Cash	101		1,200.00
	To record the payment of wages to employees with checks #1001-1006.			

Figure A-3 Sample Page in Cash Receipts Journal for the Robert Hughes HMO

		Debits	Credits				
Date	Explanation	Cash	Account	Folio	Accounts Receivable	Misc. Accounts	Service Revenue
Jan. 1	Owners' Contribution	$100,000.00	Contributed Capital			$100,000.00	
4	Services Rendered	1,000.00					$1,000.00
6	Collections from Patients	1,600.00			$1,600.00		

Figure A-4 Sample Page from the Robert Hughes HMO General Ledger

Date 19X0	Cash #101	Folio	Debits	Credits	Balance
Jan. 1		1	$100,000.00		$100,000.00
2		1		$20,000.00	80,000.00
3		1		10,000.00	70,000.00
4		1	1,000.00		71,000.00
5		1		20,000.00	51,000.00
6		1	1,600.00		52,600.00
7		1		1,200.00	51,400.00

amount of credit services, the date and amount of payments, and the current balance in each patient's account. The total of the balances in the individual patient accounts should equal the balance in the Accounts Receivable general ledger account, which is also called the Accounts Receivable control account.

Two other subsidiary ledgers usually are needed for the Accounts Payable and Payroll accounts. The information in the Accounts Payable subsidiary ledger is similar to the information in the Accounts Receivable subsidiary ledger. The Payroll ledger, on the other hand, indicates the date of the payroll and then lists each employee's gross pay and the related deductions. The total in the gross pay column should equal the wage expense for the payroll period. The totals in the other columns should indicate the amounts due in income taxes to various jurisdictions and the amounts deducted for various optional employee benefit plans. Finally, the amount in the net pay column should be equal to the total cash disbursed for the payroll. These amounts periodically are posted to the appropriate control accounts in the general ledger.

Preparing Financial Statements

The preparation of financial statements is a multistep process that not only produces financial statements, but also prepares the accounting records for the informational inputs of the ensuing period. The first step in preparing financial statements involves ruling the accounts and preparing a trial balance. In the second step, adjusting entries are made and an adjusted trial balance is prepared. After these two steps, the income statement can be prepared. However, before the balance sheet and the statement of changes in financial position can be prepared, the temporary accounts must be closed.

Ruling the Accounts and Preparing the Trial Balance

Ruling the accounts and preparing the trial balance is a fairly simple process. Ruling the accounts means calculating the balance in each account. These balances are listed in debit or credit columns next to the appropriate account names in the trial balance. The purpose of the trial balance is to check that all of the debits in the accounts equal all of the credits. The trial balance for the Robert Hughes HMO at the end of the first week of operations is shown in Figure A-5.

Adjusting Entries and the Adjusted Trial Balance

Adjusting entries are needed (1) to recognize assets or liabilities not recorded on the books of original entry, and (2) to apportion assets to expenses and liabilities to revenues, so that at the end of the accounting period all assets, liabilities, owners' equity, revenues, and expenses are stated properly. For example, when a business using the accrual basis of accounting purchases an asset, like equipment, that will be used for more than one operating period, the value at which the asset is recorded is equal to the costs

Figure A-5 Sample Trial Balance for the Robert Hughes HMO

Robert Hughes HMO
Trial Balance, January 7, 19X0

	Account Balances	
Ledger Accounts	Debits	Credits
Cash	$ 51,400.00	
Accounts Receivable	400.00	
Supplies Inventory	9,400.00	
Equipment	60,000.00	
Accumulated Depreciation—Equipment		—
Accounts Payable		$ 20,000.00
Contributed Capital		100,000.00
Service Revenue		3,000.00
Supplies Expense	600.00	
Wage Expense	1,200.00	
Depreciation Expense	—	
Totals	$123,000.00	$123,000.00

incurred to acquire it. However, since the asset will be used for more than one accounting period, the asset costs must be apportioned to the various accounting periods which receive the benefit of the asset. The systematic apportionment of asset costs is called depreciation.

Although a number of methods of depreciation are generally acceptable, health care institutions can use only a method called the straight line method of depreciation to compute reimbursable costs. Under this method, an equal portion of the asset's cost is apportioned to each accounting period. To calculate this amount, the cost of the equipment, less the amount expected to be recouped when the equipment is disposed (salvage value), is divided by the number of accounting periods in which the equipment is expected to be used. For example, assume that equipment purchased by the Robert Hughes HMO for $60,000 is expected to have no salvage value and is expected to be used for 120 weeks.[4] In this case, the weekly depreciation expense would be calculated as follows:

$$\text{Depreciation Expense} = \frac{\text{Cost} - \text{Salvage Value}}{\text{Life}}$$

$$= \frac{\$60{,}000 - \$0}{120}$$

$$= \$500 \text{ per week}$$

The depreciation expense of $500 represents that portion of the asset's cost which will be matched with the revenue generated during the week. Hence, the value of the Equipment account should decline by $500. However, the cost principle stipulates that an asset must be recorded at an amount equal to the costs incurred to acquire that asset. Therefore, a separate account, called a contra account or a valuation account, must be created to record the estimated decline in the Equipment account. In this case, the contra account is called Accumulation Depreciation—Equipment. In the financial statements, the Accumulated Depreciation—Equipment account[5] always will follow the Equipment account, and the difference between the amounts in these two accounts will be shown.

The adjusting entry to record the usage of the equipment for one week would be:

1/7/X0	Depreciation Expense	$500	
	Accumulated Depreciation-Equipment		$500

To record the depreciation expense for the week.

Depreciation is only one example of an adjusting entry. Other adjusting entries are needed (1) to record revenues or expenses that have accrued and should be recorded but have not yet been recorded in the current period, (2) to adjust revenues and expenses for amounts that have been recorded but should not have been recorded in the revenue and expense accounts this period, or (3) ot apportion the amounts in accounts that record prepaid expenses or revenues collected in advance. All of the necessary adjusting entries should be incorporated in the general journal and posted to the general ledger. Then, a new trial balance, called the Adjusted Trial Balance, which rejects the results of the adjusting process, should be prepared. The Adjusted Trial Balance for the Robert Hughes HMO appears in Figure A-6.

Preparing the Income Statement and Closing the Temporary Accounts

The income statement can be prepared directly from the adjusted trial balance. The income statement reflects the results of operations for the current operating period. Hence, to prepare the income statement, the revenue and expense accounts in the adjusted trial balance must be isolated from the other accounts. The difference between the revenues and expenses is the net

Figure A-6 Adjusted Trial Balance for the Robert Hughes HMO

Robert Hughes HMO
Adjusted Trial Balance
January 7, 19X0

	Account Balances	
Ledger Accounts	Debits	Credits
Cash	$ 51,400.00	
Accounts Receivable	400.00	
Supplies Inventory	9,400.00	
Equipment	60,000.00	
Accumulated Depreciation—Equipment		$ 500.00
Accounts Payable		20,000.00
Contributed Capital		100,000.00
Service Revenue		3,000.00
Supplies Expense	600.00	
Wage Expense	1,200.00	
Depreciation Expense	500.00	
Totals	$123,500.00	$123,500.00

income for the period. The income statement for the Robert Hughes HMO is shown in Figure A-7.

Since the income of a business increases the wealth of the owners, the net income of each period should be incorporated in an owners' equity account. The owners' equity account used to record net income usually is called Retained Earnings. This account reflects the amount of income that has been reinvested in the business (i.e., the amount not distributed to the owners) over the life of the business.

To record net income in the Retained Earnings account, the revenue and expense accounts, which are called temporary accounts because they only accumulate the effects of transactions for a specified amount of time, must be closed (i.e., reduced to zero). In the case of the Robert Hughes HMO, the temporary accounts have recorded transactions for one week. The entries required to close the revenue and expense accounts for the Robert Hughes HMO are given below:

1/7/X0	Service Revenue	$3,000	
	Supplies Expense		$ 600
	Wage Expense		1,200
	Depreciation Expense		500
	Income Summary		700

To close the revenue and expense accounts.

Once these closing entries have been made, the Income Summary account must be closed to the Retained Earnings account[6] as follows:

Figure A-7 Income Statement for the Robert Hughes HMO

Robert Hughes HMO
Income Statement
for the Week Ending January 7, 19X0

Service Revenue		$3,000
Operating Expenses:		
Supplies Expense	$ 600	
Wage Expense	1,200	
Depreciation Expense	500	
Total Operating Expenses		2,300
Net income		$ 700

1/7/X0	Income Summary	$700	
	Retained Earnings		$700

To close the Income Summary account and to state retained earnings properly.

These closing entries must be incorporated in the general journal and then posted in the general ledger. After posting the closing entries, the balances in all of the temporary accounts will be zero. Each permanent account, or each account that accumulates the effects of transactions over an indefinite amount of time, however, should reflect the value of the asset, liability, or owners' equity to which it applies.

Preparing the Balance Sheet and the Statement of Changes in Financial Position

Once the revenue and expense accounts have been closed, the balance sheet can be prepared. The balance sheet reports the values of all assets, liabilities, and owners' equity of the business at a given time. Hence, the balance sheet is merely an aggregation of the balances recorded in the general ledger. The balance sheet for the Robert Hughes HMO is shown in Figure A-8.

The statement of changes in financial position also can be prepared once the temporary accounts have been closed. This statement shows the financing and investing activities of the business for the current period, and thus gives another indication of how well the business is being managed. A complete description of this statement and the methodology by which it is prepared are given in Chapter 6.

Opening the Accounting Records in the Ensuing Period and Making Reversing Entries

Opening the accounts in the ensuing period is a fairly simple process. A notation is made in the general journal to indicate that a new accounting period has begun. After this notation, transactions are recorded in accordance with the prescribed format. In the general ledger, a notation may be made to indicate the beginning of a new accounting period, or the balance in the account may be transferred to a new page. In this case, the new page is headed with the account title and the account number. The account balance is recorded in the balance column and a check (✓) is placed in the folio column to indicate that the balance has been brought forward from the previous page.

Figure A-8 Balance Sheet for the Robert Hughes HMO

Robert Hughes HMO
Balance Sheet
January 7, 19X0

Assets		
Current Assets		
Cash	$ 51,400	
Accounts Receivable	400	
Supplies Inventory	9,400	
Total Current Assets		$ 61,200
Fixed Assets		
Equipment	60,000	
Accumulated Depreciation—Equipment	(500)	
Total Fixed Assets		59,500
Total Assets		$120,700
Liabilities		
Current Liabilities		
Accounts Payable	$ 20,000	
Total Current Liabilities		$ 20,000
Total Liabilities		$ 20,000
Owners' Equity		
Contributed Capital	$100,000	
Retained Earnings	700	
Total Owners' Equity		$100,700
Total Liabilities and Owners' Equity		$120,700

In addition to preparing the books of record for transactions of the ensuing period, reversing entries can be made at the beginning of a new accounting period to simplify recordkeeping. A reversing entry is a general journal entry made on the first day of the ensuing period that reverses an adjusting entry made to record an accrual. For example, assume that Memorial Hospital's salaried employees are paid a total of $34,580 each week. At the end of each week, the following journal entry would be made to record the payment of salaries:

Salaries Expense	$34,580	
Cash		34,580

To record the payment of salaries to employees.

Now, assume that the accounting period ends two days before salaries are to be paid. In this case, the following adjusting journal entry would have to be made to record the salaries expense associated with the last five days of the accounting period:

Salaries Expense	$24,700	
Accrued Salaries Payable		$24,700

To record salaries accrued but not paid at the end of the accounting period.

In the absence of a reversing entry, the journal entry on the day of the next payroll would be:

Salaries Expense	$ 9,880	
Accrued Salaries Payable	$24,700	
Cash		$34,580

To record the payment of salaries to employees.

However, if the following reversing entry were made on the first day of the new accounting period:

Accrued Salaries Payable	$24,700	
Salaries Expense		$24,700

To reverse the adjusting entry that recorded salaries earned but not yet paid at the end of the accounting period,

then the regular payroll journal entry could be made when the salaries were paid:

Salaries Expense	$34,580	
Cash		$34,580

To record the payment of salaries to employees.

The net effect of either alternative after the first payroll in the ensuing period would be:

	Dr	Cr
Salaries Expense	$9,880	
Accrued Salaries Payable		$ 0
Cash		34,580

Hence, reversing entries enable routine processing of certain kinds of accounting information at all times.

THE USEFULNESS OF ACCOUNTING INFORMATION

Accounting information is used (1) to evaluate the management of the business and (2) to plan the future course of the business. The three financial statements (balance sheet, income statement, and statement of changes in financial position) yield insights into various aspects of the business that are important in evaluation and planning. These statements reflect the financial position of the business at a particular time or for a particular period. In addition, comparative financial statements over a number of accounting periods can show the direction in which the business is moving over time.

NOTES

1. The method of recording transactions is discussed in detail in a subsequent section.
2. See Chapter 4 for an extensive discussion of inventory holding costs and inventory management.
3. A service revenue journal and a purchases journal also can be useful if the volume of services rendered or the volume of purchases made is large.
4. The number of periods in this case is stated in weeks because the operating period under consideration for illustrative purposes is one week. However, the life of an asset usually is stated in years.
5. A separate Accumulated Depreciation account is created for buildings.
6. The Income Summary account is used so that the net income derived in the closing process can be checked against the net income computed in the income statement before net income is closed to Retained Earnings.

Appendix B

Regression Analysis

To understand the complex relationships among organizational phenomena, management often gathers data on selected variables. In analyzing this data, it often is useful to ascertain if a functional relationship exists between the dependent and independent variables. This Appendix examines a technique—regression analysis—which translates variable observations into a function of those variables. However, before considering the derivation of the regression equation, the scatter diagram will be examined.

SCATTER DIAGRAM

The first step in performing a regression analysis is to obtain information about the nature (linear or nonlinear) of the equation which will be derived mathematically to represent the data. Management must know if the plotted relationship between (or among) variables is linear or nonlinear (see Chapter 7, Figure 7-2).

For example, to assist in scheduling the clinic staff and plan overtime, management may wish to estimate the number of clinic hours which must be worked at various levels of patient utilization. To aid in making these estimates, assume that management abstracts the following information from the payroll records and clinic patient service journals.

Month		Independent Variable: Patient Utilization	Dependent Variable: Total Clinic Staff Hours Worked
January:	X_1	120	320
February:	X_2	200	470
March:	X_3	280	520
April:	X_4	360	620
May:	X_5	380	540
June:	X_6	420	550
July:	X_7	300	440
August:	X_8	200	400
September:	X_9	600	700
October:	X_{10}	500	650
November:	X_{11}	350	480
December:	X_{12}	250	430
Monthly Average		330	510

The linearity or nonlinearity of the relationship between these two variables may be ascertained by representing these two variables as 12 points on a two-dimensional graph where utilization (the independent variable) is plotted along the horizontal axis and clinic staff hours worked (the dependent variable) is plotted along the vertical axis. In this case, these points, which are represented with an X_i in Figure B-1, seem to result from a process in which labor time and utilization are linearly related. Hence, a free-hand straight line may be drawn through the approximate middle of the 12 points.

The free-hand line in Figure B-1 intersects the clinic hours worked axis at approximately 290 hours. This intersection may be interpreted as the fixed component of clinic staffing. Therefore, at least 290 clinic hours must be worked to maintain the clinic's service potential. The line also appears to rise by approximately 65 clinic labor hours for an increase in clinic utilization of 100 (see the shaded area on the graph). Given this information, the following equation may be formulated:

$$\text{Clinic Hours Worked} = 290 + (65/100)\,X$$

where: X represents patient utilization.

Hence, if management wishes to estimate the number of clinic staff hours required to service 400 clinic patients, the free-hand line indicates that approximately 550 clinic staff hours would be required:

$$550 = 290 + .65 \times 400.$$

Figure B-1 Scatter Diagram: Monthly Clinic Staff Hours Worked and Monthly Patient Utilization

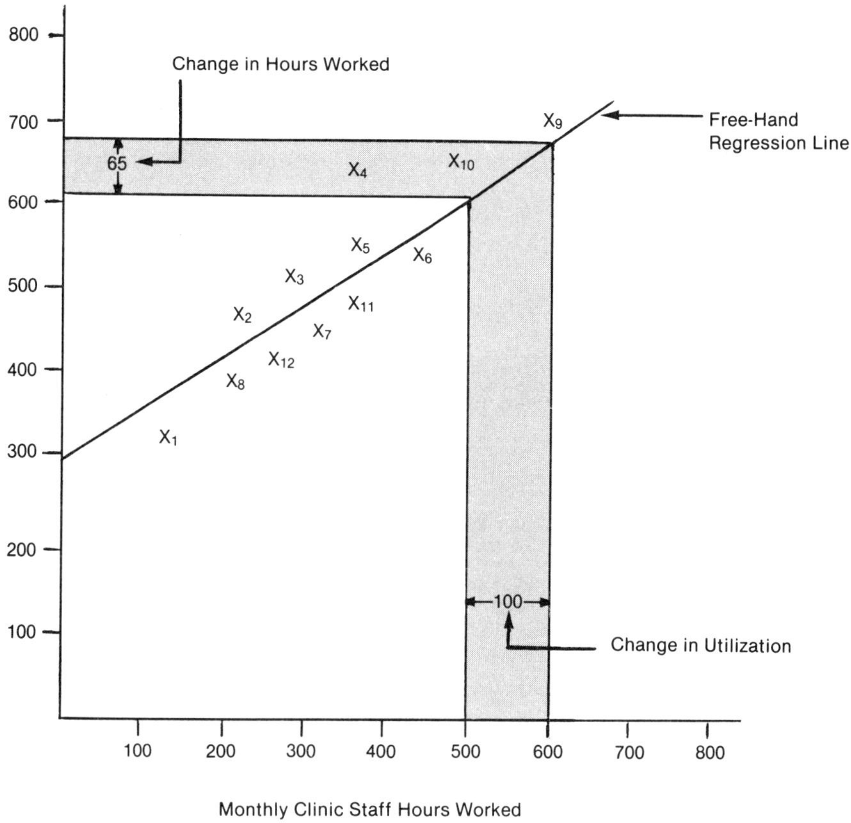

In this case, a linear regression equation would generate reasonable results because the relationship underlying the two variables, clinic staff hours and patient utilization, is approximately linear. However, assume that a scatter diagram was not constructed and a straight line was placed mathematically among the data points in Figure B-2. In this case, if management wishes to ascertain the approximate number of hours which must be worked when patient utilization is U*, the mathematically placed straight line will indicate that approximately HW_E hours are required. However, the actual number of hours which are required to service U* patients is HW_A. Hence, failure to recognize the nonlinearity between patient utilization and hours worked may cause management to plan to schedule fewer individuals than will be required to service the patient load. Therefore, when possible, the various data points should be plotted so that the functional relationship which exists (see Question B-2) between the dependent and independent variables is evident.[1]

Although the scatter diagram can be used to estimate the regression equation, its use is limited because (1) inaccurate free-hand representations give rise to poor estimates, and (2) diagramming problems with even as few as three variables is difficult. Therefore, rather than rely on a free-hand representation of the regression equation, management may use a mathematical technique known as the "least squares method" to estimate the true regression line (see Problem B-2).

LEAST SQUARES TECHNIQUE: LINEAR REGRESSION

Under the least squares technique, the regression line, noted as $\hat{Y}_i = a + bX_i$, is fitted among the plotted points in such a way that *the sum of the squared differences between the regression estimate* ($\hat{Y}_i$) *and the*

Figure B-2 Scatter Diagram: Nonlinear Relationship between Monthly Clinic Staff Hours Worked and Monthly Patient Utilization

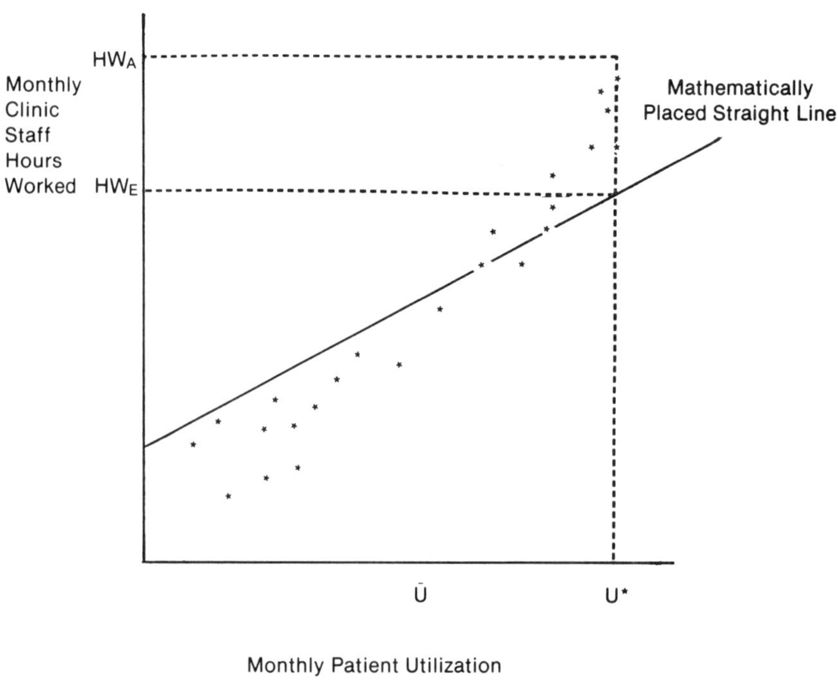

actual values (Y_i) *are minimized*. This statement may be called the equation fitting rule. The equation derived by applying this rule to the data is called the estimating equation because it is an equation used to determine the values of the dependent variable, Y_i, given values of the independent variable, X_i.

Derivation of the Estimates for a and b for the Regression Line $\hat{Y}_i = a + bX_i$

The regression equation $\hat{Y}_i = a + bX_i$ has two unknown parameters: the a and b coefficients which must be estimated from the data. These unknown parameters may be estimated from equations (called "normal equations") derived from the following mathematical statement of the equation fitting rule:

(B-1) $$\min \sum_i^n (Y_i - \hat{Y}_i)^2$$

where: Y_i represents the ith observation;
$\hat{Y}_i$ represents the regression estimate of the ith observation; and
i is an index for the total number of observations.

Equation (B-1) may be expanded as follows.

$$\min \sum_i^n (Y_i - \hat{Y}_i)^2 = \min \sum_i^n [Y_i^2 - 2Y_i\hat{Y}_i + \hat{Y}_i^2]$$

Since $\hat{Y}_i = a + bX_i$, by substitution:

(B-2) $$\min \sum_i^n (Y_i - \hat{Y}_i)^2 = \min \sum_i^n [Y_i^2 - 2Y_i(a + bX_i) + (a + bX_i)^2].$$

Then, expanding $(a + bX_i)^2$ in equation (B-2) yields:

(B-3) $$\min \sum_i^n (Y_i - \hat{Y}_i)^2 = \min \sum_i^n [Y_i^2 - 2Y_i(a + bX_i) + a^2 + 2abX_i + b^2X_i^2].$$

By performing the Σ operation on the right-hand side of equation (B-3), the following function is generated.

(B-4)
$$f(a,b) = \Sigma Y_i^2 - 2a\Sigma Y_i - 2b\Sigma X_i Y_i + \Sigma a^2 + 2ab\Sigma X_i + b^2\Sigma X_i^2$$

Equation (B-4) may be partially differentiated with respect to a and b to determine the values of the two that minimize equation (B-4).[2] The two equations which result from this operation are as follows.

(B-5)
$$\frac{\partial f(a, b)}{\partial a} = -2\Sigma Y_i + 2na + 2b\Sigma X_i = 0$$

(B-6)
$$\frac{\partial f(a, b)}{\partial b} = -2\Sigma X_i Y_i + 2a\Sigma X_i + 2b\Sigma X_i^2 = 0$$

Equations (B-5) and (B-6) are the normal equations, which usually take the following forms.

$$\Sigma Y_i X_i = \Sigma X_i a + \Sigma X_i^2 b$$
$$\Sigma Y_i = na + \Sigma X_i b$$

If the normal equations are stated as two simultaneous linear equations in the parameters a and b, by Cramer's rule these equations may be solved for b (the estimate of the slope of the regression equation) as follows:

(B-7)
$$b = \frac{\begin{vmatrix} \Sigma X_i & \Sigma X_i Y_i \\ n & \Sigma Y_i \end{vmatrix}}{\begin{vmatrix} \Sigma X_i & \Sigma X_i^2 \\ n & \Sigma X_i \end{vmatrix}}$$

where: | | indicates the determinant operation.

After computing the determinant, the slope of $\hat{Y}_i$ is:

(B-8)
$$b = \frac{\Sigma X_i \Sigma Y_i - n\Sigma Y_i X_i}{(\Sigma X_i)^2 - n\Sigma X_i^2}$$

This value may be substituted into either one of the normal equations, and after a number of simple operations, a (the estimate of the intercept of the regression equation) is determined to be:

(B-9) $$a = \frac{\Sigma Y_i}{n} - b\,\frac{\Sigma X_i}{n}$$

In summary, these values of *a* and *b* position the regression line so that the sum of the squared deviations ($\Sigma(Y_i - \hat{Y}_i)^2$) are minimized. Therefore, regression analysis provides an objective and desirable method of estimating the relationship between variables.

For example, consider the previous illustration in which patient utilization (*X*) and clinic staff hours (*Y*) are regressed to determine the clinic staff hours required for various patient volumes. The appropriate information for computing the regression equation is presented in Table B-1.

Since by equation (B-8)

$$b = \frac{\Sigma X_i \Sigma Y_i - n\Sigma Y_i X_i}{(\Sigma X_i)^2 - n\,\Sigma X_i^2},$$

the appropriate values from Table B-1 may be substituted to compute *b* (the estimate of the slope of the regression line):

$$b = \frac{(396)\,(612) - 12\,(21{,}699)}{(396)^2 - 12\,(15{,}082)}$$

$$= \frac{-18{,}036}{-24{,}168}$$

$$= .7463.$$

Similarly, since by equation (B-9)

$$a = \frac{\Sigma Y_i}{n} - b\,\frac{\Sigma X_i}{n},$$

the appropriate values from Table B-1 may be substituted to compute:

$$a = 51 - .7463\,(33)$$
$$a = 26.37.$$

Hence, the mathematically derived regression equation, which is the best estimate of the true regression equation, with *a* adjusted for the conversion from units to tens (see Question B-3), is:

(B-10) $$\hat{Y} = 263.7 + .7463(X).$$

Table B-1 Regression Computation (in Tens of Units)

Month	X_i	Y_i	X_iY_i	X_i^2	Y_i^2
January	12	32	384	144	1,024
February	20	47	940	400	2,209
March	28	52	1,456	784	2,704
April	36	62	2,232	1,296	3,844
May	38	54	2,052	1,444	2,916
June	42	55	2,310	1,764	3,025
July	30	44	1,320	900	1,936
August	20	40	800	400	1,600
September	60	70	4,200	3,600	4,900
October	50	65	3,250	2,500	4,225
November	35	48	1,680	1,225	2,304
December	25	43	1,075	625	1,849
	396	612	21,699	15,082	32,536

This regression equation indicates that the free-hand estimate was reasonably accurate because *a* was initially estimated to be 290 and the regression estimate indicates its value as 263.7; and *b* was initially estimated to be .65 and the regression indicates it to be .7463.

Furthermore, if management estimates the number of clinic hours needed to service 400 patients using the estimating equation (B-10), the estimate is:

$$562.22 = 263.7 + .7463\,(400).$$

This value also compares favorably with the free-hand estimate of 550 hours.

CONFIDENCE

In addition to estimating the hours needed to service a specific number of patients, management may wish to ascertain the likelihood that the estimate actually will occur. For example, consider the two scatter diagrams in Figure B-3. In this case, the regression equations are identical; however, a good deal of unexplained variation is associated with the regression equation in Figure B-3a because of the almost random occurrence of points from which the estimating equation is derived. Therefore, management should place little confidence in service estimates made from this estimating equation. On the other hand, the points used to generate the regression estimates $a = 263.7$ and $b = .7463$ in Figure B-3b are not random, but seem to show a real relationship between hours worked and patient volume. Hence, management would be justified in placing a good deal of confidence in regression estimates derived from Figure B-3b.

The concept of confidence in regression analysis describes the distribution of points about the estimating equation—the "tighter" the distribution of points, the more confidence management should have in the regression estimates. Two mathematical methods of ascertaining the "goodness of fit" of the regression line and the data points used to generate that line are used in regression analysis. Under one method, the coefficient of determination (r^2) is computed. Under the other method, the standard error of the regression estimate (S_e) is computed.

The Coefficient of Determination (r^2)

The coefficient of determination, r^2, represents the proportion of the total variation in the actual values (Y), which may be explained by the linear relationship existing between X and Y. Mathematically:

$$\text{(B-11)} \qquad r^2 = \left[\frac{\Sigma X_i Y_i - n\bar{X}\bar{Y}}{((\Sigma X_i^2 - n\bar{X}^2)(\Sigma Y_i^2 - n\,\bar{Y}^2))^{1/2}}\right]^2$$

where: $\bar{X}$ represents the mean of the independent variable;
$\bar{Y}$ represents the mean of the dependent variable; and
n represents the number of observations.

The range of values which r^2 may assume is 0 to 1. When the actual points lie on the regression line, $r^2 = 1$, indicating a perfect fit. When the actual points are randomly dispersed around the regression line, $r^2 = 0$.

Figure B-3 Comparison of Two Different Scatter Diagrams Which Yield the Same Regression Equation

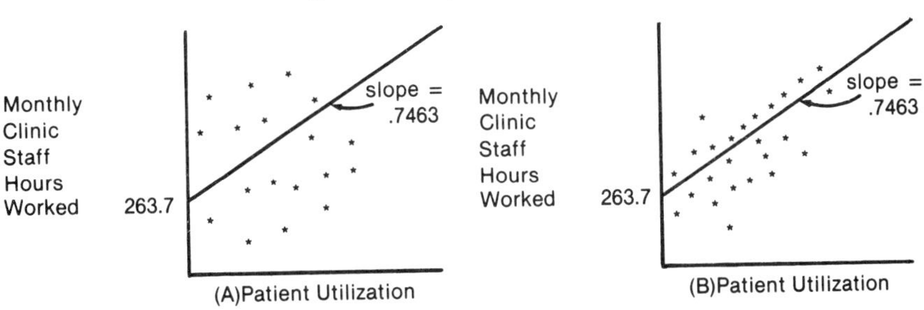

For example, consider the points plotted in Figure B-1 and delineated in Table B-1. In this case, r^2 is as follows.

$$r^2 = \left[\frac{(21{,}699 - 12\,(33)\,(51))}{((15{,}082 - 12\,(33)^2)\,(32{,}536 - 12\,(51)^2))^{1/2}}\right]^2$$

$$= (+.9204)^2 = .8472$$

This indicates that approximately 85 percent of the variation in clinic staffing hours may be explained by the linear relationship existing between clinic staffing hours and patient volume. Therefore, management may be justified in placing a high degree of confidence in the regression estimates derived with the estimating equation $\hat{Y}_i = 263.7 - .7463(X_i)$.

Correlation Coefficient (r)

Although the coefficient of determination is a valuable statistic, a related statistic called the correlation coefficient also yields valuable information. Correlation is a measure of the direction of association between variables. The coefficient of determination (r^2) is the square of the correlation coefficient (r) and the correlation coefficient has the following range.[3]

$$-1 \leq r \leq 1.$$

If the observations lie on the regression line, but are inversely related (i.e., when one variable increases the other decreases), the correlation coefficient will equal -1. If the variables are positively related (i.e., the variables increase and decrease together) and all the observations lie on the regression line, the correlation coefficient will equal $+1$. If the variables are not associated, the correlation coefficient will equal zero (see Problem B-4).

The correlation coefficient computed for the 12 pairs of points in the clinic example is relatively high, +.9204. However a correlation coefficient of .83, − .31, or .2 may or may not be sufficiently different from zero (i.e., no linear association) to warrant serious consideration of the mathematical relationships derived from the plotted points. To test the hypotheses that the correlation coefficient is different from zero, the following statistical test[4] is suggested:

(B-12) $$t_{n-2} = r/((1 - r^2)/(n - 2))^{1/2}$$

where: r represents the correlation coefficient;
n represents the number of observation pairs; and
$n-2$ represents the degrees of freedom in the t test.

The t test of the correlation coefficient derived from the data used to estimate the regression equation $\hat{Y}_i = 263.7 + .7463X_i$ is:

$$t_{10} = .9204/((1 - .8472)/10)^{1/2} = 7.5.$$

The tabled t statistic (two-tail test since r $\neq$ 0 is to be tested) for ten degrees of freedom ($n - 2$) for a confidence level of .01 is 3.169. Since the computed t value is 7.5, management is justified in assuming r is significantly different from zero and that the function $\hat{Y}_i = 263.7 + .7463(X_i)$ is an adequate representation of the linear relationship between hours worked and patient utilization.

The Standard Error of the Estimate

Since the regression line is an estimate derived from the plotted points, the actual points usually are dispersed about the regression line. The statistical measure of this dispersion is called the standard error of the estimate, S_e. The standard error of the regression estimate may be computed as:

(B-13)
$$S_e = \left(\frac{(Y_i - \hat{Y}_i)^2}{n}\right)^{1/2}$$

where: $Y_i - \hat{Y}_i$ indicates the difference between the actual values (Y_i) and the estimated values ($\hat{Y}_i$);
$\hat{Y}_i = a + bX_i$; and
n is the number of observations.

The only circumstance in which S_e equals zero is when all of the actual points lie on the regression line (see Question 7-7); in this case, $Y_i - \hat{Y}_i = 0$. The larger S_e, the more dispersed the actual points are relative to the regression line.

For the regression equation $\hat{Y}_i = 263.7 + .7463(X_i)$, the 12 squared differences are as shown in Table B-2.

As illustrated by Table B-2, the standard error of the estimate (S_e) is:

$$S_e = \left(\frac{20{,}228.79}{12}\right)^{1/2} = 41.06.$$

Table B-2 Regression Computations: 12 Squared Differences

Month		Actual (Y_i)	Regression Estimate ($\hat{Y}_i$)	$(Y_i - \hat{Y}_i)^2$
January:	X_1	320	353.3*	1108.89
February:	X_2	470	413.0	3249.00
March:	X_3	520	472.7	2237.29
April:	X_4	620	532.4	7673.76
May:	X_5	540	547.3	53.29
June:	X_6	550	577.2	739.84
July:	X_7	440	487.6	2265.76
August:	X_8	400	413.0**	169.00
September:	X_9	700	711.5	132.25
October:	X_{10}	650	636.9	171.61
November:	X_{11}	480	524.9	2016.01
December:	X_{12}	430	450.3	412.09
				20,228.79

* $\hat{Y}_1 = 263.7 + .7463\ (120) = 353.3$.
** $\hat{Y}_8 = 263.7 + .7463\ (200) = 413.0$.

Assuming that the actual data points are distributed about the regression equation with normal dispersion, the standard error of the estimate, S_e, may be used to indicate the boundaries of points for one, two, or n number of standard errors. For example, the regression line $\hat{Y}_i \pm 41.06$ distance units will be the boundary for approximately two-thirds of the actual data points, while the regression line $\pm 2S_e$ will provide a boundary for approximately 95 percent of the actual points (see Figure B-4)[5].

To illustrate how the standard error of the estimate may be used, assume that management wishes to estimate the number of hours needed to service a monthly patient demand of 120. The regression estimate would be:

$$353.3 = 263.7 + .7463\ (120).$$

Since the dispersion is assumed to be normal, two-thirds of the time the actual number of hours required will be in the interval:

$$353.3 \pm 41.06 = [312.24,\ 394.36].$$

This range is depicted graphically in Figure B-4.

Figure B-4 Regression Line with One and Two Standard Errors

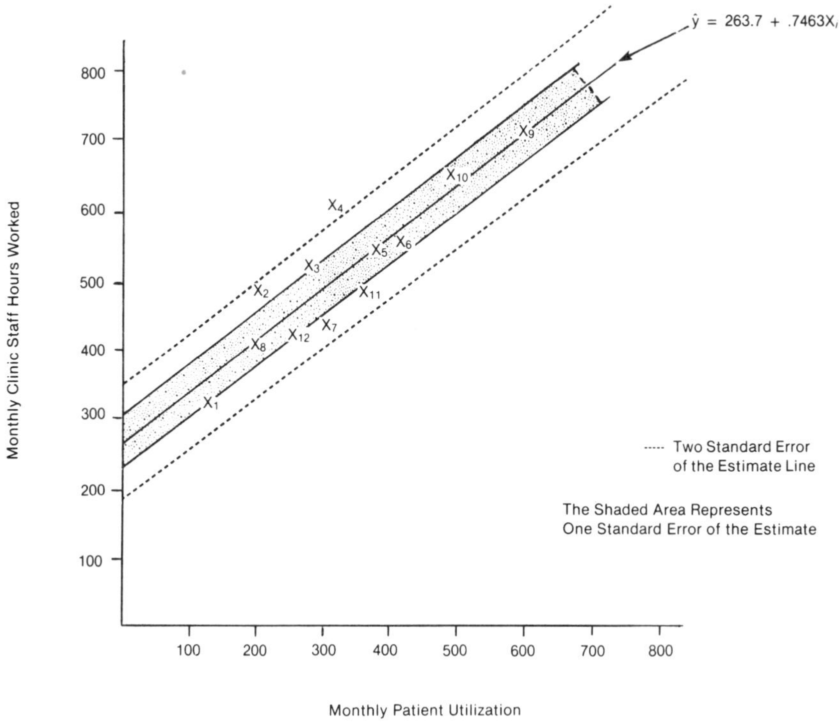

Whenever a regression line is computed in the text, the following statistical information is presented:

1. the correlation coefficient (r) and the coefficient of determination (r^2));
2. the two-tail t test level of r; and
3. the standard error of the estimate (S_e).

NOTES

1. Given a dependent variable, (Y), and multiple independent variables, ($X_j : j = 1, \ldots, m$), the linear regression equation is referred to as a linear multiple regression equation. The true regression line may be noted as:

$$\tilde{Y}_i = \alpha + \beta_1 X_{1i} + \beta_2 X_{2i} + , \ldots, + \beta_m X_{mi}$$

where: α represents the true intercept of the regression equation; and
β_i represents the true slope of the ith independent variable.

In this appendix, only the simple linear regression, $\tilde{Y}_i = \alpha + \beta X_i$ will be estimated (see Problem B-2).

2. A second order condition that $\partial^2 f/\partial a^2 > 0$, $\partial^2 f/\partial b^2 > 0$ must be satisfied for $\Sigma(Y_i - \hat{Y}_i)^2$ to be minimized. Although only the first order condition shall be examined, note that the second order condition is satisfied.
3. The correlation coefficient is formulated mathematically as follows.

$$r = \frac{\Sigma X_i Y_i - n\bar{X}\bar{Y}}{((\Sigma X_i^2 - n\bar{X}^2)(\Sigma Y_i^2 - n\bar{Y}^2))^{1/2}}$$

Note that the square of the correlation coefficient equals the coefficient of determination. However, the square root of the coefficient of determination does not equal the correlation coefficient when the correlation coefficient is in the range $[-1,0)$.

4. The t test is a statistical computation used to develop inferences regarding the likelihood of an event's occurrence. The validity of inferences derived from a statistical test depend upon the validity of the assumptions underlying the test. In this case, the t test is used to test the hypothesis that $r \neq 0$. The assumption underlying this t test is that the sample was drawn from a bivariate normal population with $\rho = 0$. When $\rho \neq 0$, the appropriate value to be used to develop inferences is:

$$Z = \tfrac{1}{2} \ln \left(\frac{1 + r}{1 - r}\right).$$

For simplicity in this text, the n sample pairs are assumed to be drawn from a bivariate normal population with $\rho = 0$. If the t test is used only to test the hypothesis that $r \neq 0$, the validity of this assumption is not as crucial as if confidence limits were to be formulated for ρ in terms of r.

5. The standard error of the estimate boundary lines represented in Figure B-4 are only approximations of the actual boundary lines. The actual standard error of the estimate boundary lines are hyperbolic concave to the estimating equation when individual observations, Y_i, are to be estimated. However, when the extrapolations are not extensive, one may use the standard error of the estimate adjusted to correspond to the population standard error of the estimate to provide reasonably accurate information. The adjusted standard error of the estimate would be

$$\hat{S}_e = S_e \times (n/(n - 2))^{1/2}.$$

Questions and Problems

Question B-1. When the slope of the regression equation is negative, what is the sign of the correlation coefficient? The coefficient of determination?

Question B-2. The scatter diagram is a useful technique to ascertain the type of regression equation which should be fitted to the observations (i.e., linear or nonlinear). However, for practical purposes, the scatter diagram is limited to cases with one dependent and one independent variable. Discuss how the coefficient of determination (r^2) provides the same information as the scatter diagram regardless of the dimension of the problem (i.e., one dependent variable and multiple independent variables).

Question B-3. The intercept, *a* (equation (B-10)), was restated to reflect the proper unit magnitude. Why was a restatement of *b* unnecessary?

Problem B-1. Assume the following information has been collected for a service population:

Nursing Services

Region 1		Region 2		Region 3	
Percent Y	(000) X	Percent Y	(000) X	Percent Y	(000) X
36	86	20	92	35	92
32	93	18	96	46	101
40	102	32	105	49	108
38	105	34	112	47	108
31	107	37	113	55	117
46	107	35	117	62	123
45	110	30	120	50	135
		30	121	51	137
				53	138
				57	142

where: *Y* represents the percentage of uncollectable accounts (the dependent variable; and
X represents the number of individuals (the independent variable).

Required:

a. Determine the regression equations and correlation coefficients for the nursing services in regions 1, 2, and 3.
b. Assume that the population of all three regions combined is expected to increase by 3.73 percent. What is the regression prediction of the bad debt percentage?

Problem B-2. The regression line is determined by minimizing the following expression:

(B-1) $$\sum_{i}^{n} (Y_i - \hat{Y}_i)^2.$$

Recall that in equation (B-1), $\hat{Y}_i = a + bX_i$; however, in Note 1 the simple regression equation is stated as:

$$\tilde{Y}_i = \alpha + \beta X_i.$$

Why is there a difference between the two statements of the dependent variable? How are α and β related to the a and b derived from the normal equations (B-5) and (B-6)?

Problem B-3. Verify the standard error of the estimate calculations for the information provided in Tables 7-1 and 7-2.

Problem B-4.

a. If the variables X and Y are not linearly related, the coefficient of determination may be approximately zero even though a functional relationship exists between X and Y. In this case, the standard error of the estimate may be used to decide which functional form represents the best regression equation to estimate. In order to demonstrate this, compute the standard error of the estimate for equation 7-7. Compute the linear regression equation for the profit figures represented in Table 7-3. Contrast the standard error of the estimate of the linear profit regression equation with the standard error of the estimate of $\pi = -1238 + 6.29X - .0054X^2$.

b. Your computations in part (a) should indicate that a second order regression better represents the data in Table 7-3 than a linear regression equation. Using the actual data points in Table 7-3 as the X variables and the regression points generated with equation 7-7 as the Y variables use equation B-11 to compute r^2. Now use as the Y variables the regression points generated with the linear regression equation estimated in part (a) and compute r^2 using equation B-11. Contrast the two values of r^2 computed and discuss the relationship between this information and the information generated in (a).

Appendix C

Evaluating Data Processing and Information Systems Consultants

Most control systems rely on information generated by the institution's management information system. However, the computer and systems technology required to keep the institution's management information system operating with relative efficiency is modified constantly, resulting in numerous data processing alternatives. Unfortunately, health care institutions rarely have the expertise to select, evaluate, and compare these data processing alternatives. Consequently, management often solicits the information to analyze these alternatives from data processing and information systems professionals. In general, individuals in health care institutions have been justifiably dissatisfied with the results of their interaction with these systems professionals. Whether this dissatisfaction arises because the health professionals develop unreasonable expectations or because the systems professionals fail to understand the unique nature of the health care conversion process is subject to argument.

Interactions between health professionals and systems professionals most frequently arise when medical or administrative management becomes involved in a project that in some way affects the institution's data processing and management information system. To give proper attention to all aspects of the project, project teams are created, and a project manager is appointed to coordinate their various activities. Usually one of the project teams is responsible for the information systems aspect of the project.

A well-balanced information systems project team should include (1) the project manager, (2) an information systems coordinator who is chosen from management by the project manager to be responsible for the data processing or management information systems aspects of the project, (3) a systems consultant who is engaged by management to render expert opinions on the information systems aspects of the project, and (4) a representative from an information systems vendor, once one is selected. The consultant's role on this team is often critical in the planning, execution, and implementation stages of the project. Hence, the duties and responsibilities of the consultant should be well defined.

CONSULTANT RESPONSIBILITIES

Generally, eight basic responsibilities are delegated to the consultant. These responsibilities can be divided into three major categories: (1) planning responsibilities, (2) vendor selection responsibilities, and (3) followup responsibilities. Specifying these responsibilities not only lets the consultant know what is expected, but also provides the project manager and management with a basis for evaluating the consultant's work on the project.

Planning Responsibilities

The consultant's planning responsibilities begin with aiding management in developing (1) specific statements regarding the purposes of the project, (2) the anticipated control and evaluation systems changes required by the project, and (3) the data processing systems activity required to support the project. This information enables management to anticipate the complex systems interactions necessary to develop an implementable project.

The consultant's second planning responsibility is to assist in preparing a project work schedule. The consultant must collaborate with the information systems coordinator to prepare this document, which outlines the estimated work schedule from the beginning to the completion of the project. The major categories on this work schedule should include vendor selection, information systems forms design (input and output), systems development, systems testing and implementation, and project documentation.

Vendor Selection Responsibilities

The next phase in the consultant's work involves providing information regarding the selection of an information systems vendor that can provide the best technical support to meet the needs of the project. The role of the consultant in this phase of the project is crucial because the consultant acts as the mediator and interpreter between the institution and the information systems vendors.

The first of the consultant's vendor selection responsibilities is to encourage competitive bidding among the vendors interested in providing their service. The consultant also should encourage the information systems coordinator and appropriate administrative personnel to derive criteria by which the vendor bids can be evaluated. However, the consultant should not develop these criteria or provide the management with a checklist, because such lists often erroneously imply that all criteria have equal weight. In order for the organization to make an informed decision, the information systems coordinator and the appropriate administrative personnel should derive the evaluation criteria, and thereby develop a sense of the unique weighting of each criterion. Table C-1 includes a list of possible evaluation criteria.

The consultant's second vendor selection responsibility involves gathering useful technical information about the vendors. Each prospective vendor should be given a bidding document prepared by the management which clearly states (1) the project overview, (2) the project objectives, (3) the subcontractor responsibilities, and (4) the criteria by which the bids will be evaluated. This bidding document is essential if comparable vendor proposals are to be developed. After examining the vendor reactions to the

Table C-1 Possible Criteria by Which Vendor Bids Could Be Evaluated*

A. Costs of:
   1. Development
   2. Testing and operation in a demonstration mode
   3. Future operations (assuming responsibility for input, processing, and output)
   4. Subsequent modification and system maintenance
B. Anticipated clerical cost savings
C. System operating characteristics, including:
   1. Ease of operation
   2. Flexibility
      - New output reports
      - Modification of input data
      - Response to ad hoc inquiries or special evaluation studies
   3. Timeliness of reports
   4. Data input characteristics
      - Verification
      - Validation
   5. Data security provisions
D. Transferability of the system to other departments or institutional contexts
E. Transferability of the system to other computational facilities
F. Timing
   1. Systems development
   2. Testing and operation in a demonstration mode

*These criteria are not listed in order of priority.

bidding documents, the consultant should require the vendors to detail the technical aspects of their proposal in a formal contract so that vendor responsibilities can be definitively ascertained. Then the consultant should put the contractual information presented by each vendor into perspective relative to the project. In addition, the consultant should make sure that additional information supporting each vendor's ability to perform on the proposed contract is being gathered from (1) vendor financial statements, (2) legal opinions regarding the proposed vendor contract, (3) meetings with members of the vendor's staff who will execute the contract, (4) discussions with current vendor clients, and (5) the vendor's credit rating. Discussions with current vendor clients usually provide insights to the vendor's ability to deliver on the claims presented in the contract, while information on the vendor's credit rating provides insights on the vendor's long term performance potential.

The consultant's third vendor selection responsibility involves obtaining and evaluating the vendor's work schedules. The consultant should request each vendor to submit an estimated computer or systems project schedule which details the vendor work schedule for beginning and completing various aspects of the work. These vendor schedules may be evaluated in terms of the overall estimated project work schedule. After examining the vendor work schedules, the consultant should indicate to the information systems coordinator and the appropriate administrative personnel which vendor activities are critical to the successful completion of the project.

The consultant's final vendor selection responsibility is to render an opinion regarding the vendor proposals. At the time the vendor is to be selected, the consultant, the information systems coordinator, the project manager, and the appropriate individuals from administration should meet to discuss the pros and cons of each proposal. The consultant should respond only to the specifics of the proposed contracts, and not attempt to guide the decision to a particular vendor or decide which vendor contract is approved. This point is critical because the consultant is not responsible for the project; responsibility lies with management.

Followup Responsibilities

Once the vendor has been selected, the consultant's vendor selection responsibilities have been completed and only two followup responsibilities remain. The first of these is to review vendor progress. The consultant should meet with the vendor periodically to review the vendor's progress. Based upon the information derived from these reviews, the consultant should inform the administrator of any delays that might occur in the overall project work plan due to delays experienced by the vendor. The second followup and last of the consultant's responsibilities involves setting up a program for reviewing feedback from the project routinely. The consultant should emphasize the necessity for the information systems coordinator to review feedback from those involved in developing or implementing the new system.

Conclusion

Each of these eight basic responsibilities is equally important. Failure to perform adequately on any of them may cause serious problems in successful completion of the project. Hence, these guidelines can be useful in the ongoing evaluation of the consultant. However, they cannot be used to select a consultant.

SELECTION OF A CONSULTANT

Five characteristics may be useful in selecting an individual to fill the role of consultant. First the consultant should have a knowledge of and an interest in the project. A statement from the consultant regarding the project may be useful in evaluating this interest and enthusiasm. Second, the consultant's work plan should show cognizance of the eight basic responsibilities discussed above. Of course, management must require the submission of a work plan to evaluate and select a particular consultant. Third, the consultant should have the ability to draw upon expertise without having to subcontract for it. For example, if statistical questions arise in conjunction with the consultant's work and the consultant cannot provide answers, he or she should be able to secure the necessary advice without subcontracting for it (unless, of course, the consultant pays for the subcontract). Fourth, the consultant should have the education and experience to recognize her/his limitations. Further, if the consultant expresses a research interest in the project, management may be able to extend the consultant's productivity beyond the monetary aspects of the contract. Finally, the project should not be the consultant's sole source of income.

Answers and Partial Solutions to Selected Questions and Problems

Chapter 2

Problem 2-1.

Memorial Hospital
Bank Reconciliation
July 31, 19X1

Per Books		Per Bank		
Beginning balance	$5,451	Beginning balance		$6,180
Additions:		Additions:		
Transposition error	9	Deposit in transit		42
Proceeds of Note Collection	636			
	$6,096			$6,222
Deductions:		Deductions:		
Bank service charge	12	Outstanding checks	$58	
NSF check	10		72	130
		Transposition error		18
	22			148
Correct Adjusted Balance:	$6,074	Correct Adjusted Balance:		$6,074

The required journal entry is:

Cash	$623.00	
Accounts Receivable (·)	$10.00	
Service Charge	12.00	
Wage Expense		$9.00
Notes Receivable		600.00
Interest Revenue		36.00

Problem 2-2.

a. Corrected balance	$17,674.25	
b. Accounts Receivable (·)	$ 196.80	
Service Charge	97.01	
Collection Charge	121.73	
Cash	1,656.45	
Miscellaneous Expense		$.99
Notes Receivable		1,900.00
Interest Income		171.00
c. Bank Receipts	$10,309.65	
Bank Disbursements	2,455.15	
Book Receipts	7,894.41	
Book Disbursements	6,908.85	
Book Balance, 11/30/19X1	15,032.24	

Problem 2-3.

Correct Adjusted Balance	$ 2,780.00

Problem 2-4.

a(i) Petty Cash	200.00	
Vouchers Payable		$ 200.00
To set up the petty cash fund.		
(ii) Miscellaneous Expense	$ 60.81	
Accounts Receivable (E. Greene)	40.00	
Vouchers Payable		$ 100.81
To replenish the petty cash fund.		

b. Item 6 should be sent to the bank it is drawn upon. If it is paid by the bank, the $80 in cash will be included in the petty cash. If it is not paid, the following entry should be made:

Accounts Receivable (employee)	$ 80.00	
Vouchers Payable		$ 80.00.

Problem 2-5.

Correct Adjusted Balance $5,216.84

Problem 2-6.

Balance in the Purchase Discounts Lost account:	$355.71
Balance in the Purchase Discounts Taken account:	$ 72.83

The minimum cost payment was $44,907.22.

Problem 2-8.

The amount of theft must be at least $198.38 per month.

Chapter 3

Problem 3-1.

a. Patient Accounts Receivable (C. Jones)	$ 173.50	
Treatment Revenue (D)		$ 173.50
b. Change in the subsidiary ledgers		
: Increase the account of K. C. Jones by $46.77		
: Decrease the account of C. Jones by $46.77		
c. Bad Debt Expense	$ 8,070.01	
Allowance for Bad Debts		$ 8,070.01
d. Allowance for Bad Debts	$ 126.73	
Patient Accounts Receivable (C. Jones)		$ 126.73
e. Cash	$ 130.53	
Allowance for Bad Debts		$ 126.73
Interest Revenue		3.80

Problem 3-2.

12/31/19X1		
Bad Debt Expense	$ 9,167.06	
Allowance for Bad Debts		$ 9,167.06
During 19X2		
Patient Accounts Receivable (·)	$187,247.31	
Patient Revenue (D)		$187,247.31
During 19X2		
Cash	$213,597.20	
Patient Revenue (D)		$ 8,427.04
Patient Accounts Receivable (·)		205,170.16

During 19X2		
Allowance for Bad Debts	$ 6,397.21	
Patient Accounts Receivable (·)		$ 6,397.21
12/31/19X2		
Bad Debt Expense	$ 5,185.37	
Allowance for Bad Debts		$ 5,185.37

Problem 3-3.

a. $37,020.80

Problem 3-7.

a. 12/31/19X1		
Collection Fees Receivable (·)	$ 5,790.00	
Collection Fees Revenue		$ 5,790.00
b. 1/30/19X2		
Cash	$95,790.00	
Patient Accounts Receivable (·)		$93,000.000
Collection Fees Receivable (·)		$ 2,790.00
d. Cash	$25,000.00	
Patient Accounts Receivable (·)		$25,000.000
Allowance for Bad Debts	$ 375.00	
Collection Fees Receivable (·)		$ 375.00

Problem 3-8.

a. $24,877.73

b. (i) Bad Debt Expense	$14,202.16	
Allowance for Bad Debts		$14,202.16

Chapter 4

Problem 4-1.

a. 138 units

b. Periodic

PERIODIC

	Inventory	Cost of Goods Used	Inventory Shrinkage
LIFO	$1,281.42	$ 997.09	$70.64
FIFO	$ 685.86	$1,609.81	$53.48
AVERAGE	$ 991.39	$1,300.29	$57.47

c. Either FIFO periodic or FIFO perpetual.

Problem 4-2.
Direct Storage Costs: Item A

$$\frac{3763 \times \dfrac{715}{16{,}800}}{\dfrac{159}{2}} = \$2.01$$

Cost of Funds: Item A

$$\$9.24 \times .15 = \$1.39$$

Total Direct Storage Costs

$$\$1.39 + \$2.01 = \$3.40$$

Direct Cost: Purchase Order

$$\frac{\$6{,}469.45}{1623} = \$3.99$$

$$\text{EOQ} = \left[\frac{2 \times \$3.99 \times 11{,}000}{\$3.40}\right]^{1/2}$$

$$= 161 \text{ units}$$

Problem 4-3.

a. $$\text{TC} = \text{M} \times (1 - \text{D}) \times \text{EYU} + \text{P} \times \frac{\text{EYU}}{\text{I}} + \text{C} \times \frac{\text{I}}{2}$$

$$= \$2{,}400.00 + \frac{\$3{,}614.40}{\text{I}} + \$.865 \times \text{I}$$

b. $$\text{dTC}/\text{d}_I = -\frac{\$3{,}614.40}{\text{I}^2} + \$.865 = 0$$

Since a necessary condition for a minimum is $\text{dTC}/\text{d}_I = 0$, I may be solved for, yielding:

$$\text{I} = 65 \text{ units}$$

Problem 4-4.

c. \$9.8791103

Problem 4-6.

Gross Price Method
(a) New Recorded Cost = \$49.40657
(b) New Recorded Cost = \$49.231258

Problem 4-7.

a(i), a(ii)

	Value of Medical Supply			
Case	A	B	C	AGGREGATE
I	$9.86	$18.11	$5.32	$33.71
II	9.86	18.53	5.03	33.71
III	9.31	18.10	5.32	33.17
IV	9.86	18.53	5.12	33.71

b(i) Case I:	Inventory Shrinkage	$276.78	
	Inventory (B)		$276.78
Case II:	Inventory Shrinkage	$142.97	
	Inventory (C)		$142.97
Case III:	Inventory Shrinkage	$573.77	
	Inventory (A)		$290.40
	Inventory (B)		283.37
Case IV:	Inventory Shrinkage	$ 98.60	
	Inventory (C)		$ 98.60

Problem 4-8.

Revised SS_1 = 19 units
Revised SS_2 = 106 units
Revised SS_3 = 19 units

Problem 4-9.

EOQ = 279 units

$$TC_{EOQ} = (M \times EYU) + \left(\frac{EYU}{I} \times P\right) + \left(\frac{I}{2} \times C\right) - (M \times D \times EYU) = \$73{,}689.84$$

Chapter 5

Question 5-1. The bond financing would be economically preferable in both cases. Given the financing requirement of $500,000, bond financing yields a return to the owners of 8.6 percent, while equity financing yields a return to the owners of 7.2 percent.

Problem 5-1.

a. Expected interest rate: .08 = .4 × .085 + .4 × .06 + .2 × .11
Price of bond: $3,187.50 × 17.292033 + $75,000 × .30831867 = $78,242.26

b. 1/1

Cash	$61,374.61	
Discount	13,625.39	
Bonds Payable		$75,000

7/1

Interest Expense	$ 3,641.68	
Cash		$ 3,187.50
Discount		454.18

Problem 5-3.

a. Cash received	$ 99,908.09
b. Interest expense (8/1/X1)	$ 4,553.96

Problem 5-4.

a. The HMO should retire the bonds.
b. Approximately 32 percent.

Problem 5-5.

The amount of the annuity is $13,278.93.

Chapter 6

Problem 6-1.

VISITING NURSES SOCIETY
Statement of Changes in Financial Position; Working Capital Basis
for the Year Ended June 30, 19X2

Sources of Working Capital		
From operations:		
Net Income	$ 300	
Add (deduct) adjustments for income transactions not affecting working capital:		
Depreciation expense	3,000	
Gain on sale of equipment	(1,000)	
Amortization of bond discount	500	
Total working capital from operations		$ 2,800

From other sources:		
Sale of equipment	$ 3,000	
Sale of land	8,000	
Issuance of bonds	4,700	
Philanthropic contribution (Note 1)	1,400	
Total working capital from other sources		$17,100
Total sources of working capital		$19,900
Applications of Working Capital		
Construction in Process on the Maternal and Infant Care Clinic	$19,900	
Total applications of working capital		$19,900
Net change in working capital		$ -0-

Working Capital Accounts	Balances : December 31 19X2	19X1	Working Capital Increase (Decrease)
Current Assets:			
Cash	$ 1,100	$ 3,400	($2,300)
Accounts Receivable	7,000	2,000	5,000
Allowance for Uncollectables	(2,000)	(300)	(1,700)
Inventory	2,600	1,200	1,400
Total Current Assets	$ 8,700	$ 6,300	$2,400
Current Liabilities:			
Notes Payable	$ 6,000	$ 5,000	($1,000)
Accounts Payable	7,000	6,000	(1,000)
Accrued Interest Payable	3,400	3,000	(400)
Total Current Liabilities	$16,400	$14,000	($2,400)
Working Capital	($ 7,700)	($ 7,700)	$ 0

Note 1: Philanthropic contribution was a $1,400 contribution from the Ladies Aid Society on January 24, 19X2.

VISITING NURSES SOCIETY
Statement of Changes in Financial Position; Cash Basis
for the Year Ended June 30, 19X2

From operations:	
Sources of Cash:	
Revenues	$90,100

Add (deduct) adjustments to convert revenues to a cash basis:		
Accounts receivable increase	(5,000)	
Cash generated from revenues		$85,100
Expenses	90,800	
Add (deduct) adjustments to convert expenses to a cash basis:		
Depreciation expense	(3,000)	
Allowance for uncollectables increase	(1,700)	
Inventory increase	1,400	
Notes payable increase	(1,000)	
Accounts payable increase	(1,000)	
Accrued interest payable increase	(400)	
Amortization of bond discount	(500)	
Cash disbursed for expenses		$84,600
Total cash from operations		500
From other sources:		
Sale of equipment	3,000	
Sale of land	8,000	
Issuance of bonds	4,700	
Philanthropic contribution (Note 1)	1,400	
Total cash from other sources		17,100
Total sources of cash		$17,600
Applications of Cash:		
Construction in process on the Maternal and Infant Care Clinic	$19,900	
Total applications of cash		$19,900
Decrease in cash during the period		$ 2,300

Note 1: Philanthropic contribution was a $1,400 contribution from the Ladies Aid Society on January 24, 19X2.

Problem 6-2.

a. Increase $12,500
b. Increase $11,000
c. Decrease $102.88
d. Increase $93.47
e. Decrease $30
f. Decrease $5,000

Problem 6-3a.

Working Capital Accounts	Balances : December 31 19X2	19X1	Working Capital Increase (Decrease)
Current Assets:			
Cash	$ 37,000	$ 46,000	($ 9,000)
Accounts Receivable (net)	70,000	92,000	(22,000)
Inventory	55,000	53,000	2,000
Total Current Assets	$162,000	$191,000	($29,000)
Current Liabilities:			
Accounts Payable	$ 27,000	$ 36,000	$ 9,000
Notes Payable	30,000	20,000	(10,000)
Total Current Liabilities	$ 57,000	$ 56,000	($ 1,000)
Working Capital	$105,000	$135,000	($30,000)

b. Partial Solution. Depreciation on building $46,300.00.

Problem 6-4.

Partial Solution

a. January 2, 19X1

Cash	$123,322.94	
Discount on Bonds Payable	6,677.06	
Bonds Payable		$130,000.00

Since only current assets and current liabilities affect working capital, the debit (increase) to cash (an asset) is the only part of the transaction which affects working capital. Thus, working capital is increased by $123,322.94.

b. December 31, 19X1

Bond Interest Expense	$ 5,858.85	
Discount on Bonds Payable (6,677.06 ÷ 20)		$ 333.85
Accrued Interest Payable		5,525.00

The only working capital account in this transaction is Accrued Interest Payable. Since accrued interest payable (a liability) is being increased, working capital is decreased by $5,525.00.

Problem 6-5.

Partial Solution

Cash	Working Capital	Net Income
a. Increase $15,340	Increase $153,400	Increase $153,400
b. Uncertain	Decrease $55,700	Decrease $90,700

Chapter 7

Question 7-12.

a. Either the average revenue per unit was approximately $18.00 for that month, possibly due to a disproportionate amount of free care, or errors were made in crediting the radiology unit with the proper revenue. In this particular case, the hospital and the radiology department chose not to investigate this apparent discrepancy.

Problem 7-1.

a. (i) $\pi = 2{,}413 - 3.36X$

a. (ii) $\pi = -73 + 22.06X - .9X^2$

b. (i) 718 units

b. (ii) 4 units and 21 units

Problem 7-3.

b. $\pi = -110.8 + 27X - .2X^2$ and $\pi = -409.7 + 42.7X - .4X^2$

c. {4, 131} and {11, 96}

f. 68 and 53

Problem 7-4.

a. $R(X) = 1{,}320 + 9.6X$

b. The cost of a fixed cost alteration which would make the administrator indifferent is $1,834.12.

The cost of a variable cost alteration which would make the administrator indifferent is $17,723.52.

Problem 7-6.

The point of indifference is 848 = (449.69/.53). The manager would never choose to alter fixed costs because over the range of patient volumes for which altering costs is cost beneficial, altering variable costs is more economical than altering fixed costs.

Chapter 8

Problem 8-1.

Break-even volume 19X1 = 11,600 units.

Problem 8-2.

a. 350 patients

b. $575 profit

c. Clinic would offer $MC_{su} = AVC_{su} = \$5.00$

d. Service unit would demand $P = \$5.00 + \$450/350 + \Pi$, but in theory they would only receive $5.00

e. 350 patients

f. $1,025 profit

Chapter 9

Question 9-14.

The controller is right. Other factors equal, an investment with a longer life will have a lower VA_{IRD} than an investment with a shorter life. However, this is to be expected, since the VA_{IRD} represents the value of the annuity that must be invested annually to renew the investment. Other factors equal, an investment with a longer life will have a lower annuity than an investment with a shorter life. However, the VA_{IRD} is only one statistic which may be used to evaluate an investment. It is by no means the only statistic that should be used in selecting capital investment alternatives.

Problem 9-4.

a. $$RAR = (1 + .48)\left(\frac{\$250{,}000 - \$43{,}000}{7}\right)\left(\frac{(1 + .11)^7 - 1}{.11}\right)$$

$$(1 + .11)^3 + \$43{,}000.$$

$$= \$628{,}581.$$

ERC (.04, − .02) = $304,749.
ERC (.12, + .04) = $1,102,859.

Problem 9-5.

a. A = $15,250
RAR_{MDU} = $224,334
ERC_{MDU} = $816,584

b. $\gamma \approx .2747$. This means that additional financing must be secured to cover $(1 - \gamma)$ percent of the cost of renewing the MDU. In this case 75.53 percent additional financing must be secured at the end of the eighth year.

Problem 9-6.

a. IRD_{MDU} = $183,958

b. RAR_{MIC} = $197,370
IRD_{MIC} = $180,568

c. Other factors equal, the MIC should be selected since its financing requirements are smaller.

d. $VA_{IRD_{MDU}}$ = $13.401
$VA_{IRD_{MIC}}$ = $20,628

Problem 9-9.

$$IIE_2 = [7{,}750 - (1{,}155 - 620)] \times .08 = \$577$$

$$IIE_{10} = [2{,}059 - (1{,}155 - 165)] \times .08 = \$\ 86$$

Problem 9-10.

a. RAR = \$11,487.
   ERC = \$20,102.
   VA_{IRD} = \$562.

Problem 9-12.

Case A

VA_{IRD} = \$9,406

Case B

$$RAR = 32{,}000\,(1.07)^4 + 25{,}600\,(1 + .07)^3 + 19{,}200\,(1 + .07)^2 + 12{,}800\,(1 + .07) + 6{,}400 + 4{,}000 = \$119{,}385$$

VA_{IRD} = \$8,542

Case C

$$RAR = \$40{,}000\,(1.07)^4 + \$24{,}000\,(1.07)^3 + \$14{,}400\,(1.07)^2 + \$8{,}800\,(1.07) + \$8{,}800 + 4{,}000 = \$120{,}535$$

VA_{IRD} = \$8,342

Chapter 10

Problem 10-1.

(a)

		Variance Analysis	
	Total Variance	Efficiency	Rate
Physician	\$171.00 A > E	234.00 E > A	\$405.00 A > E
Nurse	\$4633.50 E > A	4248.75 E > A	384.75 E > A

Problem 10-2.

(a) Year 19X1, $11,997.69, Year 19X2, $11,702.51 to the Service Categories I and II; and $207,703.11, $209,302.65 to other Service Categories in Years 19X1 and 19X2, respectively.

(b)

Service Category	Year X1	Year X2
I	$8,158.76	$7,089.74
II	$3,838.93	$4,612.77

(c) Year 19X1, 4 minutes; Year 19X2, 7 minutes.

Chapter 11

Problem 11-1.

a. [2/3, 1/3]

b. [.28, .33, .39]

c. [1/3, 1/3, 1/3]

d. [.44, .49, .07]

e. [.69, .23, .08]

Problem 11-2.

a. 2.0 b. 5.45 c. 3.0 d. 3.013 e. 3.0

Problem 11-4. Consistency Measures:

a. 0 b. .344 c. 0 d. .0018 e. 0

$1 - \theta_j^i$ Adjustment:

a. 1.0 b. .656 c. 1.0 d. .9982 e. 1

Appendix B

Question B-1. The correlation coefficient will be negative since:

$$b = r\frac{(\Sigma(Y_i - \bar{Y})^2)^{1/2}}{(\Sigma(X_i - \bar{X})^2)^{1/2}}.$$

Therefore if $r < 0$, b will be negative. Similarly, if $r > 0$, b will be positive.

Problem B-1.

		Regression Equations	Correlation Coefficients (r)
a.	Region 1	$Y = 5.4576 + .3237X$	.4831
	Region 2	$Y = -23.5266 + .4843X$	.7593
	Region 3	$Y = 16.3051 + .2847X$	.6869

REFERENCES

Cathcart, R. H. "Including the Community in Hospital Governance," *Hospital Progress,* October 1970.

Ferguson, C. E., and Saving, T. R. "Long-Run Scale Adjustments of a Perfectly Competitive Firm and Industry," *American Economic Review* LIX: 774–83.

Harman, H. H. *Modern Factor Analysis.* Chicago: The University of Chicago Press, 1976.

Hildebrand, F. B. *Introduction to Numerical Analysis.* New York: McGraw-Hill, 1974.

Katz, S.; Ford, A. B.; Moskowitz, R. W.; Jackson, B. A.; and Jaffe, M. W. "Studies of Illness in the Aged: The Index of ADL, A Standardized Measure of Biological and Physiological Function," *Journal of the American Medical Association* 185: 914.

Katz, S.; Ford, A. B.; Downs, T. D.; Adams, A.; and Rusby, D. *Effects of Continued Care: A Study of Chronic Illness in the Home* Washington, D.C.: U.S. Government Printing Office, 1972 (HEW No. 73-3010).

Levitan, M. S. "The Impact of 'New Generation' Proprietary Hospitals on Health Care," *Hospital Progress*, July 1970.

Lusk, E. J. "Hospital Investment Evaluation," *Journal of Accounting and Business Research*, Autumn 1974.

Lusk, E. J. "A Bipolar Adjective Screening Methodology," *Journal of Marketing Research*, May 1973.

Lusk, E. J. "The Relationship between Judgmental Inconsistency and (λ_{max}-n)/(n-1)," Working Paper, Philadelphia, Pa.: The Wharton School, University of Pennsylvania, 1977.

Novick, David. *Current Practice in Program Budgeting (PPBS).* New York: Crane, Russak, 1973.

Pindyck, R. S., and Rubinfeld, D. L., *Economic Models and Economic Forecasts*, New York: McGraw-Hill Book Co., 1976.

Ofer, A. R., "Third Party Reimbursement and Evaluation of Leasing Aternatives," *Topics in Health Care Financing* 3:1976.

Osgood, C. E.; Suci, C. J.; and Tannenbaum, P. H., *The Measurement of Meaning.* Urbana: University of Illinois Press, 1957.

Saaty, T. L., "A Scaling Method for Priorities in Hierarchical Structures," *Journal of Mathematical Psychology* 15:1977.

Index

A

C

J

L

M

Q

R